Ethics of Health Care

An Introductory Textbook

THIRD EDITION

Ethics of Health Care

An Introductory Textbook

THIRD EDITION

Benedict M. Ashley, O.P.
Kevin D. O'Rourke, O.P.

Georgetown University Press / Washington, D.C.

Georgetown University Press, Washington, D.C.
© 2002 by Georgetown University Press. All rights reserved.
Printed in the United States of America

10 9 8 7 6 5 4 3 2 1   2002

This volume is printed on acid-free offset book paper.

Ethical and Religious Directives for Catholic Health Care Services, Fourth Edition. Copyright © 2001 United States Catholic Conference, Inc., Washington, D.C. Used with permission. All rights reserved.

Nihil Obstat
Reverend William P. Grogan, M.A., M.St., J.D., S.T.L.
Censor Deputatus
December 31, 2001

Imprimatur
Most Reverend Raymond E. Goedert, M.A., S.T.L., J.C.L.
Vicar General
Archdiocese of Chicago
January 3, 2002

The *Nihil Obstat* and the *Imprimatur* are official declarations that a book is free of doctrinal and moral error. No implication is contained that those who have granted the *Nihil Obstat* and *Imprimatur* agree with the content, opinions, or statements expressed. Nor do they assume any legal responsibility associated with publication.

Library of Congress Cataloging-in-Publication Data

Ashley, Benedict M.
    Ethics of health care : an introductory textbook / Benedict M. Ashley, Kevin D. O'Rourke.—3rd ed.
      p. cm.
    Includes bibliographical references and index.
    ISBN 0-87840-375-2 (pbk. : alk. paper)
    1. Medical ethics. 2. Medicine—Religious aspects—Catholic authors. 3. Christian ethics—Catholic authors. 4. Pastoral medicine—Catholic Church. I. O'Rourke, Kevin D. II. Title.

R724 .A738 2002
241.642—dc21   2002190228

Contents

Introduction | ix

1 *Methods in Health Care Ethics* 1
The Enlightenment and New Ethical Systems 1
Hume's Contribution to Other Systems 3
Other Ethical Systems in the United States 6
The Moral System of the Catholic Church 7
Summary 12
Questions 12
Cases 12

2 *The Content of Catholic Health Care Ethics* 15
Is There a Catholic Ethics? 15
What Is an Ethical Principle? 17
Principles of Christian Faith 17
Principles of Christian Love 23
Principles of Christian Hope 25
Summary 30
Questions 30
Cases 30

3 *The Person Seeking Health* 31
The Notion of Person 31
The Person and Community 34
Developing Common Values 36
Priorities in Needs and Values 38
Summary 40
Questions 41
Cases 41

4 *Defining Human Health* 43
Concepts of Health and Disease 43
Disease and Illness 45

Biological Health   47
Higher Levels of Health   49
Integrating Human Functioning   51
Summary   52
Questions   52
Cases   53

5   *Personal Responsibility for Health*   55
The Individual's Quest for Health   55
Preventive Medicine and Lifestyle   58
Creative Stewardship of Health   59
Developing a Well-Formed Conscience   60
Concrete Application of Moral Norms   65
Elements of Informed Consent   66
Choosing a Physician   67
Summary   69
Questions   69
Cases   70

6   *Responsibilities of Health Care Professionals*   71
What Is a Profession?   71
Ideals of the Medical Profession   74
The Christian Health Care Professional   76
Personalizing the Health Care Profession   77
Professional Communication   81
Peer Relationships and Professional Discipline   83
Summary   85
Questions   85
Cases   86

7   *Social Responsibility for Health Care*   87
Models of Health Care   87
Gospel Principles of Social Organization   91
Functionalism   93
The Health Care Team   96
Health Care Ethics and Public Policy   98
The Catholic Health Care Facility   100
Summary   102
Questions   103
Cases   103

8   *Human Research and the Allocation of Resources* 105
Human Research   105

Norms for Research on Human Subjects   108
Allocating Resources: Micro and Macro Issues   115
Summary   118
Questions   119
Cases   119

9   *Sexuality and Reproduction*   121
The Meaning of Sexuality   121
Human Sexuality   124
Abortion   129
Disputed Cases: Ectopic Pregnancy and Anencephalic Infants   131
The Morality of Contraception   132
Natural Family Planning   134
Surgical Sterilization   135
Care of Rape Victims   136
Pastoral Considerations   137
Summary   139
Questions   140
Cases   140

10 *Reconstructing Human Beings*   141
Human Dominion over Nature   141
Surgical Procedures   143
Manipulation of Embryonic Cells   148
Genetic Manipulation   154
Summary   157
Questions   157
Cases   158

11 *Mental Illness: Medical and Psychiatric Therapies*   159
Mental Illness   159
Therapies for Mental Illness   161
Ethical Issues in Psychotherapy   168
Addiction   172
Summary   175
Questions   176
Cases   176

12 *Death and Dying*   179
The Mystery of Death   179
Determining the Moment of Death   181
Telling Truth to the Dying   186
Euthanasia and Suicide   187

Allowing a Person to Die   189
Pain and Dying   197
Care for the Corpse and Cadaver   198
Summary   201
Questions   201
Cases   202

13 *Spiritual Ministry and Health Care*   203
The Purpose of Pastoral Care   203
Spiritual Counseling   204
Celebrating the Healing Process   206
Baptism and the Eucharist   210
Summary   212
Questions   213
Cases   213

Epilogue   215

Appendix 1: Ethical and Religious Directives for Catholic
    Health Care Services   217

Appendix 2: The Universal Declaration of Human Rights
    of the United Nations   243

Sources   247

Index   251

Introduction

In the summer of 2001, the interest of the nation was consumed as never before with an issue of health care ethics: All agreed that it would be worthwhile for the country to sponsor research using human stem cells, but the means of obtaining these stem cells was intensely debated.

Should stem cells be harvested from the remains of aborted fetuses, from fetuses still living but temporarily frozen, or from adults? The arguments put forward by both sides for and against the use of stem cells from aborted fetuses will be considered later in the text. The significant fact for our consideration is the intense interest shown by all segments of society in this issue. For many years, health care ethics and the problems involved in the practice of medicine were considered the proper domain of health care professionals. It is now clear, however, that they are the concern of all citizens because of their effect upon the common good of society, and they will continue to be of intense concern as procedures such as germ cell manipulation become possible. Solving the ethical issues associated with and arising from health care will be a national need for years to come. Every concerned citizen in our society should be able to contribute intelligently to this dialogue or at least understand the constituent elements of the various ethical problems. Rather than refer to the discipline that enables people to discuss problems in medicine and health care as "bioethics," we prefer the term *health care ethics* because it has a wider purview and includes social as well as clinical issues arising in the practice of medicine and the provision of health care.

We believe that the Catholic tradition in ethics or morality has something important to contribute to this dialogue. The Catholic tradition is founded upon the belief that the Three Persons of the Trinity offer us their friendship and that the doctrine that will enable us to acquire this friendship is presented in the conclusions of natural law theory and the teaching of the Catholic Church. The *Ethical and Religious Directives for Catholic Health Care Facilities* (National Conference of Catholic Bishops 2001; see appendix 1) is the main compendium of Catholic teaching for Catholic health care institutions and professionals in the United States. This volume is in accord with the *Directives*, but it seeks to consider some of the theoretical issues not contained therein, such as the social teaching of the church and a more complete theological explanation for some of the individual directives.

This book stresses the Catholic tradition in health care ethics, but it does not seek to separate this tradition from the broader Christian tradition, or even from the humanistic approaches to the significant problems in health care prominent in our society. Certainly, Catholics are not the only citizens of the United States who are concerned about the ethics of medicine, health care, and death and dying. Hence, we seek to stress as a common ground for mutual understanding the *Universal Declaration of Human Rights of the United Nations* (appendix 2). We also realize that, in our pluralistic society, the Catholic concept of the dignity of the human person does not receive full adherence. Moreover, the pragmatic approach to ethical issues in health care, which is common in the scientific community, often separates the Catholic tradition from the "commonsense" answers of secular ethicists and scientists. Thus, although our approach is ecumenical, it is not overly irenic in the sense that we would gloss over the problems that separate the Catholic tradition from more popular opinions.

Since the second edition of *Ethics of Health Care* (1994), many developments in Catholic theology and the provision of medicine and health care justify this third edition. In the field of theology, the Catholic Church has issued several significant teaching documents, such as *The Splendor of Truth* (*Veritatis Splendor*), *The Gospel of Life*, (*Evangelium Vitae*), *Faith and Reason* (*Fides et Ratio*), and the *Catechism of the Catholic Church*, and a revised version of *Ethical and Religious Directives* (appendix 1), to mention just a few. These documents clarify many teachings of the church with regard to theory and specific issues.

Several changes in the provision of health care and in clinical practice have taken place since the previous edition: Managed care has become the prominent method of providing health care, most surgery is performed on an "outpatient" basis, therapy for mental illness has changed considerably as the result of the use of pharmaceuticals in addition to "talk therapy," the Human Genome Project has identified many sources of genetic anomalies, and hospice care for the terminally ill has become an integral element of health care. These changes and more have also led to revisions to the second edition.

The presentation of material in this volume is different from the two previous editions. We begin with a short history of contemporary ethical theories in an effort to present the various methods of attacking issues in health care ethics in our society. Then we focus upon the content of Catholic ethical tradition, discussing the derivation and meaning of ethical principles, and presenting a selection of the main ethical principles derived from the teachings of Christ and human experience associated with ethical fulfillment. After these historical-theological presentations in chapters 1 and 2, we examine the meaning of the term "human person in community." Because fulfilling the needs of persons is the touchstone of ethics, we examine the needs or goals of the human person, citing humanistic as well as theological sources, in chapter 3. Chapters 4 through 7 present the context of the U.S. health care system within which human persons seek health; thus, we examine the meaning of health, the personal responsibility for health, the responsibility of health care professionals, and the responsibility of the various human communities involved in providing health care. Next, we consider various contemporary ethical issues in medicine using the principles discussed in chapter 2 as a leitmotiv for more detailed discussions. Hence, chapters 8 through 12 discuss research upon persons, issues in sexual ethics and human reproduction, reconstructing and modifying human beings, mental illness and therapeutic methods, and death and dying. Last, in chapter 13 we present some thoughts on pastoral care, not seeking to present an entire tract on spirituality, but rather discussing in general the main concerns and opportunities of patients, health care professionals, and chaplains.

We have retained the following pedagogical methods that were introduced in the second edition: Each chapter begins with an overview, the conclusions are stated at the end of each section, and chapters end with short summaries, questions, and cases. We have kept citations and endnotes to a minimum, and we encourage readers to use the Internet to find additional information on any topic. Information on documents quoted in the text may be found in the sources section.

We thank the professors of health care ethics who have sent us observations and suggestions resulting from their use of the previous editions of this book. Finally, we thank Donna Grace Troy for her industrious efforts in preparing this volume for publication.

1

Methods in Health Care Ethics

OVERVIEW: What system of ethical reasoning should be used to determine whether certain values are worthwhile to pursue or what constitutes good or bad human actions? At present, several different systems of ethics are being followed in the United States. This chapter presents the best known of these systems, cites their historical sources, and contrasts them with the system of ethical determination followed in the Catholic community.

This chapter explains the system of the Catholic Church for making ethical decisions, that is, the form of ethical decision making. Chapter 2 will investigate the content of this system, that is, the matter of ethical decision making. The remainder of this volume will be devoted for the most part to applying these principles to contemporary ethical issues in health care.

1.1 THE ENLIGHTENMENT AND NEW ETHICAL SYSTEMS

By the end of the seventeenth century, controversy and wars between Catholics and Protestants and among the reformed churches caused great scandal and religious skepticism among the European intellectual elites. Moreover, in the fifteenth and sixteenth centuries, nations and peoples never before known challenged the possibility of ethical norms that would apply to all people. Added to this confusion in ethical thinking was an emphasis upon legalistic morality among Catholic theologians that brought discredit to the contemporary methods of doing ethics. As a result of these controversies and discoveries, philosophers and leading thinkers lost their faith in the ability to use human nature as a measure of ethical behavior, and in the contribution of religious thought to creating a just and orderly society. From this loss of faith in natural law reasoning and divine revelation arose the so-called Enlightenment, which sought to replace the teaching of various churches with a "religion of reason," which it was hoped would transcend religious quarrels and offer a unified understanding of human behavior. The religion of reason was not the result of a reasoned dialogue. Rather, it arose from a conviction on the part of philosophers, which was never defended by objective reasoning, that the power to discern good and evil was intuitive and present in every person. For example, the founders of our republic, who were largely products of the Enlightenment, justified their revolution from England by asserting in the Declaration of Independence that it is a "self-evident truth that all men are created equal and have been endowed by their Creator with certain inalienable rights, including life, liberty, and the pursuit of happiness." The power of Enlightenment thinking is shown by the fact that no argument was offered to prove that these truths were "self-evident" or that they justified revolution.

In contemporary times, the Enlightenment worldview has indeed taken control of the economic system, the universities, public schools, and the public media in the form of "secular humanism." Although these entities at times pay lip service to religious sources of truth by quoting the Bible or other documents of revealed religion, for the most part they consider the teaching of revealed religion as "outside" the realm of human knowledge and prefer to relegate religious thought to the sidelines of human life.

It is characteristic of the value systems descended from the Enlightenment that they reject any unified, official formulations of ethical theory as inimical to freedom of speech and conscience, which are considered as unassailable values and the basis of all human progress. This attitude leaves coherent formulations of Enlightenment "faith" up to various formulations of philosophers. Historically, most of the ethical philosophies of the Enlightenment stem from the questions concerning human knowledge raised by David Hume (d. 1776), who was a member of the Scottish school of philosophy.

Hume doubted that we can have objective knowledge through experience (*skepticism*) and though he maintained the concept of moral obligation, he held that one cannot go from the "is" of human experience to the "ought" of ethical norms by means of human reason. With Jean-Jacques Rousseau (d. 1753) and Francis Hutcheson (d. 1746), he maintained that human beings have an intuitive faculty for discerning moral good and evil that is not rational, but rather is emotional, the result of feelings. Thus, moral imperatives are basically subjective. Rousseau argued that if people would free themselves from prejudice acquired by bad education and return to their natural feelings, they would make much better ethical judgments. Such thinking seems to be the basis for our American confidence in the common sense of the people. We take opinion polls because we believe that what most people "feel is right" probably *is* right. The difficulty with this approach is that it provides no method of public, objective discussion but leaves problems to rhetoric and passion. Whose instincts are sound, just, accurate, or true?

1.2 HUME'S CONTRIBUTION TO OTHER SYSTEMS

From Hume's speculations have arisen the three major ethical systems of the past 300 years: *emotivism, formalism,* and *utilitarianism* (or *consequentialism*). Emotivism was Hume's own solution. In this system, it is granted that one cannot go "from the is to the ought" by means of human reason but only by means of an emotional faculty. Hence, emotivism concludes that values have no rational basis for determining good and evil actions and are prompted only by emotional experience when making such decisions. It is certainly true that at the beginning of most ethical discussions, people express emotional attitudes. Fortunately, some ethical discussions progress beyond this phase. But we cannot rest content with the initial impasse arising from emotions. Feelings are not sufficient criteria for ethical behavior, no matter how sincere they might be, because we differ in our emotional reactions and cannot find a common norm for acting from this source of human behavior. People are often led to do things by their feelings, which are often destructive of their own good or the good of others. How can we distinguish a feeling or emotion that is transitory and held only by a few from what is universal and consistent?

Consequently, as Aristotle (d. 322 B.C.E.) long ago taught in *The Nicomachean Ethics,* emotion is to be trusted only when it has been refined, educated, and disciplined by virtue (*right reason*). Recently, ethicists have emphasized that good decisions are not possible by merely following rules. We need *character* to meet the crisis of ethical decision making in medical affairs. Decisions made by people who have a respect for persons, reverence for life, and compassion for the suffering are likely to be good decisions, whereas decisions made by people who are insensitive and lack empathy are likely to be morally bad, no matter how much knowledge and skill they might possess.

In view of the foregoing, it is helpful to realize that sound ethical decisions will never be made in a purely rational manner. We are all emotional beings. Ultimately, all ethical decisions do involve a degree of moral sensitivity, fairness, and compassion. Yet we also realize that the emphasis upon pure emotion, no matter how sincere a person might be, is not a valid source of ethical decision making because it is too subjective and erratic. *Existentialism,* an ethical theory resembling emotivism that was popular in Europe during the middle of the twentieth century, maintains that every ethical decision is made in new circumstances. No doubt, each ethical decision is made in different circumstances, and this requires intelligent creativity, not mere conformity. But human nature is constant and consistent, and without general norms derived from human reason, people cannot act together for the common good.

Formalism, the second major ethical system, was developed by Immanuel Kant (d. 1804), who read the work of David Hume and stated that "it awakened him from a dogmatic slumber." Kant sought to overcome Hume's skepticism and reliance upon emotion as the basis for ethical obligation by presenting a complete system proposing his view of both speculative and practical (ethical) thinking. His *Critique of Pure Reason* is beyond the purpose of this study, but we shall consider the main ideas proposed in *The Critique of Practical Reason*, because this work influences many American ethicists today, even though few follow it exclusively.

Kant sought to develop a new type of ethics based not on our unknowable human nature but upon logical categories that he claimed are innate and preexisting in our minds. Reasonable persons of good will, he surmised, should agree on a consistent value system that would make a stable society possible. He was a deontologist in the sense that, in accord with his pious Protestant background, he thought that morality is a matter of obeying the moral law. But he did not posit any content for the moral law, providing only a formalistic procedure for decision making. Hence, his theory is called formalism.

Kant believed that for human beings to be truly free and truly moral they ought not to obey some external (*heteronomous*) law outside the human conscience but only a purely interior (*autonomous*) law legislated by the conscience of each individual. It might seem that self-legislation could end in the crudest form of egotistical emotivism. Kant, however, being well aware of this danger, insisted that people cannot claim to be ethical or moral unless they legislate for themselves in a rational way, free of all self-interest. Thus, his system is sometimes called "ethical rationalism" or "altruism." He argued that truly moral norms must follow the "categorical imperative": Act so that you are willing that your act should be a norm for all other agents. Thus, I must not steal or lie, because I do not want you to steal from me or to lie to me. But this does not tell us *why* stealing or lying is ethically wrong. Thus, formalism, although it aims to be the very opposite of emotivism, does risk degenerating into it, so that rationalism easily turns into sentimentalism, as it did for the romantic wing of the Enlightenment in the eighteenth century.

Undoubtedly, Kant saw the categorical imperative as a secular form of Jesus's saying, "Do unto others as you would have them do unto you." But Jesus indicates that his Golden Rule has a definite content, namely the Ten Commandments, the Beatitudes, and the right motive of love of God and neighbor. Kant's categorical imperative is an abstract mental form that provides no ethical content; nothing is right or wrong in itself, but only after the categorical imperative is invoked.

Today, Kant's theory in its original form is usually rejected as unrealistic, because pure disinterested formalism demands a morality devoid of human emotion. Nor is it clear how formalism can produce nonarbitrary concrete rules. Hence, some modern ethicists seek to maintain a "duty ethics" by adding principles or maxims that supplement the categorical imperative from the original theory of Kant. A well-known version of formalism was proposed by John Rawls, who bases morality upon an implied contract by which human persons agree to protect each other's rights. Beauchamp and Childress (1994), in their attempt to design a "common morality" of medical ethics, have outlined four principles—autonomy, fairness, beneficence, and nonmaleficence—which have no other justification than that they help us reach a consensus in a consistent manner. Such a method, however, is open to the objections of Kantian thinking: (1) It does not provide nonarbitrary concrete rules; (2) consistent behavior does not mean consistently good behavior; and, (3) it gives no objective, transcultural criteria for what makes behavior good or bad except the redundant concept of universalizability (i.e., common or customary morality).

Utilitarianism or consequentialism, the third major ethical system, was developed by Jeremy Bentham (d. 1832), who was also influenced by Hume. Bentham refined Hume's thought by stating that a person's emotional acceptance or rejection of a human act as good or bad is founded upon an estimation of how much pleasure or pain it gives the person performing the act. In some forms of utilitarianism, the pleasure or pain is considered from an *individualistic point of view*. This view seems the very opposite of Kant's ethics, which are based on the idea that any self-interested action is immoral by definition, but perhaps it is more realistic. Certainly, each person has the responsibility to care for his or her needs and interests. Even Jesus in giving us the great commandment to "love God and neighbor" added that one must love one's neighbor "as oneself."

Few ethicists have accepted a purely personal utilitarianism. Rather, they oppose Kantian duty ethics by insisting that ethical choices be made for the "greatest good for the greatest number of people." In this form, utilitarianism is often called consequentialism, because it abstracts from the morality of the action itself and focuses upon the consequences of the action for a number of people. Its model is economic exchange, in which gains and losses can be calculated in terms of monetary measures. But evil can be done if a greater good is to be achieved. In American society, this system of ethical decision making is common, from the dropping of the atomic bomb upon undefended civilians in Japan, to the consideration of sources of human stem cells for research or therapy. Thinking of this kind is in accord with our computerized logic and the pragmatism of American scientists. If the actions to which consequences give rise are not subject to ethical determination, it is clear that utilitarianism or consequentialism does not result in objective norms, nor does it offer criteria for judging human actions aside from the pain or pleasure they might cause. The *first conclusion* of this chapter: The Enlightenment gave rise to many ethical systems, based mainly upon belief in intuition as opposed to reason as the main source of moral decision making.

1.3 OTHER ETHICAL SYSTEMS IN THE UNITED STATES

In addition to the three foregoing methods derived from the Enlightenment thinkers, several other systems are followed in the United States, some of which predate Enlightenment thinking. These systems are often used in conjunction with the three systems we have already discussed.

Legalism or Positivism

Many people tend to think of morality or ethics in terms of a code of laws. If the laws are from secular law, or from custom, we have *legalism or positivism,* that is, ethics or morals resulting from positive civil law. According to this theory, which is propagated by many sociologists and anthropologists, morality or ethical behavior is determined by conformity to accepted social standards of a particular culture. This leads of course to *moral relativism* because different cultures have different moral norms. If the source of the positivistic norm for moral behavior is law, then the moral norms will change whenever the law changes. Thus, before the decisions of the U.S. Supreme Court legalizing abortion, most people considered abortion an immoral act. But after the decision, many people considered it moral because it was now legal.

Human laws or accepted customs are not the ultimate criteria for human morality for three reasons: (1) Legal morality is always broad and unrefined, so in personal life, the law must be supplemented by more particular standards. (2) Human laws, which might be just to begin with, often become unjust due to changed circumstances, so it becomes necessary to criticize them, try to change them, or even occasionally refuse to obey them. (3) Some laws, like those of Hitler's Third Reich, require behavior that is really criminal.

Religious Legalism

If the laws that form the basis of moral norms are derived from religion, such as the Ten Commandments, or the Qur'an, the result is *religious legalism.* Many theists ground ethics in a direct appeal to the will of God, who is the ultimate authority and who determines what is right and wrong. Jews, Christians, and Muslims believe that God has revealed His will in the Bible or the Qur'an. This is often called *divine command morality,* and before the Enlightenment, it was a predominant form of framing moral or ethical norms, especially for religious communities.

Today, this type of moral mandate remains common among some Christians, and it predominates among Protestants. Although there are many different Protestant approaches to ethical theory, most of them teach that because of the fall of Adam into sin, human beings are blinded to moral truth by our self-righteousness. People can be freed from this blindness only when confronted with the righteousness of God as revealed in the Word of God, especially in the Incarnate Word, Jesus Christ. Even with biblical revelation, the will of God remains essentially mysterious to us, so we ought simply to obey Him in absolute trust.

Catholics generally have not favored this approach because the emphasis on blind submission to God does not seem to do justice to the biblical doctrine that human beings are made in the image and likeness of God; that is, we have an intellect and will. True, this image of God has been profoundly distorted by sin, so that without God's help we could never arrive at a true knowledge of our human nature and destiny. Only by the grace given us in Christ are we able to achieve the goal of eternal life with God. But it is also true that, in spite of sin, we retain the image and likeness of God.

This indelible likeness to God constituted by the gifts of intelligence and freedom opens all human beings to God's call to friendship. After we are reborn through grace, we are able to obey God not blindly, but intelligently and freely, recognizing that God has forbidden or commanded certain behavior. God's will does remain a mystery, but it is not arbitrary, and its reasons should be explored. Thus, Catholic moral theology seeks to go beyond *religious legalism* to an ethics that insists that God wants us to understand His wise purposes and to use our own intelligence and experiences, enlightened by grace, to carry them out in our daily lives. The *second conclusion:* One form or another of legalism is a common method of decision making for many people in the United States.

1.4 THE MORAL SYSTEM OF THE CATHOLIC CHURCH

The moral or ethical system of the Catholic Church is a combination of truths accepted on Divine Faith as revealed by God and natural law reasoning. Although "revelation ended with the death of the last Apostle" (*Catechism of the Catholic Church* 1997, n. 66), the church develops a more explicit, clear, and certain knowledge of the truths of revelation, either by penetrating this teaching more thoroughly over the centuries, or by applying this teaching to contemporary ethical issues. Revelation teaches us about many different aspects of human behavior, but we often summarize the moral teaching of revelation by citing the Ten Commandments or the moral teaching of Jesus, which includes the Ten Commandments and the Beatitudes and which is summarized in the one Great Commandment, "Love God with all your heart and mind, and your neighbor as yourself" (Mt 22:34).

Catholics believe that the church has the right and responsibility to teach with authority the truths of the Gospel that are necessary for our salvation— whether these truths are stated explicitly in Scripture or are supported implicitly by the truths contained therein. In addition, the church can teach principles of natural law with authority, when necessary. The method of church teaching is a complex topic. Recently, the teaching authority of the church has sought to make this doctrine more understandable through the document *To Defend the Faith* (*Ad Tuendam Fidem*; Congregation for the Doctrine of the Faith 1998). We shall say more about this teaching in chapter 5.

Natural law, an important element of church teaching, is often misunderstood. Natural law is "natural" because the goals and major values human beings seek are innate; that is, they are from nature and are not selected freely by individual persons or communities. (See chapter 3 for an examination of these natural goals or values.) Because human nature does not change, the basic goals are constant and thus basic morality does not change. Choosing actions to achieve these goals is open to human freedom, but not the choice of the goals themselves.

Although the basic goals are common to all human persons, there are also acquired goals, which are the result of the culture in which one lives. Acquired goals are associated with basic goals because they bespeak ways in which basic goals can or should be pursued. For example, human beings have a basic goals of seeking knowledge, but the manner in which they seek it varies according to the culture in which they live. In Western culture, knowledge is acquired through schooling. Hence, schooling is mandatory and is also considered a right.

Natural law is "law" because by reasoning about our innate goals and values we can determine actions, which we phrase in norms or laws that will enable us to achieve these goals. Thus, we have an innate desire to prolong life, and we determine that eating healthy foods and avoiding the use of tobacco will dispose for a longer life; thus, we formulate norms or "laws" concerning healthy habits or behavior. Because human nature does not essentially change, these basic goals remain constant, and the safe and sure methods of pursuing these goals also remain constant. Hence, natural law is not a moral instinct but rather a type of reasoning that enables us to know what is right and wrong in most situations of life.

The norms of natural law, however, are not "deontological," that is, merely based on obedience to law, but rather "teleological," that is, based on the choice of means suitable to achieve the true goals of human life. Conclusions derived from natural law are accepted because of the intrinsic nature of the reasoning process used to reach conclusions or because the norms of natural law are sometimes confirmed by the teaching authority of the church. The proximity of natural law reasoning to revelation is evidenced by the fact that the Ten Commandments express the principles of natural law (*Catechism of the Catholic Church* 1997, n. 2070).

The natural law method of seeking moral norms and evaluating human acts has a long history in the Catholic community. Saint Thomas Aquinas (d. 1274), building on the ethics of Aristotle—who knew nothing about the

Christian faith and wrote purely on the basis of reason and human experience—in the *Summa Theologica* outlined a method of ethical decision making. Pope John Paul II, in turn, utilized this method in the encyclical *The Splendor of Truth* (*Veritatis Splendor*) in 1993. We shall use these sources as we present the Catholic tradition in ethical decision making.

The natural law method of reasoning used in the Catholic community presupposes first of all that human beings should be dedicated to achieving the ultimate purpose of human life, their ultimate goal. According to Catholic teaching, the ultimate purpose of human life is happiness, which is found only in friendship with God and our neighbor. Second, we seek to determine through natural law reasoning whether the specific and individual actions we perform are proper means to fulfilling the ultimate goal of life, friendship with God and our neighbor. The most important element in this process of specific determination is the moral object or the goal of the action, called in Latin the *finis operis*. As Pope John Paul II stated in *Veritatis Splendor*, "The morality of the human act depends primarily and fundamentally on the 'object' rationally chosen by the deliberate 'will'" (John Paul II 1993, n. 78).

The moral object, not to be confused with the physical activity associated with human action, is the purpose that the act accomplishes in the moral order. The moral object can be described as the intention inherent in the action that one is actually performing; what you are here and now doing on purpose. It specifies the human act and is the purpose that the act accomplishes as a means to the ultimate goal of life. Saint Thomas and Pope John Paul II refer to the moral object as the "proximate end" of the moral act (*Summa Theol.*, Aquinas 1947, I-II, q. 1, a. 4, ad. 2; *Veritatis Splendor*, John Paul II 1993, n. 78). If I give money to the poor, I am performing an act of charity, a good human act judged by its moral object or the intention inherent in the act.

Although the moral object or *finis operis* is the fundamental element in discerning the morality of a human act, it is not the only element. The circumstances of the act must also be considered in order to evaluate the total moral act (*Summa Theol.*, Aquinas 1947, I-II, q. 18, a. 3). Many circumstances can be enumerated, depending upon the moral act in question. Thus, we might ask "when," "how much," or "in what manner," depending upon the elements that might influence the morality of the action being considered. But one circumstance that is present in every moral act, and that has a significant role in determining the morality of the totality of human action, is the circumstance of "why."

This circumstance of "why" is the most important circumstance. Human motivation is often mixed. Besides the fundamental intention of the object that makes it a moral and not just a physical object, this fundamental intention (the *finis operis*, or essential character of the moral object) may be qualified by other motives. These other accidental or secondary motives qualify the essential intention by making the act better or worse. This secondary motivation, the *finis operantis*, is only a circumstantial intention, and no matter how good it might be, it cannot make the essential intention of the moral act good if that essential intention is intrinsically immoral (i.e., contrary to the true goal of human life). That is why we may not "do evil for good to come of it" and why "the end does not justify the means."

Consider the case of a physician who injects a debilitated patient with a fatal dose of drugs to end his suffering. The moral object of the act (what the physician actually intends to do) is to kill the patient, and it is this intention that makes the physical act of the injection a moral evil. The circumstances of the physician's act (e.g., the time, place, and condition of the patient) cannot make this a good act, nor can his circumstantial or secondary intention (e.g., ending the patient's suffering). The ultimate reason that determines the moral goodness or badness of an act is the intention of the act as a means to true happiness both of the agent and of the common good. Thus, killing an innocent person to help relieve pain cannot be justified.

Notice that the term *intention* has been used to refer to three different elements involved in human acts: the ultimate end, the moral object (*finis operis*), and the motive of the agent (*finis operantis*). When engaging in an ethical discussion, it is important to specify which sense of intention is meant. Too often, people speak as though the intention of the agent—which is really an accident, insofar as the moral object is concerned—determines the morality of the human act. However, as Pope John Paul II pointed out in *The Splendor of Truth* (*Veritatis Splendor*), the intention of the action is the primary specification of morality, and the intention of the agent is only ancillary to the original determination of morality (John Paul II 1993, n. 79).

In addition to considering the moral object of the action (*finis operis*) and the total motivation of the agent (*finis operantis*), other circumstances that could influence the morality of the act must be considered (*Summa Theol.*, Aquinas 1947, I-II, q. 7, a. 4). As was indicated above, only the circumstance of why is significant in every human act. At times, however, other circumstances may become important; for example, stealing is morally wrong, but it makes a difference in the overall morality of the act whether I steal pennies from a rich man or hundreds of dollars from a poor man. Stealing a chalice makes a simple theft a sacrilege, thus changing significantly the moral character of the total action.

It follows from the above that some actions that are evil by reason of the moral object can never be made good by the intention of the agent. These actions, which are called *intrinsically* evil, are incapable of being ordered to God because they radically contradict the good of the person made in the image and likeness of God. They are always wrong, quite apart from the intention of the one acting. Pope John Paul II listed several of these actions in *Veritatis Splendor*: "Whatever is hostile to life itself, such as homicide, genocide, abortion, euthanasia, voluntary suicide, and whatever violates the integrity of the human body" (John Paul II 1993, n. 80).

In sum, to make an ethical decision, one must do three things:

1. Act toward the right ultimate goal, that is, friendship with God and neighbor.
2. Choose an effective means to achieve that goal. Thus, acts that are intrinsically evil must be rejected. Help in selecting good actions and in avoiding bad actions is offered in the various moral codes of the church; e.g., Ten Commandments and *Ethical and Religious Directives*.
3. If the act chosen is an appropriate means to the ultimate end, then one must have an honest intention, and all other circumstances must contribute to the good moral object.

According to this natural law tradition of discerning the morality of a human act, all three criteria that we have discussed must be good in order for the act to be considered morally good. The traditional slogan is: "Good from an integral cause, evil from any defect."

In the second half of the twentieth century, several Catholic moral theologians who were seeking a teleological revision of legalistic ethics proposed a new system of moral decision making called Proportionalism. It was based on an alleged principle of proportionalism, according to which no act could be judged intrinsically evil simply by reason of its moral object. Moral decisions should be made by taking the moral object, the circumstances, and the secondary intention together. If on this basis the "pre-moral goods" outweighed the "pre-moral evils," the acts could be judged good. As we have shown above, this theory fails to make the important distinction between the primary and essential intention of the moral object and accidental and secondary intentions that could somewhat qualify the fundamental intention. Only after the goodness or badness of the primary intention has been determined do any secondary or circumstantial intentions become relevant.

The reason that Proportionalism enjoyed considerable popularity—until it was rejected by Pope John Paul II in the encyclical *The Splendor of Truth* (*Veritatis Splendor*)—was that it permitted exceptions to all moral norms, because in weighing so-called pre-moral values against negative values, with a little ingenuity one could always imagine some circumstances and some good intentions that would seem to outweigh the disvalues and permit one to do what is pragmatically convenient. Thus, in the example given above, a physician might justify "mercy killing" by arguing that he has a good intention of relieving suffering and in the circumstances life is not worth living. In fact, the moral object of his act is to directly kill an innocent person, whereas his intention of relieving suffering is secondary.

A system so arbitrary is open to rationalization and abuse, and hence John Paul II calls it "teleogism"—not a truly teleological method of decision making. He shows that this is contrary to Catholic tradition, which has always designated certain acts, such as killing the innocent, as "intrinsically evil" by reason of their moral object, whatever the circumstances, including good secondary motivations.

SUMMARY

Several methods of ethical decision making are utilized in the Western world. As the first part of this chapter indicates, most of these systems share the conviction that emotion, not reason, is the fundamental element of ethical decision making. Because emotions are such a changeable element in human decision making, however, it is very difficult—if not impossible—to frame moral norms using these systems, which are unchangeable or which pertain to all persons. Equally deceptive are moral systems that depend on legal norms, because legal norms do not of themselves indicate why an action is morally good or bad. If natural law and revelation are used as the basis for ethical decision making, general ethical norms can be formulated that will be applicable to all persons insofar as basic goals and moral norms are concerned. The Ten Commandments, for example, which have meaning in very diverse cultures, can be derived from the basic principles of natural law.

QUESTIONS

1. Describe the reasons why so many different ethical systems are utilized in the United States.
2. The Catholic method of ethical reasoning assumes that all human beings have the same human nature and thus that some general ethical norms can be formulated for all people. Is this logical?
3. How do the Supreme Court decisions on abortion reflect the diversity of moral decision making in the United States?

CASES

1. A few years ago, two federal circuit courts approved the practice of physician-assisted suicide. The Supreme Court of the United States, however, reversed both decisions. Was this fundamentally a disagreement over legal reasoning or ethical norms?
2. Several ethics committees or boards have been instituted by the federal government in the past thirty years. For the most part, they have not been successful, because the members have different ethical

assumptions. Can you describe a method that might allow these agencies to consider constructively some of the difficult ethical issues of our time?

3. Sam maintains that Catholics, because they are a minority in the United States, should not try to influence the ethical decisions that affect people who are not Catholics. Rather, they may live according to their own ethical norms, but not try to influence public policy in accord with these norms. Would you be able to debate Sam on this issue? If so, what would your argument be?

2

The Content of Catholic Health Care Ethics

OVERVIEW: Chapter 1 considered the form that several contemporary ethical theories follow and contrasted them with the Catholic tradition in this regard. In this chapter, we consider the content of the Catholic moral tradition, especially as it is concerned with questions of health care ethics. Before presenting the various principles or truths that constitute the content of Catholic health care ethics, however, we present some basic ideas concerning the content of Christian ethics: "Is there a Christian ethics?" and "What is the meaning of a principle in ethics?" These questions are especially important for those who adhere to Catholic health care ethics because it depends upon the natural law reasoning that causes some to maintain that Catholic ethics is not really Christian. Moreover, Catholic ethics uses the word "principle" in a much different sense than other ethical systems now in use in the United States. The remaining chapters of this book will be guided by the principles elucidated in this chapter.

2.1 IS THERE A CATHOLIC ETHICS?

Certainly, the moral values contained in the Bible or in the teaching of the Catholic Church are found also in other philosophies of life. We have already illustrated this fact by referring to the *Universal Declaration of Human Rights of the United Nations* (1948), to which all nations of the world, no matter what their ideology, have subscribed. Moreover, natural law values and principles may be utilized to some extent by any method of ethical theory. But when people agree on a set of values, they may differ on which values are more important than others. Thus, there is always a hierarchy of values. Are the priorities of Christians different from the priorities of others who ascribe to the *Universal Declaration of Human Rights*?

Christians summarize their priorities as the *theological virtues*: faith, hope, and charity. These virtues are primarily concerned with pursuing an intimate friendship with God and neighbor and secondarily with pursuing other goals that fulfill the individual human person. The Christian tradition has also recognized the need for four other principal virtues: prudence, justice, fortitude, and temperance, which are called *moral virtues,* and which support our pursuit and practice of the theological virtues. These moral virtues give us balance in pursuing our individual goals and in recognizing and protecting the rights and needs of others.

Thus, though it is true that the reasoning of Christian ethics may at time use some of the same norms and reasoning process as natural law theories (e.g., do not kill innocent people), the entire context within which these principles are applied is different for the Christian than for the person who is merely trying to follow the law, whether natural or positive. The Christian is first of all striving for friendship with God, and to achieve this goal, faith, hope, and charity are necessary. Moreover, in response to the love that God has for each person, one strives to love one's neighbor as oneself; for this goal, faith, hope, and charity also are necessary. To facilitate the practice of faith, hope, and charity, Christians need to cultivate the virtues of prudence, justice, temperance, and fortitude.

It is important to understand that faith, hope, and charity, as Christians use these terms, are not mere feeling or sentiments, but rather are rooted in faith in the Incarnate Word of God, Jesus Christ, who tells us who God is and what our relations with him and our neighbor must be. Thus, Christian faith moves people from an emotional to a rational level of ethical understanding, because rather than a blind trust, faith is a genuine understanding of God's purpose for us, an imperfect but real share in God's wisdom. Christian faith, therefore, moves beyond a duty ethics of mere obedience to God's will to a means–end level of intelligent free choice.

For Saint Paul, the primary virtues of faith, hope, and charity derive from his conviction that a fully human life can be achieved only through a personal union with God by incorporation into the risen Christ. For Catholic moral teaching, therefore, Jesus provides the supreme model of Christian character marked by these seven virtues. Secular humanists might agree that these seven virtues are significant, but they would not agree on the priority given them. The difference in evaluation often results in striking differences in moral decisions. This does not mean that Christians have a monopoly on the true God or his grace, but only that the gracious God has made himself most fully, explicitly, and intimately known to humanity in Jesus Christ. The *first conclusion:* The gifts of faith, hope, and charity work toward the satisfaction of our deeper needs. Saint Paul writes of these three virtues: "So faith, hope, and love remain, these three; but the greatest of these is love" (1 Cor 13:13). Hence, they can well serve to classify a set of ethical principles that are explicitly and exclusively Christian and that can be applied to ethical issues in health care.

2.2 WHAT IS AN ETHICAL PRINCIPLE?

To reach any conclusion, including the practical conclusions involved in ethical reasoning, we must go from the more well known to the less well known. An ethical principle is a general norm or statement that helps us do this. Thus, we have an ethical norm that we should respect the rights of others. In applying this norm, we first seek to understand what a right is, and then consider whether allowing people to make their own decisions about health care procedures is a right. If so, it is clear that we should allow people to make such decisions.

The principles that we present in this chapter are derived from objective experience. They are general norms derived from the experience of human beings as they have pursued happiness through the centuries. They present the wisdom of theology, "what works" if we are to effectively pursue the goals of life in an integrated manner. They are not a priori forms in the mind that pre-exist our experience or are the result of an intuitive faculty, as many of the Enlightenment philosophers and their modern-day followers maintain. Thus, as we state principles gathered from experience, we affirm that we know things as they exist in reality, not merely our own thought. Other more particular principles of moral action could be stated. But the twelve principles we present here are especially important guides to human happiness.

What we seek through the use of these principles is an understanding of what it means to be human. Our model for this effort is Jesus Christ. But we must remember that Jesus did not hesitate to express his moral teaching in principles or norms, which we find throughout the Gospels. The *second conclusion:* The principles we present are derived from human experience, enlightened by the teaching and example of Jesus. Because the theological virtues of faith, hope, and charity are central to Catholic moral tradition and teaching, we shall cluster our principles of Catholic health care ethics around these virtues, and we shall point out how the moral virtues of prudence, temperance, fortitude, and justice are instrumental in helping persons develop these theological virtues and seek fulfillment in life.

2.3 PRINCIPLES OF CHRISTIAN FAITH

Faith in God, especially in the person of Jesus Christ, is a "free assent to the whole truth that God has revealed" (*Catechism of Catholic Church* 1997, n. 150). One aspect of the truth revealed through faith is to give us definite goals to pursue: friendship with God and love of neighbor. These goals are pursued by practical acts of intellect and will, inspired by grace. Once we freely assent to the teaching of Jesus, we not only believe certain truths about God, but we have certain practical goals to strive for and norms that guide our pursuit. Thus, the practical aspect of divine faith is pursued through a series of human acts forthcoming from the virtue of prudence.

Christian prudence (often called "wisdom" in the Bible) is faith in its practical aspect, as it enables us to be open to the guidance of Christ's spirit as we pursue the purpose of life. Although prudence is often synonymous with caution in the contemporary world, in the sense used to denote a virtue, it implies the correct selection of a means to a goal. Thus, prudence as a virtue is involved in all of our decisions of intellect and will as we pursue the ultimate or intermediate goals of human life. The first five principles of health care ethics, which we cluster around the virtue of faith, are all concerned with perfecting the choice of a means to an end, or faith in action. If our faith is to be practical, we must take care to inform our own conscience (*principle of well-formed conscience*) and respect the right of others to do the same (*principle of free and informed consent*).

At times, the actions we perform may be difficult to discern ethically. They may have two effects, one in accord with our proximate intention (*finis operis*), and one contrary to our proximate intention. To discern that our action is truly in accord with our proximate intention, we use the *principle of double effect*. Or when cooperating with other people as we strive for a goal, we may find that we are contributing to another person's immoral action; to be assured that our actions are not willfully or significantly contributing to an evil action of another person, we use the *principle of cooperation*. Finally, the moral "person" (actually, institution) that is responsible for ethical health care is a complex of persons needing accurate information. The whole network is in need of good communication; hence, the *principle of professional communication*.

The Principle of a Well-Formed Conscience

To make a prudential ethical decision, a person must make four determinations. First, the person must proceed on the basis of a fundamental commitment to God and the authentic dignity of persons, including themselves. In every person's life, there is a commitment to some goal that has priority and that influences the choice of subordinate goals. This fundamental commitment or option is the source of all morality; the general intention that gives unity and pattern to one's whole life. Jesus said, "Seek first the Kingdom of God" (Mt 6:33). He realized that, unfortunately, many people have no clear idea of their purpose in life, no fundamental commitment, and so he referred to them as "sheep without a shepherd."

Second, among possible actions that might seem able to achieve a proximate goal, the person must exclude all that is contradictory to loving God and neighbor as oneself—that is, all actions that are intrinsically evil. Human freedom is given to help us pursue the good, not to choose between good and evil. From the beginning, then, we should exclude actions that are intrinsically evil, not only because we wish to reject what is harmful, but also because we are willing to listen to the teaching of Christ as presented to us through the church.

Third, the person must analyze the moral object of the action (essential or primary intention, or *finis operis*), his or her circumstantial motives (secondary intentions, *finis operantis*), and the other circumstances of the action, to assure that the action is in accord with striving for friendship with God, the person's own integral well-being, and the well-being of others (ultimate and subordinate goals).

In making these three determinations, a person needs accurate information, which is available through his or her own experience and other sources, especially through divine guidance from Christ, who said, "I am the way, the truth, and the life" (Jn 14:6). It is true that in giving us human intelligence God expects us to think intently and creatively about how we are to journey toward him, but he has not left us alone in the dark. In this regard, the person in health care has the explicit guidance of the church in such documents as the *Ethical and Religious Directives* (see appendix 1) and the *Catechism of the Catholic Church* (1997).

Fourth, the person must act in accord with his or her well-formed conscience. Prudence is sometimes described as a process by which we see, judge, and act. Too often, people have a well-formed conscience but do not follow through with the act. In social settings, people are often influenced by the attitudes of others. Certainly, the thoughts and feelings of others should be considered in creating a well-formed conscience. But once one's conscience is formed, it may be necessary to act contrary to the attitudes of others to practice prudence. Thus the virtue of fortitude is often needed to activate decisions of prudence.

The Principle of Informed Consent

The principle of informed consent is really a corollary of the principle of a well-formed conscience. If, as a health care professional, I must act with an informed conscience, it would be unethical for me to ask others to cooperate with me unless I share with them the relevant information required for ethical decisions. If the person from whom consent is required is incompetent, then another person, a proxy, must offer the necessary consent. We treat this topic at greater length in chapter 5 because of its pivotal role in clinical situations.

The Principle of Double Effect

The principle of double effect is an important element of Catholic theology. Saint Thomas Aquinas introduced the concept into theological discourse when he stated: "Nothing hinders one act from having two effects, only one of which is intended, while the other is beside the intention. Now moral acts take their species according to what is intended, and not according to what is beside the intention, since this is accidental" (*Summa Theol.*, II-II, q. 64, a. 7).

Thus, if a woman who is pregnant is found to have a cancerous uterus, a surgeon could remove the cancerous uterus in order to save the woman's life, a good moral object. The surgeon would realize that removing the gravid uterus will result in the death of the fetus, but this effect is beyond the intention of the woman and the surgeon; thus, it is not a moral effect but a physical effect of the act. If they could, they would both counteract the cancer and save the child, but the evil effect is inextricably connected with the good effect.

This principle is rejected by many contemporary ethicists of the proportionalist and utilitarian schools because they maintain that if you foresee that an evil effect, even if it is beyond your intention, you are still morally responsible for it. It seems this opinion follows from their conviction that humans must perform moral evil and that a morally good act is one that in light of its effects inflicts as little evil as possible. This theory does not comprehend the actual situations of the moral life.

There are four conditions for invoking this principle. First, the directly intended object (*finis operis*) of the act must not be to intrinsically contradict one's own fundamental commitment to God and to neighbor, or to oneself (i.e., it must be an action judged to be good by reason of its moral object).

Second, the intentions of the agent (both primary and circumstantial) must be to achieve the good effect and to avoid the harmful effects in so far as possible, i.e., the evil effect is only indirectly intended. Third, the foreseen beneficial effects must not be achieved by means of the evil effect. For instance, in the above-mentioned example, it would be unethical to kill the fetus directly (as the moral object) to make it easier to remove the uterus.

Fourth, the benefits of action must be equal or greater than the foreseen harmful effects. In a certain sense, only the first condition is necessary, because the other conditions are commonsense methods of assuring that the first condition is fulfilled. Some Catholic ethicists have erroneously maintained that the principle of double effect allows a person to choose "the lesser evil," but it is contradictory to claim that it can be ethical to choose what is evil or unethical in itself, even under duress. True, it may happen that in some situations when a person is determined to do evil, that another might counsel this person to avoid a greater evil, and as a result of this counseling the person being counseled chooses "the lesser evil," but this is very different from choosing an evil for which one is personally responsible or approving of an evil in itself.

The Principle of Cooperation

Sometimes people cooperate with a person doing evil by approving what the person does, or by willfully and knowingly partaking in the evil action. Thus, I may join freely with another person in robbing a bank. This is *formal cooperation* in an unethical act, and it is always wrong. Conversely, I may cooperate with another person, not because I freely approve or cooperate in the evil action, but because I am coerced into cooperating for one reason or another. Coercion, whether physical or moral, is often called duress. When the duress is present, the cooperation is known as *material cooperation*, and it may be of two different kinds. If one cooperates in an evil act by performing something that is essential for the performance of the evil action, then it is *immediate* material cooperation. If one cooperates in an accidental or nonessential manner in the evil action, then it is called *mediate* material cooperation.

For example, if one works at an abortion clinic only because one needs a job to support one's family, this is material cooperation. But the type of material cooperation will depend upon the manner in which the person cooperates with the person responsible for the evil action. If one operates the vacuum machine that aborts young fetuses, one is doing something that is essential for performing the evil of abortion, Thus, it would be immediate material cooperation. Immediate material cooperation in the evil act of another is not ethical, even if there is duress present.

However, if one nurses people after they have had abortions, or cuts the grass at the abortion clinic, it would not contribute anything essential to the act of abortion and would be an act of mediate material cooperation. Finally, the possibility of scandal could prohibit acts of even mediate material cooperation because, even though the moral object of the act is good, it may lead another into sin (*Catechism of the Catholic Church* 1997, n. 2287). Because it is often difficult to determine whether one is contributing something essential or accidental to the evil action, and whether true scandal might be present, it is often difficult to apply this distinction correctly.

Mediate material cooperation should be avoided if at all possible. But mediate material cooperation may be performed if there is a sufficient reason. This is an application of the principle of double effect. Thus mediate material cooperation may be justified if there is a serious reason for it because the action of the cooperator is fundamentally good.

When some theologians discuss the principle of legitimate cooperation, they prefer to distinguish formal cooperation as explicit or implicit, and to identify only one type of material cooperation. This is a valid method of distinguishing the possible ways of cooperating with another in sinful actions, even though it is not as traditional as the terminology used above.

However, only one set of distinctions should be used at one time. Recently, some Catholic theologians maintained that if duress were present, a Catholic health care corporation could manage a hospital where direct sterilizations were performed, if the sterilizations were performed by employees of the non-Catholic hospital. But managing an institution is an essential participation in the work of the institution, and the form of cooperation in the direct sterilizations would be immediate material cooperation or implicit formal cooperation.

In a recent edition of *Health Care Ethics* (Ashley and O'Rourke 1997), we pointed out that the appendix of the *Ethical and Religious Directives for Catholic Health Care Services* of 1994 was misleading because it seemed to allow cooperation in actions that are intrinsically evil if "duress" were present. To eliminate this misconception, the *Directives* have been revised (2001); the appendix has been eliminated, and a new directive has been added (directive 70) that explicitly rejects cooperation in actions that are intrinsically evil, even if duress could be alleged.

The Principle of Professional Communication

Truth cannot be arrived at simply by an individual effort. The moment a patient enters a health care facility, a process of history taking, testing, and chart keeping begins. Moreover, because the institution is an administrative network of cooperating personnel, problems of interpersonal relations arise between the staff and the patients themselves.

This whole network depends upon *good communication*, which is impossible without (1) trust, (2) contact among the people who have information, (3) clear articulation and expression of information, and (4) continuous feedback to correct failures in communication. Modern communication theory has shown that this work of communication depends upon good emotional relations among the communicators, because emotional conflict is a powerful barrier to exchange of information and brings into play all sorts of unconscious factors. It thus becomes a serious moral duty in every institution to promote an emotional openness between the staff and the patients. The *principle of professional communication* can be formulated as follows:

1. to strive to establish and preserve trust at both the emotional and rational levels;
2. to share the information one possesses that is legitimately needed by others to develop an informed conscience;
3. to refrain from lying or giving misleading information, and
4. to keep secret information that is not legitimately needed by others, but that if revealed might harm either the patient or others or destroy trust.

The Christian specification of this principle arises from the understanding of trust and forgiveness. Jesus is represented as dealing with individuals in a way that won their trust and confidence, even though he recognized their sinfulness. For the Christian, therefore, professional confidentiality is not only professional, but expresses respect for the dignity of the human person, whom only God has a right to judge. Hence the *third conclusion:* Both reason and Christian faith convince us that all persons are created in God's image as intelligent, free, morally responsible agents. Consequently, they must strive to base their free decisions upon accurate information and must truthfully share this information with patients and coworkers, at the same time respecting the privacy and the consciences of others.

2.4. PRINCIPLES OF CHRISTIAN LOVE

Having considered how norms that guide faith are rooted in our basic need for truth, we consider another basic need, the need for society, which is the result of love. Our fundamental motivation for loving God, ourselves, and our neighbor is the love that God shows us all. This divine love disposes us to self-fulfillment through relationships with other human beings and above all with the three divine Persons: Father, Son, and Holy Spirit (*Catechism of the Catholic Church* 1997, n. 1822).

Love is not only a kind of feeling but also the practical will that leads one person to be concerned about another and that person's true needs. Furthermore, love motivates people to help others fulfill these needs by sharing with others the values they themselves enjoy. Love, however, degenerates into sentimentality unless it is assisted by the virtue of justice, which is the consistent will to respect the rights of others. Although love presupposes justice, it goes beyond justice to meet the needs of people, even if they are undeserving.

The principles of love related to health care are threefold: (1) Every person must be valued as a unique, irreplaceable member of the human community (the *principle of human dignity*). (2) Every person must be encouraged to play a part in the human community and fully share in its benefits (the *principle of common good*, sometimes called the *principle of participation in community*). (3) All persons must be helped to realize their full potential (the *principle of the totality and integrity of the human person*).

The Principle of Human Dignity

The root cause of all unjust discrimination is the failure to understand that human dignity is not based on physical or mental health, any more than it is upon money or education, but upon the single fact that a human person is made in the image of God. Once this principle is firmly held, there is no shame or personal inferiority in being blind, crippled, homosexually oriented, poor, or illiterate. All are equally persons, have the same human rights, and have the same claim to justice and dignity. Thus, it is contrary to the Gospel to refuse to respect the rights of others because of their nationality, race, sex, age, or physical or mental impairment. The health care professions, in their best tradition, have always sought to help people on the basis of need, not because of social status.

Jesus said; "Treat others the way you would have them treat you: This sums up the law and the prophets" (Mt 7:12). Thus, we formulate the principle of human dignity as follows: All ethical decisions in health care must aim at human dignity, that is, the maximal integrated satisfaction of the innate and cultural needs—biological, psychological, ethical, and spiritual—of all human persons, as individuals and as members of both their national communities and the world community.

The Principle of Common Good and Subsidiarity

The principle of common good and subsidiarity is also called the principle of participation in community. The principle maintains that human communities exist only to promote the common good of their members, and that each person or social group has a right and a responsibility to participate in this effort. Insofar as health is a concern of the human community, when discussing the responsibility for each person to strive personally for health, and to depend upon the community when personal effort is not enough, we demonstrate the meaning of this principle (chapters 5 and 7).

The word subsidiarity is often used to describe one aspect of this principle, the aspect that calls upon each person or lower social unit to be given the opportunity to exercise the responsibility to achieve the goals proper to it. But the principle also calls for a dependence of individuals and lower social units upon higher units of society, which will provide assistance that lower groups or individuals within society cannot acquire for themselves.

The principle can be formulated at follows. Human communities exist to promote and share the common good among members, "from each according to ability, to each according to need." First, then, decision making rests vertically primarily with the person, and then with the lower social levels and (horizontally) with functional social units.

Second, the higher social units intervene only to supply the lower units with what they cannot achieve for themselves, while at the same time working to make it easier in the future for the lower units and individuals to satisfy these needs by their own efforts. Notice how this principle—if applied to our national health programs—would change the manner in which health care is allocated. At present, for the most part we allocate health care to those who can pay for it, not according to the need of the persons in the community.

The Principle of Totality and Integrity

The principle of totality and integrity applies the principle of human dignity to oneself. To promote human dignity in community, all persons must care for and develop their natural functions in two ways. First, bodily and psychic lower functions are never sacrificed except for the better functioning of the whole person, and even then with an effort to compensate for this sacrifice.

Second, the basic capacities that define personhood are not sacrificed unless it is necessary to preserve life. This principle makes explicit another aspect of the principle of human dignity by requiring self-respect as well as respect for others. Unless we respect our own integrity, which includes our natural bodily and psychic integrity, and seek to preserve and protect our own gifts, we do not fulfill our needs as social beings. Both person and community depend upon each other, but they are radically different. A person is a natural primary unit, an organism whose parts depend upon the whole and exist for the sake of the whole. On the contrary, a community is a system made up of primary units—persons—and so exists for their sake, not merely as isolated individuals, but as sharers in a common interrelated life. But the parts—the persons—do not exist simply for the power of the state or its leaders. When a state preempts the rights of individuals, it is totalitarian.

Insofar as individuals are concerned, there is a hierarchy of personal powers, which we described in chapter 3. The creative and social values have higher priority than the psychological and biological values, but such priority must not be understood dualistically, as though the lower could be sacrificed for the higher whenever a person wished to enhance the function of the higher power. We are human not only because we think and love, but also because we eat and procreate; the lower powers can be sacrificed only to preserve the life or moral integrity of the person, although one can die for the sake of another or one's community (Jn 15:13).

Hence, the *fourth conclusion:* Three particular norms help to define the content of truly human and Christian love and the justice it presupposes: (1) Every person must be valued as a unique, irreplaceable member of the human community. (2) Every person must be encouraged to play a role in the common life of the community and to share fully in its benefits. (3) All persons must be helped to realize their full potential. These principles are not specific to medical ethics, but they do provide the fundamental motivation for the work of the health care professions.

2.5. PRINCIPLES OF CHRISTIAN HOPE

Hope is the Christian virtue by which we desire the Kingdom of Heaven and eternal life, placing our trust in the promises of Christ and the grace of the

Holy Spirit (*Catechism of the Catholic Church* 1997, n. 1817). Clearly, hope is concerned with pursuing difficult and even mysterious goals, goals that lead beyond human life. For this reason, Christians live a more rigorous discipline of their natural drives for pleasure and the avoidance of pain and of their fears and aggressive tendencies than might seem reasonable if their only goals were temporal happiness.

Christian hope is assisted by the two cardinal virtues of temperance, or moderation in the use of food, drink, and sexual pleasure, and fortitude, or courage in the endurance of suffering and risk taking to attain the goals that are proposed by hope. In health care, this sense of hope is the source of all healing, so that to be a health care professional is constantly to affirm the possibility of turning suffering into a victory over disease and death.

Four ethical norms are related in a special way to Christian hope. First, as intelligent and free human beings we seek to achieve control over our world through science and technology. We can do so constructively only if we cultivate the gifts of nature, including our own bodies, with a profound respect for nature and ecology. To do this, we are guided by the *principle of stewardship and creativity*. Second, one of the greatest obstacles to this right use of our own bodies is our too common pursuit of compulsive pleasures. These often deprive us of a rational use of our gift of freedom. Consequently, we need a *principle of inner freedom*, which helps us avoid the snares and bad habits that impede our progress toward our life's real goals. This principle has social implications with regard to drug addiction and other addictive behaviors.

Third, some of the most dangerous pitfalls on this path toward happiness result from the misuse of human sexuality, which through its creation of the basic social unit, the family, is also the source of great hope for the future; hence, the need for a *principle of personalized sexuality*. Fourth, what if the dangers in life are unavoidable and we are immersed in suffering? It is then that our hope enables us not only to endure the suffering of life courageously, but to grow stronger as persons through this experience, as shown by the *principle of growth through suffering*.

The Principle of Stewardship and Creativity

The concept of "stewardship and creativity" is basic to the ethics of using technology to satisfy human needs in such a way that protects the rights of future generations to the earth that God gave us. Thus, we formulate the principle of stewardship and creativity as follows. The gifts of multidimensional human nature and its natural environment should be used with profound respect for its intrinsic teleology. The gift of human creativity, especially, should be used to cultivate nature and environment with a care set by the limits of our actual knowledge and the risks of destroying these gifts.

This principle requires us to appreciate the two great gifts that a wise and loving God has given: the earth with all its natural resources, and our own human nature (embodied intelligent freedom) with its biological, psychological, social, and spiritual capacities. Recently, we have come to recognize that our earthly environment is a marvelously balanced ecological system without which human nature would never have evolved. We must take the utmost care to conserve our ecological system unpolluted and unravished and to recycle raw materials and energy supplies. Similarly, our own bodies and minds are wonderfully constructed. We must work to prevent defects in our bodies through medical innovations but with the greatest respect for what we already are as human beings.

Consequently, a technology based on the false principle, "if it can be done, it should be done," is a misuse of creative intelligence. Rather, we should ask first, "Should it be done?" and bring the effects that any new innovation would have upon the environment and upon human nature into consideration. Our creativity should be a co-creativity with the Creator, not a reckless wasting of his gifts.

The Principle of Inner Freedom

Self-control with regard to pleasure and pain is an element in human behavior and needs to be stated as an ethical principle because it is of great importance in helping people seek human fulfillment. Certainly, we cannot live a truly human life without some physical pleasure; but as we shall explain in chapter 11, when the pursuit of pleasure or flight from pain becomes obsessive, the person becomes an addict. Addiction and phobias waste human energies. They reduce the freedom of the victims and hence their moral responsibility, because freedom of choice depends upon our capacity to make prudent choices.

Yet addicts and phobics cannot be wholly excused from moral responsibility. All programs that are designed to overcome addiction or phobias demand some response on the part of the victims, which leads them to ask for help. The first step to freedom is usually the humility to admit that we need help. The virtues of temperance and fortitude help overcome the excessive pursuit of pleasure and the fear of attempting difficult remedies.

We can formulate the principle of inner freedom as follows. To be free to follow our conscience, we must avoid actions that may cause addiction to immoderate physical pleasures or obsessive fears that could result in a loss of rational control of our behavior. If such a loss occurs, one must seek therapy and the help of others, who have an obligation to intervene and support recovery.

The Principle of Personalized Sexuality

The gift of sexuality must be used in keeping with its intrinsic human teleology. Personalized sexuality is based on an understanding of sexuality as one of the basic traits of a person and must be developed in ways consistent with enhancing human dignity. A more detailed discussion of sexuality is contained in chapter 9. Here it is sufficient to answer the common charge that the Catholic Church has an obsession with sexual morality. The reason for the emphasis on sexual morality in the teaching of the church is because this element of human character leads so often to a loss of dignity and an inability to pursue the truly fulfilling goals of human life.

Genuine Christian teaching on sexuality is clear enough in the Scriptures and was given an even richer, more accurate expression in the Second Vatican Council and the documents issued by Pope Paul VI and Pope John Paul II afterward. Genesis 1–3 teaches that God created persons as male and female and blessed their sexuality as a great and good gift. Jesus confirmed this teaching, and perfected it by affirming that men must be as faithful in marriage as women (Mk 10:2–21; 1 Cor 7:10). Nevertheless, Jesus also taught that although sexuality is a great gift, its use in marriage is only a relative value, which can be freely sacrificed for the sake of higher values, "for the good of the Kingdom." Thus, for the Christian, the celibate or single life, with its freedom from domestic cares to be of service to others, can be as personally mature and fulfilling as married life (1 Cor 7:25–35).

In the Jewish-Christian tradition, which is based on the first chapters of Genesis, human sexuality is always seen in relation to the family as the basic community into which we are born and educated and on which the larger community is built. Hence, sexuality is not only a private matter, although it involves the most intimate of relationships. It also concerns the common good of society and requires its public support and defense as the basic social institution.

The church's moral teaching on sex, therefore, can be understood primarily as support for the family. When the church opposes certain kinds of sexual behavior, it is not because the church is antisexual but rather because the church is convinced on the basis of centuries of experience that such behavior undermines the family institution and deprives children of their right to a secure family life. Moreover, most men and women find their fulfillment in this mutual commitment of their love through their children. Thus, it is only in the family that the different values of sexuality can be realized in their profound interconnection.

The principle of personalized sexuality may be stated as follows. The gift of human sexuality must be used in marriage in keeping with its intrinsic, indivisible, specifically human teleology. It should be a loving, bodily, pleasurable expression of the complimentary, permanent self-giving of a man and woman to each other, which is open to fruition in the perpetuation and expansion of this personal communion through the family they beget and educate.

The Principle of Growth through Suffering

Suffering is the great paradox of human life. In any teleological ethics, the ultimate criterion of morality is true happiness. An action is morally good because it leads to happiness for persons. People sometimes fail to realize, however, that not all that appears to lead to happiness actually does so. The only authentic happiness is that which satisfies the whole person at his or her deepest needs, and permanently. Thus, from an ethical point of view, it is essential to realize that true happiness can not be measured by physical pleasure, comfort, or freedom from anxiety and guilt. These factors are good and desirable, but they are secondary signs and not the proof or measure of real human achievement or happiness.

In this life, experience teaches us, the pursuit of our goals will involve difficulty and suffering. Only by overcoming suffering can we hope to attain happiness and the intermediate goods that lead to ultimate happiness. Suffering is a violation or subversion of a person's bodily integrity or psychic stability. Death is the complete and ultimate violation of the human person.

The Christian faith looks on suffering and death in two distinct but related ways. On the one hand, suffering is evil because it is a violation of the human person, ultimately resulting from sin, our own or that of others. On the other hand, suffering can be a liberating and grace-filled experience if the proper motivation is present. These two views are not contradictory; rather, they are complimentary. Suffering and death, joined to the suffering and death of Christ, represent not dissolution but growth, not punishment but fulfillment, not sadness but joy. God allows suffering and death to enable us to live with Christ now and forever.

The principle of growth through suffering, which is supremely exemplified in the Cross of Christ, is rooted in the basic human need to preserve life and may be expressed as follows. Just as bodily pleasure should be sought only as the fruit of the satisfaction of some basic need of the total human person, so suffering and even bodily death, when endured with courage and united to the suffering of Christ, can and should be used to promote personal growth in both private and communal living.

Hence, the *fifth conclusion* concerns the four norms flowing from Christian hope: Four ethical norms are related to human and Christian hope. Our hope enables us to endure the suffering of life courageously and to grow as persons through this experience. Hope also enables us to have an inner freedom that avoids addiction and the misuse of physical pleasure, so that we can pursue the goods of marriage or celibacy in a grace-filled manner, promote and participate in the goods of human society in a way that builds families and communities and fosters ecological respect for the earth and our environment.

SUMMARY

Catholic moral theory gives rise to several principles, which are enunciated above. More principles could be stated, but these principles are the basic ones insofar as pursuing a life characterized by the theological virtues of faith, hope, and charity is concerned. In the following chapters, we shall apply these principles to particular questions that dominate the provision of health care in the United States.

QUESTIONS

1. What is the purpose to the theological virtues of faith, hope, and charity, and how do the moral virtues contribute to the practice of the theological virtues?
2. Of the twelve principles discussed in this chapter, how has one been used in your life?
3. Does the principle of double effect allow us to choose evil for its own sake?

CASES

1. Ingrid maintains that the Christian faith does not have to be divided into principles that would aid its practice and development. In fact, she believes that such theological speculation will weaken the assent of faith to the person of Jesus Christ. Describe the basis for her thought, and analyze whether it is a sufficient interpretation of the material presented in this chapter.
2. When discussing health care for the many U.S. citizens who are not covered by any private or public insurance plan, many people maintain that the poor have no right in justice to health care if they cannot pay for it. Some of the same people, however, would state that the poor should be cared for out of charity. Is there any coordination between charity and justice?

3

The Person Seeking Health

OVERVIEW: Ethics is concerned with fulfilling the needs of human persons in an integrated manner. To have a solid basis for the study of health care ethics, therefore, we must have a thorough knowledge of the needs of the human person, that is, what it means to be human (chapter 3). One need of the human person is health, and thus we shall consider what it means to be healthy (chapter 4). In chapter 3, which concerns the meaning of being human, we consider the qualities that make one human, and the role of the community in helping people strive for human fulfillment. Moreover, we consider the values that lead to human fulfillment; the possibility of discerning these values; and the basic needs of a person, which when fulfilled in an integral manner enable one to be truly human. In this chapter, we mainly are concerned with the principles of human dignity and of common good and subsidiarity.

3.1 THE NOTION OF PERSON

Ethics concerns the needs and values of human persons. Nothing is more human, more personal, than the common concern we call "health." Concern about health goes far beyond physical well-being. The World Health Organization has declared that health is a state of complete physical, mental, and social well-being and not merely the absence of disease or infirmity. Although this description of health has been criticized as being too general, at least it indicates that there is more to health than physiological function. In this book, "health" is generally used in the more restricted sense of physical health, that is, the optimal functioning of the human body, including the effects of bodily functions on human psychology.

To make ethical decisions that will enable us to strive for health, we must be aware of the true worth and dignity of persons. Today, there is much confusion about what it means to be a person. We live in a technological age and in an artificial environment. We view the world through scientific eyes. Scientific training equips us to deal well with facts, but it does little to clarify the meaning of values. Yet in making ethical decisions, we are always concerned with values or goods that lead to our fulfillment as persons.

Perhaps the best way to find a working definition of person in the ethical context, and in a way that goes beyond questions of fact to questions of value, is to begin with the notion of human need. The human being is not definable merely as a static entity, but rather as a dynamic system of needs. Although humans have many of the same needs as plants and animals, they also have distinctively human needs, some of which are acquired through nurture and culture, and others of which are genetically innate. Anything that fulfills a human need, whether that need is innate, such as food, or created by us, such as a car for transportation, is called a good or a value. Pursuing something that does not truly fulfill a human need is a disvalue.

Hence, a good human act is one by which we pursue or achieve a value. For example, nutritious food is a value, because it meets a basic human need; however, so is a symphony concert for one who has learned to enjoy classical music. Junk food and music out of time and tune to sensitive ears are disvalues. Faithful friendship is a value; treachery is a disvalue.

It is not always easy to distinguish those human needs and capacities that are basic or genetically determined and common to the whole human species from those that have been created by human culture (which are often called acquired needs). But it is obvious that human beings stand out among all animals in their capacity and need to use symbols, to invent tools, to communicate by speech with a variety of invented languages, to create and modify social and political systems, and to understand and control the world through science and technology. We human beings actually create some of our own values as we create needs, yet we do so because creativity, through which needs are created, is a value we did *not* create for ourselves. Creativity is a value *innate* to human persons. We are creative animals and so, unlike any other animals, we have developed culture.

Satisfying Needs

We are indeed bodily, biological, animal beings with inherent needs for food, shelter, and reproduction, but our intelligence makes it possible and even necessary for us to choose from a vast range of ways to satisfy these needs. Culture is only the expression of our nature, which is to be intelligently free from fixed patterns of behavior, free to create our own lives of intelligent choices from among many options. This *embodied intelligent freedom*, by which we create some needs and choose the ways to satisfy needs, defines us as human and gives unity and continuity to the human family across time and space. When we discuss needs and values in relation to other members of the human family, we speak about rights. By insisting upon a recognition of rights, we make it possible to pursue our own needs and values as well.

Because we are beings who make intelligent, free, and creative choices about the methods of fulfilling human needs, and because we live with other human beings, we are ethical beings. Ethics is the discipline that helps human beings and human communities to fulfill innate or created needs wisely. Thus ethics determines which values are truly human, that is, which actions or things help us fulfill truly human needs (whether innate or acquired) and help us decide what to do when values seem to be in conflict. Above all, ethics helps us distinguish true values or goods from values or goods that are only apparent. When we begin to consider how to protect our ability to pursue needs and how to respect the ability of others to do the same, we move into the field of rights and law. Law, then, is based upon ethics, not vice versa, because rights are based upon human needs.

Personhood

When we talk of human needs and human rights, we have to ask: Who is a member of the human family? Is personhood a quality derived from being human or is it conferred by society? When considering whom the human family comprises, some philosophers today raise the question: Is every human being a human person? Or is every member of the human species, as science defines that species factually, necessarily a human person?

Some modern philosophers prefer to define a person as a moral agent— a human being mature enough to make free moral decisions. Others want to add qualifications such as "conscious," "able to form interpersonal relations," or "having feelings." Therefore, many modern philosophers conclude that an infant is only potentially a person, and a severely defective infant who will never be a moral agent, or a senile or irreversibly comatose adult who will never recover the ability to be a moral agent, is considered by some ethicists to be a human being but not a person. Because rights belong only to persons, according to this view, such immature, defective, or senile humans have no inalienable rights.

The main confusion concerning personhood consists in saying that a child or a retarded adult is only potentially a person, when what is really meant is that he or she is actually a person, but a person whose full potentialities have not developed. Of course, none of us has yet realized our full potential for growth and learning, but this does not mean that we are only potentially persons. Only a very static conception of personhood overlooks the fact that to be a person is to be always in the process of growth, unless that growth is pathologically hindered. We ought to maintain, therefore, that every human being is a person at every stage of maturation or dying, and that personhood is attributed to humans by reason of their nature, not because society approves of them as persons and then grants them rights.

The Christian View of the Person

The Christian view of the worth of the human person is based on the biblical teaching that each human being is created by God in his own image and likeness, differing from the animals in the possession of a spiritual intelligence and free will (Gn 1:26–31). Although God produces the human body through the cooperation of human beings, the creation of the human soul is a direct act of God (Gn 2:7; 2 Mc 7:22–23), which calls each person into existence in relation to God himself (Ps 22:10–11). Each person is unique and irreplaceable (Mt 10:29–31), and all are called not only to maturity but to eternal life (1 Tm 2:4). Differences of sex, race, or individual talents in no way detract from this basic equality of all human beings (Rom 2:11; Gal 4:7; Eph 6:9).

The worth of human persons was confirmed when God sent his Divine Son to take on human nature and to share our life with us, including the miseries wrought by human sin (Heb 4:14–16). In recalling us to our dignity and restoring to us the hope of perfect happiness, which God intended when he created us, Jesus Christ worked miracles of healing (Mk 1:32–39) to encourage us to use God's gifts for the health care even of the most neglected and powerless members of society (Mt 26:31–46).

Our *first conclusion:* A human person is a being with a radical capacity for embodied intelligent freedom, whether that capacity is still undeveloped or has been frustrated by accident, disease, or neglect, and thus has inalienable rights that should be ethically respected, including those rights that relate to health care.

3.2 THE PERSON AND COMMUNITY

Every ethical problem about health care ultimately is reduced to our conception of what it is to be human and to actualize personhood. This vision of personhood, however, must not lead to either of the opposite errors of collectivism or individualism. Aristotle, who first formulated the definition of a human being as a rational animal (i.e., having embodied intelligent freedom) also insisted that a human being is a political animal (i.e., a being who needs the company of other people). No person can exist long apart from the human community. Each of us has parents, and no one can develop either physically or psychologically without constant human relationships. The human brain cannot develop fully without language, and language is a cultural, social creation.

This correlation of person and community is not merely superficial. People need a community not only because it supplies them with certain instrumental needs (food, housing, clothing, defense), but also because their personalities can be fulfilled only in the act of communication and sharing. If personhood is embodied intelligent freedom, it can be fulfilled only in the free acts of knowing and loving. This means that a health care professional cannot understand a patient or diagnose his or her ailment as if the patient were a thing, because the patient is a person whose whole mode of health or sickness is relational.

In our contemporary world, there are two predominant views about the relation of a person to community, and they are in constant competition. One is *collectivism*, which is characteristic of communist governments, such as the government of China. Generally, collectivism favors an economic system in which the state closely regulates the production and distribution of wealth. Collectivism teaches that the welfare of individual persons must be strictly subordinated to the welfare of the total community, and thus the rights of persons can be sacrificed to the interests of the nation.

The other theory, *individualism*, begets a system that is characteristic of democracies in the Western world. We often hear individualism called the "democratic way of life." For many people, it is identified with the free-enterprise system "capitalism," in which the economic system is regulated by the free market, but which in practice often means competition between a few private corporations. Many argue that the goal of government is to protect maximum individual freedoms from the influence of collectivism, so that any restrictions on freedom, including any regulation of the economy, are believed to be an attack on the survival of the nation. Radical or exaggerated individualism is identified by many as a serious detriment to personal and community fulfillment.

The Christian point of view, which also has support in many other religions and philosophies of life, rejects both collectivism and individualism. Christianity repudiates collectivism, because the community should exist to serve persons and not persons to serve the community as if the community were a superperson. Christianity also renounces individualism, because Christianity teaches that the highest and most important goods of the person are not private property but spiritual goods, which can be achieved and fully enjoyed only by sharing with others. Because modern states, both collectivistic and individualistic, are oriented to maximizing material goods and economic power rather than maximizing spiritual goods, the struggle between person and community has become chronic.

The Christian point of view is neither idealistic nor altruistic. The words of Jesus are "Treat others in the way you would have them treat you; this sums up the law and the prophets" (Mt 7:12); and "You shall love your neighbor as yourself" (Mt 22:39). According to this teaching, we are not asked to love our neighbor and *not* love ourself, but to love our neighbor *as* ourself. In other words, if we really love ourself—not selfishly, but intelligently—we will realize that we cannot be happy in isolation, because we were created as social beings. We can be truly happy only by sharing in a community of happy people, and that means that we each must not only respect the rights of others in a negative sense, but must be actively concerned to promote each other's welfare. Therefore, both collectivism and individualism are self-defeating.

The social teaching of the Catholic Church, which is derived from the teaching of Jesus, insists therefore that the human community, including its governments, must be actively concerned to promote the health and welfare of every one of its members, so that each member can contribute to the common good. This concern cannot be a matter of a mere trickle down by which the weak live on the leavings of the powerful, but must be aimed directly at enabling the weak to share in the goods of life. The Christian remembers that God has called us all to share in his own life, the community of Father, Son, and Holy Spirit, in which there is nothing that is not common to all (1 Jn 1:3).

Thus, our *second conclusion:* The human community and its governments exist to promote the welfare, including the health, of all. Moreover, each member of the community, according to one's abilities and resources, must contribute generously to this common welfare or common good.

3.3 DEVELOPING COMMON VALUES

Human community is difficult when there is no agreement on values or goods that all hold in common. At least there must be the possibility of dialogue toward common values. The Second Vatican Council, in the document *The Pastoral Constitution of the Church in the Modern World* (Flannery 1975b), insisted that the spirit of dialogue must extend beyond the Christian family to other world religions. The monotheistic religions Judaism and Islam, like Christianity, affirm the dignity of the human person.

The religions of China and India are becoming more popular in American life. At first sight, their outlook might appear incompatible with the Christian emphasis on the dignity of the human person in relation to a personal God, because they teach that the individual, after a series of reincarnations, is absorbed into the unity of the Absolute. Closer study, however, reveals that this Absolute is not subpersonal or impersonal, but superpersonal. Thus, it becomes possible for monotheists to join with believers in these Eastern religions in a common search for authentic spiritual selfhood. Americans are beginning to appreciate how much these religions, with their meditative disciplines, can contribute to personal integration and total health. Thus, Christians can learn a great deal from other world religions about ethical dialogue and the pursuit of true health.

Catholics also should realize that they have something in common with humanists. According to the well-known "Humanist Manifesto" (1933), signed by a group of distinguished American thinkers under the leadership of the famous philosopher John Dewey:

Religion consists of those actions, purposes and experiences which are humanly significant. Nothing human is alien to religion. It includes labor, art, science, philosophy, love, friendship, recreation—all that is in its degree expressive of intelligently satisfying human living. . . . Religious humanism considers the complete realization of human personality to be the end of man's life and seeks its fulfillment and development in the here and now. This is the explanation of the humanist's social passion. (p. 13)

In 1980, some humanists renewed their creed in *A Secular Humanist Declaration* (Council for Secular Humanism 1980). Most Christians would ascribe to eight of the ten principles in the new document, but the document belittles religion and divine guidance. In the opinion of many observers, humanism today is rapidly replacing Protestant Christianity as the predominant religion in American culture. While recognizing the shortcomings of the secular humanistic value system, Christians must respect the goodwill of humanists and seek common values that will enable all to build a peaceful, even though pluralistic, society.

Many Catholics are under the impression that the Catholic Church, because it opposes communism, favors capitalism. They are unacquainted with the fully developed social teaching of recent popes, which must be considered in any Catholic approach to today's ethical problems, including those in the medical field. The popes urge us to work for a world community based on spiritual goods or values and economic cooperation. They link human health and world poverty as the most fundamental ethical problems of our time, problems that in the United States are often ignored by ethicists and health care professionals alike while attention is devoted to secondary problems such as eugenics and heart transplants.

Thus the Kingdom of God begins here on earth with social justice, as modern popes have constantly preached, and no one will gain heaven who has neglected to work for social justice on earth. Jesus said, "I was hungry and you never gave me food . . . insofar as you neglected to do this to one of the least of these, you neglected to do it to me" (Mt 25:31-46). In the parable of Lazarus and the rich man (Lk 16:19–31), he taught the same lesson.

Consequently, genuine Christian ethics cannot be conceived from the viewpoint of the status quo, which in a sinful world tends to reflect the materialistic spirit of domination and possessiveness. It must also view the world from the side of the oppressed, whose needs have been ignored and neglected. Thus, Jesus pointed to his preaching of the Gospel to the poor as the best sign of the authenticity of his own mission (Mt 11:5). A Christian politics of health care must then be based on an option for the poor.

Christians, therefore, must join in a common effort with all those who are sincerely concerned about human needs and human rights, including the right to health. This ecumenical and interfaith search for an ethical consensus on needs and rights has its solid legal and political foundations in the *Universal Declaration of Human Rights of the United Nations* (United Nations

1948; see appendix 2), which was signed by most countries of the world and supported by all the major religions, as well as by humanists and Marxists. Catholics have been urged by all the recent popes to support this declaration as a sound basis for social justice.

Thus, in contemporary times, there are grounds for a basic consensus on the fundamental ethical values on which world peace and community must be based and on which health for all human beings must be sought. The aim of this book is to take that consensus very seriously—without, however, glossing over the profound differences that continue to divide the Christian and secular communities and that challenge us to further research and dialogue.

Thus, the *third conclusion:* If human needs and rights, including the right to health, are to be well served, we must strive through research and dialogue to broaden the consensus on ethical principles that teach respect for the dignity of the human person.

3.4 PRIORITIES IN NEEDS AND VALUES

The fact that the nations of the world at least nominally agree on a list of human needs, values, and rights is an important step toward making possible an ethical consensus. But it is only a first step. Human beings must not only list agreed-upon needs or values, but they must also deal with the question of priorities. Which goods or values are more important? Which values or rights are most important? These are key ethical questions. Some will reply that these questions of emphasis and priorities are a wholly subjective matter, about which rational discussion is impossible. Whether this is the case can be decided only if the concept of need-value and its relation to objective facts is examined more closely.

We defined ethics above as a study of the free choices persons make to satisfy their needs, whether innate or created. Persons are able to make free choices because they are intelligent and free social beings. Anything that satisfies a human need is a good or a value. Thus a given good or value is always correlative to a human need; that is, it is a desire to satisfy the need. Conversely, a negative value, or disvalue, is inimical to human need, and a neutral value neither satisfies nor obstructs a need. A value, therefore, can be something as trivial as a cup of coffee to satisfy physical thirst or as sublime as the truth of Plato's philosophy to satisfy thirst for meaning in the cosmos. The basic or the more important human values correspond to the basic human needs.

In accord with ancient and modern philosophers and the psychologist Abraham Maslow (1964), we can identify four basic human needs. First are *biological needs* (Maslow's physiological needs). Human beings share with all living organisms the need to maintain themselves homeostatically in a dynamic relation with their environment, to grow and mature to full biological development as individuals, and to continue the species through reproduction. This is the level of need dealt with by physicians.

Second are *psychological needs* (Maslow's safety needs, and also his belongingness and love needs in their more emotional aspects). Human beings are psychic organisms who sense, imagine, and feel. This is the level of need generally dealt with by experimental psychologists and psychotherapists.

Third are *social needs* (Maslow's esteem needs, as well as the belongingness and love needs in their more developed aspects). This is the level of human free choice within the limits of an existing culture. It comprises the need of the individual both for self-control and for social relationship beyond those determined by the family. This is the level dealt with by lawyers, political leaders, and clergy acting as moral counselors.

Fourth are *spiritual and creative needs* (Maslow's need for self-actualization, including needs to know and understand, to contemplate, and to create). Although many refer to this level as spiritual, we add the word "creative" because too many people confine the meaning of the word "spiritual" to our friendship with God. Actually this is the level of function where we also relate to other human beings. The function that enables us to think, love, reflect on the past, and plan for the future is the level of commitment, creativity, and transcendence at which persons not only live within a culture, but also criticize it, transcend it, and contribute to it. It includes all activity with a creative element—in art or science or political innovation—and religious activity as it extends to ultimate, cosmic meaning. This is the level dealt with by the inspiring teacher and spiritual guide.

Each of these levels contains a complex of natural and cultural needs—the cultural needs being rooted in the natural needs but greatly expanding them. It cannot be emphasized too strongly that these four levels of needs are not stories in a building but dimensions of the human person that can no more be separated from one another than can be the length, breadth, and height of a cube. Every human act or event has all four dimensions. A human spiritual activity—whether it is a creative, scientific, or artistic activity or the graced acts of faith, hope, or love—is at the same time a biological, a psychological, and an ethical event.

Moreover, the reciprocity between these levels of the organization and function of the human personality are hierarchically ordered. Thus, spiritual or creative activities are the deepest, most central, and the most integrating. Biological activities are the least unified and the most peripheral. And psychological and social activities have intermediate positions. Yet the higher activities in this hierarchy are rooted in and depend on the lower ones in a chain of interrelations. Nevertheless, because each level has a certain genuine autonomy and differentiation in its structure and modes of functioning, each must be served respectively by the professions of medicine, psychotherapy, ethical counseling, and spiritual direction, using different healing and helping techniques.

In addition to the list of needs described by Maslow, Saint Thomas Aquinas gave a somewhat different and simpler classification of basic needs (*Summa Theol.*, Aquinas 1947, I-II, q. 94, a. 2):

1. the need to preserve health and life;
2. the need to procreate the future generation;
3. the need to live in society; and
4. the need to know the truth.

These needs are similar to those stated by Maslow and maybe used as another set of criteria for evaluating human actions.

The *fourth conclusion:* Persons are to plan their lives and to make decisions in such a way that all these basic needs are satisfied in an integrated and consistent manner. This obviously requires the adjustment of priorities with regard to both aims and objectives and of the practical steps to be taken to fulfill these needs. Moreover, it demands the subordination, and even sacrifice, of less important needs to greater ones. The exact mix or proportion will depend on both the culture and the individual. As was indicated above, this is the meaning of ethics: to make accurate decisions about which actions and objects truly fulfill human needs, whether the needs are innate or acquired.

SUMMARY

Humanity differentiates human health from mere animal or vegetative health and from the functioning of a well-oiled machine. Our discussion on health and what it means to be a human person can be summed up in four statements. First, health care must serve persons. Human health is the physical, psychological, social, and spiritual well-being of a living organism of the human species, distinguished from other animals by its personhood—that is, by its capacity for intelligent freedom or ethical judgment, which can be actualized only in a truly human community.

Second, a truly human community must be based primarily on the sharing of human values—the communication of truth and love—and only instrumentally on material values. The physical and mental health of persons, however, is a necessary basis not only for the acquiring and sharing of material, but also of spiritual values. The human community exists to enable its members to achieve all these values, and each member of the community is ethically obliged to share what he or she achieves with others.

Third, to be truly human, the global community must not be restricted on the basis of nationality or race but must extend to the whole human family resting on a consensus about basic human values. The existing basis for such a consensus is the United Nations' *Universal Declaration of Human Rights*, which is founded on the principle of human dignity. This consensus must be broadened and rendered practical by continuing patient research and dialogue.

Fourth, all ethical decisions, including those in health care, should satisfy both the innate and cultural needs (biological, psychological, ethical, and spiritual) of every human person in each of the world's political communities.

QUESTIONS

1. How would you explain each of the three terms in the definition of the human person: *embodied, intelligent, freedom*? How do the differences between the anatomy of a human being and a chimpanzee show evolutionary adaptation to the free, intelligent mode of human behavior? If we can approximate the capabilities of a human being by a computerized humanoid robot, what differences will remain between the human and the robot?

2. Does human society exist to serve its members, or do the members exist to serve society? Debate both sides of the question and then try to resolve the question.

3. Debate the issue of whether the community confers personhood. How would you resolve this issue?

4. It is often said that "law should not impose morality" and that "religious groups should not impose their morality on others." In what sense are such statements valid and invalid?

CASES

1. Saint Roch's Children's Hospital is engaged in research in chemotherapy for leukemia in children. Experimental drugs are tested first on monkeys to determine possible side effects and then, if they prove relatively safe, on human subjects with leukemia. A laboratory assistant notices that the monkeys are made very ill by some of these drugs, suffer a good deal, and finally die. In other cases, they are permanently crippled. He wonders why it is ethically justifiable to cause this suffering to animals in order to help children who do not seem to suffer any more than the animals. Do not animals also have rights? What answer would you give him?

2. Dr. Meyer attempts to persuade the Clarks to give permission for a blood transfusion for their child, who is to undergo dangerous surgery. The Clarks are Jehovah's Witnesses, whose religious views forbid blood injections as a form of "eating blood" denounced in the Old Testament. The Clarks point out to Dr. Meyer, who is Jewish, that he has had his two sons circumcised, even though recent studies have shown that this ritual practice involves some medical risk. Dr. O'Brien enters the argument by saying that the risk of circumcision is not very great, whereas the risk arising from refusing a transfusion can be very great. The Clarks reply by asking Dr. O'Brien, a Catholic, whether he would perform an abortion on a woman with a heart condition for whom continued pregnancy is a serious risk. If you were involved in this discussion, how would you deal with these conflicts of value systems and the relation between medical and ethical values?

3. Samuel is a concert pianist who has suffered a serious accident to his left hand. He has consulted two physicians, who differ in their opinions. Dr. A recommends immediate amputation, not only because he predicts that the hand will be useless but also because it might develop life-threatening necrosis, symptoms of which seem already to be present. Dr. B agrees that the situation is very grave, but he would like to try a new and experimental therapy that has some promise of saving the hand and giving an opportunity for successful rehabilitation. Samuel says, "I would rather be dead than to give up my career. It is my whole life!" How would you help him make a decision?

4

Defining Human Health

OVERVIEW: We are engaged in the study of the ethics of health care. But health is an analogous concept; that is, the word may be used with several different meanings. This chapter explains the various different meanings of the term "health." It also examines the concept of disease or illness, which inhibit, limit, or nullify the capacity to be healthy. Biological health, emotional health, and moral health are different aspects of human health but should be integrated for a person to be truly healthy. In this chapter, we shall be applying the principles of human dignity and of totality.

4.1 CONCEPTS OF HEALTH AND DISEASE

Many health care professionals know a great deal about disease, but often they are not able to define health. Unless one knows the meaning of "health" or of "illness," which indicates an absence of health, one will be unable to discuss the human values involved in health care and thus will not be able to make clear and accurate ethical decisions. The word "health" is related etymologically to the Anglo-Saxon word from which are derived not only "healing" but also "holiness" and "wholeness." The root of the word "health" denotes completeness.

Wholeness or health can be considered statically, as when a structure has all its parts, each properly proportioned and all parts in their places. Thus, a disabled person lacks wholeness or perfect health because some part of his or her anatomy is missing or deformed. Conversely, health or wholeness can be considered dynamically as a functional whole, in which all the functions present are acting cooperatively and harmoniously. In this concept of health, the person who is crippled may lack some function, but those he or she does possess are acting harmoniously. Thus some sicknesses do not involve any lack of an organic part or its deformity, but rather a dysfunction of a part. That is, some needed function is suppressed, or there is a lack of harmonious balance between functions—for example, if a person has diabetes or hyperthyroidism, his or her function is impaired, even though no organs are missing. Combining the static and dynamic perspective of the human person, health may be defined as "the state of being in which an individual does the best with the capacities he or she has, and acts in ways that maximize his or her capacities."

In the practice of medicine today, health is most commonly defined in terms of only one function, the physiological. Moreover, when evaluating physiological function, only standard physiological parameters are considered, that is, the vital signs, the presence of various chemicals in the blood, and electro-neurological readings. In medical circles, therefore, health is often defined by a model of what is physiologically usual or normal. But what is normal or usual for one person (e.g., weight) may not be normal or usual for another.

Because of the anomalies associated with the normal-average evaluation in a limited physiological sense, health is better defined as the optimal functioning of the whole person, rather than as correspondence to "normal" standards. This implies that each organ and organ system is functioning well and that together they form a single life process. This concept of health is a consequence of considering a human being as an organism, a system, that is, a living whole composed of functionally differentiated parts. A system is a complex of interacting elements. A living system is dynamic or open, that is, capable of maintaining homeostasis (dynamic stability) in relation to its environment by regulating the input and output of matter and energy. The whole system cannot be reduced to the behavior of its parts.

Obviously, a definition of health in terms of the optimal functioning of an open system must include the input–output of that system. A living thing cannot maintain itself in static existence; it must interact with the environment so as to modify it in its own interests. Thus animals build shelters and nests, fertilize plants on which they feed, and rid their environment of enemies. In fact, the present terrestrial environment is largely the product of living things themselves, which have modified both the soil and atmosphere in ways favorable to life.

Because humans have cultural as well as physiological capacities, their interaction with their environment is highly creative. Even more significant is the fact that human creativity is not limited to interaction with an external environment. Humans create not only external things, but also mental and emotional symbols to fulfill needs that cannot be fulfilled by what is merely objective, that is, outside consciousness. Ultimately, human beings need to assimilate subjectively the whole order of the external environment. Thus, to understand the universe, scientists are constantly striving to re-create, as it were, the entire external cosmos in the form of symbols. The great importance of this human life process, from a personal point of view, is that such symbols provide communication between persons in the form of language.

Human society is ultimately formed by communication with others within the same symbol universe.

In view of this more complete concept of human functioning, we can see that human health means not only the capacity of the organism to maintain itself in its environment, but also its capacity to create functions within itself. This involves an interrelated, well-balanced, and ever-expanding culture. In the broad sense of the term, then, health is the optimal functioning of the human organism to meet its biological, psychological, social, and creative needs.

The health care professions, however, are concerned with health in the narrower sense of the term, as the optimal functioning at human biological and psychological levels. Yet even in this narrower sense of health, the goal of integrating all four levels of human need is of paramount importance (see chapter 3). Even though physicians specialize in biological or psychological functions, they must never neglect or ignore the social and creative needs of their patients if they wish to be truly concerned about human health in a manner that respects the humanity of their patients.

Our *first conclusion:* Human health in the broad meaning of the term is optimal and integrated functioning of the person to meet biological, psychological, social, and creative needs. In a more limited sense of the term, and the way in which it is commonly used in medicine, health is concerned with the optimal functioning of persons with regard to their physiological and psychological needs.

4.2 DISEASE AND ILLNESS

Given the concept of health as the structural and functional wholeness of the human organism in relation to itself and to its environment—a wholeness that extends even to the social and creative functions—the notion of disease can be more precisely defined. The World Health Organization definition maintains that disease and infirmity are not the exact contrary of health. Health, as we have defined it, is optimal functioning. It is possible for an organism to fall short of optimal functioning without actually being diseased or infirm because the organism can be healthy in a narrow sense without actually reaching its full capacity. However, less than optimal functioning soon leads to dysfunction. A man can be healthy in this narrow sense and yet be lazy and half-alive, lacking the full use of his capacity for living; but he will not stay healthy even in this minimal way for long because his faculties will atrophy.

The terms *disease, illness, sickness, malady, ailment, disorder, complaint,* and many more synonyms have different connotations. Some seem to be more subjective; that is, they designate the feelings of the person (illness, sickness, complaint); others are more objective (disease, malady, ailment, disorder). We use the term *disease* or *illness* to denote the opposite of health defined as optimal functioning.

In the history of medicine, the pendulum has constantly swung between two concepts of disease: the ontological and the physiological. The ontological concept regards diseases as separate entities (contagions, morbid matters, bacteria, genetic defects, neuroses, psychoses) that can be classified and named like plants and animals. These entities attack the person and weaken or destroy human function. This view of disease supports the theory that the organism constantly fights to throw off diseases as alien invaders that disturb its homeostasis. Those who think in these terms tend to diagnose diseases as clearly classified and labeled entities and to treat them by seeking specific remedies (e.g., drugs or surgical procedures).

The opposite of the ontological concept, the physiological concept, views disease as a breakdown of the internal harmony of the organic system due to the hyperfunctioning or hypofunctioning of an organ. Thus dysfunction opens the organism to attack by external agents such as bacteria, but the bacteria are not the primary cause of the disease. If the organism were functioning properly, it would resist such bacteria because of the defenses present in a human system that is functioning optimally.

The central tradition of medicine (usually identified with that of the Greek physician, Hippocrates) has always tried to reconcile the ontological and physiological concepts of disease. From the ontological concept, traditional medicine borrows the concept that there are limits to the power of self maintenance, or homeostasis, and thus the functioning person may be attacked successfully by objective entities. From the physiological concept, traditional medicine borrows the realization that regimen and lifestyle are more helpful than drugs and surgery insofar as the overall well-being of the patient is concerned. Moreover, traditional medicine seeks to overcome disease by concentrating upon the function of individual organs, as befits the physiological concept. But it also realizes, in accord with the ontological concept, that the various parts can only be understood in the context of the system in which they exist. The eye, the kidney, the cell, and even the molecular gene cannot be understood except in the context of the whole organism of which they are parts.

Having defined human health as optimal functioning and having understood this as the satisfaction of innate and cultural needs, or the realization of all human potentialities, we reach our *second conclusion:* Disease or illness may be conceived as an ontological entity that only causes sickness or even death, if the organic system of the person cannot resist the ontological entity. Thus, our concept of disease and illness is a combination of the ontological and physiological concepts. A mechanistic concept of disease is valuable only if integrated with the concept of the human person as a dynamic system of interacting elements. Having considered the generic notions of human health and disease, we shall now consider the various parts of the human organism upon which integrated human health depends.

4.3 BIOLOGICAL HEALTH

This book cannot present even a sketch of the specifics of the biological level of human functioning. Biological and medical science are constantly making new discoveries about the chromosomes, genes, cells, organs, and secretions that constitute the human body; their chemical composition, structure, and functional interrelations; and the control of their differentiation, development, and modification by environment and through individual life cycles. We, however, are concerned with discussing general biological function insofar as it contributes to integrated human behavior, and thus is an essential component of health in the more complete sense of the term.

The important question for health care ethics is how the biological level of functioning can be considered truly human and personal, that is, as having ethical and creative significance. Dualistic theories of the human being have been present in all cultures throughout history. According to these theories, body and soul are in essential conflict with each other (i.e., the biological and psychological levels of human functioning are in conflict with the ethical and creative levels). Generally, the body is regarded as the negative factor and the soul as the positive factor.

Underestimating the attractiveness of dualistic anthropology is a mistake. The body is frequently experienced as a burden, as something negative, for two reasons. First, people cannot voluntarily control much of what goes on inside them physiologically. Biological life, which is often uncontrollable, becomes deranged and fails human purposes. People find themselves weary and exhausted and unable to do what they would like to do. When people suffer from pain and disease, they are acutely conscious that the body becomes subject to age and ultimate failure in death. Thus the body appears as a burden, a liability.

Second, the basic biological drives are urgent, constant, and inescapable—the need for sleep, the fear of insecurity, the demands of hunger and thirst, and the tension of sexual desire. They are so insistent that people feel them as compulsions, limiting their freedom and sometimes overwhelming them against their will.

Because the dignity of human personhood consists essentially in self-knowledge and freedom, we find it profoundly humiliating to be the helpless victims of our own bodies, with their limited energies, liability to pain, and urgent and deterministic demands that arise from unconscious depths and disorganize our self-possession and freedom of action. Sexual drives have especially seemed demonic.

Thus it is understandable that dualism is so widespread. It is essential to certain religious systems (Buddhism, Gnosticism, Manichaeism) and has affected all of them (the Neoplatonic influences in Jewish, Christian, and Muslim theologies). It might seem though that such dualistic views are no longer common, because modern society emphasizes the value of sensual pleasure, the dependence of psychic functions on the body, and the equality of male and female. But some ethicists maintain that human biological structure and function, such as the body–soul unity, have no moral significance. Rather, these objective biological facts receive their moral meaning only from culture, that is, from subjective human choice.

Certainly it is fallacious to argue that the moral character of human behavior can be settled simply by asking biologists what is natural or unnatural to animals or even to human beings. The morality of any act must be considered in the context of the activity of the person as a whole, because the biological level of function is only one level of the total system. Conversely, however, this consideration means that the ethical meaning of a human act cannot be indifferent or neutral to its biological character. Every human act is an act of the whole person, involving creative, social, psychological, and biological dimensions. Every human biological function has human (and therefore creative and social) significance; and, conversely, even the most creative activities involve the body and must respect the structure and functioning of the body.

Theologians of all the great monotheistic religions (Judaism, Christianity, Islam) have insisted that body–soul unity is a necessary implication of the doctrine of the creation of the human person by God and of the resurrection of the body. These theologians also have rejected the notion of reincarnation found in polytheistic religions because it seems to imply that the human person is a purely spiritual being and the body only its prison or a garment to be changed. Christianity goes even further by insisting on the Incarnation (through which God becomes truly a human being in bodily existence) and on the indwelling of the Holy Spirit in the human body as its temple, through which believers become members of the Body of Christ. This same principle leads to the sacramental concept of the human body, through which the basic biological functions become signs of spiritual events; birth is reenacted in baptism, eating and drinking in the Eucharist, and sexual union in the sacrament of matrimony.

Catholic theology, however, recognizes a certain measure of truth in body–soul dualism. The seeming dualism arising from body–soul conflicts may be overcome only by discipline and a sane asceticism. Such asceticism does not imply that the human body in its biological functions is evil or of little value, but rather that it shares in the spiritual dignity of the total person and therefore needs to be integrated with the other dimensions of human personality. Hence the body cannot be suppressed or ruthlessly sacrificed to higher values or even trivialized as of no moral significance. Catholic theology has always been concerned to find a middle way between the dualistic extremes of asceticism and antinomianism, thus respecting the intrinsic teleology of bodily structures and basic biological functions. Therefore, the *third conclusion:* Biological health and biological function are integral elements in the health of the person, because there is a dynamic unity and interaction between body and soul. The body has an integral role in determining ethical behavior, or the fulfillment of human capacity.

4.4 HIGHER LEVELS OF HEALTH

The development of modern psychotherapy and of psychosomatic medicine leaves no doubt that mental health, although it is intimately connected with physical health, is not identical with physical health. Mental disease is not describable in terms of physiological malfunction but only in terms of impairment of the characteristic human ability to deal with the environment through *symbolic* activity and communication. Human beings far surpass animals in their capacity to use symbols (images, feelings, words) that stand for realities but that can be combined and ordered in many ways different from the relatively fixed order of real things.

The images and concepts by which people represent their world do so only imperfectly, but they can be verified and refined by using them as tools to change the world. Physical disease, especially dysfunctions of the central nervous system, can impair this symbolic activity; but the activity also can be disturbed by social and educational factors within the symbolic realm itself. For example, a physiologically healthy child can acquire prejudiced ways of perceiving reality and neurotic ways of reacting to it because of his or her social environment.

At this level of symbolic or psychic activity, however, there are differentiated levels of health and disease that are too often lumped together. To reduce human psychic health to emotional adjustment and maturity is a common fallacy today; a fallacy that we call *psychologism.* Psychologism assumes that a physically healthy person, who also is free from mental illnesses that are considered within the purview of psychotherapy, is entirely healthy.

To avoid psychologism, one must realize that psychotherapy has the modest goal of helping patients acquire that degree of self-understanding and emotional integration that will free them from unconscious psychological determinisms that interfere with practical daily life. Psychologically healthy persons are "in touch with their feelings." They perceive the world of ordinary activity as most people do—without manifestly absurd illusions or projections. They are free to choose between practical alternatives, do not have unrealistic expectations, and are willing to assume responsibility for the consequences of their actions.

At this point of freedom from psychological determinisms, a whole new level of human activity opens up: the level of free, responsible moral activity. Psychotics are incapable of moral action because they are not free, at least within the area of the psychosis, and neurotics are severely limited in their freedom and responsibility. Only the free man or woman is a person fully capable of either moral good or evil.

It is also possible to fall into still another fallacy—that of *moralism.* This error reduces mental or physical disease to the victims' sins and attempts to heal them with moral exhortations. A more subtle form of this same fallacy is the assumption that the highest wholeness in the human personality is achieved at the level of practical ethical life. Some people identify the good person with the responsible, law-abiding, decent man or woman.

This fallacy ignores the deepest, most central fact of the human personality: its spiritual, intuitive, and creative aspects. To deal with this spiritual-creative level of human existence on its own terms is the task of neither the psychologist nor the moralist, but of the spiritual guide. Spiritual health and disease, therefore, cannot be reduced simply to moral or psychological terms.

Even at this spiritual level, it is possible to fall into the fallacy of what the philosopher Jacques Maritain (1929, 54) called "angelism"—treating human persons as bodiless angels, or pure souls, as Plato and Descartes considered the true human self. Human problems cannot be treated in purely spiritual terms, in which the lower levels of human functioning—physiology, symbolic activity, and practical responsibility—are ignored. It would seem that this fallacy has influenced those mystical and religious enthusiasts who attempt to heal all bodily, psychological, and moral ills with purely spiritual means.

Hence our *fourth conclusion:* Trying to understand the fullness of human health requires being on guard against those reductionist fallacies that ignore the many dimensions of the human person. Because human persons are a complex of various elements, health may be predicated of any one of the elements. But realizing that these various elements are intimately united in the human person, health at any one level of human function must not be predicated as the basis for total human health. Hence, simply because a person's physiological function is healthy does not mean that the person as such is healthy. Before the person as such is deemed to be healthy, other functions of the person must be considered, and the integration of functions that occurs at the spiritual-creative levels must be considered.

4.5 INTEGRATING HUMAN FUNCTIONING

Human nature is an open system in which several hierarchical orders of functioning are integrated in the healthy person. The term *integrity* indicates that in a perfect whole each part must be fully differentiated and developed. Furthermore, each part must be fitted into the whole and harmonized with it by correct interrelations and interactions with the other parts of the whole. Integrity is lacking when a part is suppressed or unduly inhibited in function or when one part is hypertrophied because of the injury of others.

In a hierarchical order, some parts are said to be higher because they are necessary for the unification and integration of the whole in the performance of its most complex and specific functions (e.g., the central nervous system). Other parts are said to be lower because their functions are more integrated than integrating. Yet the lower parts may be essential for the higher parts to function at all (e.g., the liver and kidneys). This concept is expressed in the saying, "He lives to eat, but should eat to live," which means that engaging in higher activities (living) requires eating. Consequently, eating is integral to human life. But eating is a lower activity, a means and not an end. When eating becomes an end, an absolute not measured by something higher, it destroys the integrity of human functioning.

It would be a mistake, however, to think that only the higher values in this hierarchy are human personal values. People share biological and psychological needs with other animals, but they share social and creative needs only with other persons. Nevertheless, all these needs and their correlative values, whether they are generically animal or specifically human, are equally needs and values of the human person, none of which can be destroyed without destroying personhood. People are human not only because they need love, but also because they need food.

This hierarchical yet interdependent ordering of the four levels of human functioning is true for any subsystem within each level. At the biological level, the human body is divided into organ systems and then into organs, each having specific functions. The organ systems are identified as:

1. Nervous
2. Endocrine
3. Skeletal and muscular
4. Integumentary (skin)
5. Alimentary
6. Respiratory
7. Circulatory
8. Excretory
9. Reproductive

These systems are interrelated in very complex ways and not in any simple, linear hierarchy. Yet the nervous system (along with the intimately related endocrine system) obviously coordinates the others and is the most directly involved in the psychological and higher functions. Also, the reproductive system has a special importance (1) because it is directly involved in the evolutionary process by which the human species came to be and is continued and (2) because it is the source of the family and hence of the communal character of the human person.

Greater unification of function occurs at the psychic level of personality. Yet psychic life is also composite. The external senses are differentiated by their organs; psychological functions, such as feelings and emotions, have some kind of localization in various parts of the brain, although they also involve other centers and the endocrine system as well.

At the rational and ethical levels, still greater integration and unification of functions into the self-aware, conscious, free, self-controlling subject or person take place. Even at this level, what have been traditionally called the reason and the will are differentiated as distinct but ultimately correlative functions. Our *fifth conclusion:* Although there is a consistent human desire for integration and unity, only at the spiritual level do the intellect and will come together in the top of the mind or heart (in the biblical, metaphorical sense) of the human person, in which peak experiences and basic decisions, commitments, and fundamental choices from among options complete the total integration of the person.

SUMMARY

Health is an analogous concept and applies to things and persons in different ways. But human health has a definite meaning: It is the optimal functioning of the human organism to meet and integrate biological, psychological, social, and spiritual-creative needs. Disease is the weakening or absence of optimal functioning. Hence human health involves much more than disease-free biological functioning.

QUESTIONS

1. If you were asked to select five men and five women who were the most healthy physically and mentally from a specific population, what criteria would you use? If you were asked to select from this same population those who "ought to see their physician," what criteria would you use?

2. If you were interviewing a person "with a problem," what questions might you ask to determine whether the person should be referred to a physician, a psychologist, a lawyer, an ethicist, or a spiritual director?

3. What are some examples of *psychosomatic* illnesses? Within the psychic realm, give some examples of how spiritual, ethical, and psychological factors can affect health and are affected by it.

4. Many medical ethical controversies today make use of the concept of "quality of life." What criteria would you use to evaluate the quality of life of an adult, a child, and a very old person?

CASES

1. In the United States, persons are heavier for their height and body build than the average persons in Japan, where fewer people suffer from cardiovascular disease. How would you define *normal* weight? *Normal* types of diet? *Normal* exercise?

2. Saint Augustine of Hippo, whose physical health was often poor, is considered one of the great saints and doctors of the church. He is famous for his creative work as a theologian and for his remarkable dedication, courage, self-sacrifice, and compassion for the suffering. He also had extraordinary mystical experiences. Psychoanalytical studies based on his intimate *Confessions* have explained his career in terms of his Oedipus conflict and his love-hate attachment for his mother, Monica. Can you posit other reasons to explain his dedication and compassion? Was he a healthy human being?

3. In the United States, people are concerned about their cholesterol count, as well as about their blood pressure. As we well know, these are both physiological signs. What relationship do these signs have with physiological health? Do they have any relationship with social or spiritual health? Defend the concern for physiological health insofar as the purpose of a person's life is concerned.

5

Personal Responsibility for Health

OVERVIEW: With all the discussion of a fair and just health care system that has occupied the attention of the American public for the past ten years, we sometimes forget the one principally responsible for health: the individual person. In this chapter, we analyze the quest for health as a personal moral endeavor, pointing out the various aspects of ethically responsible free choice and formation of an informed conscience concerning free decisions of health care. The chapter is concerned mainly with the principles of human dignity, a well-formed conscience, informed consent, and totality and integrity.

5.1 THE INDIVIDUAL'S QUEST FOR HEALTH

The primary responsibility for a person's health rests with the individual, not the community. This principle follows upon the intensely personal character of health in all its dimensions. Thus, the main ethical principle for health care ethics is that one must seek to preserve and maintain one's own health insofar as is possible. Biological health concerns that which is most individual and private to me, namely, my own body. My body, by its very materiality, its space-time limitations, is mine and mine alone. It identifies me as *not* anybody else. Someone can share a room with me, a table, a bed, even my clothes; but that person cannot share my body. Ultimately, it is by reason of my body that I am alone in myself; yet it is also by reason of my body that I am in the world of things and persons.

My body is profoundly subjective, not only because I possess it as my own and know it as myself, but also because it is incommunicable. Much of what goes on in my body is hidden even from me; and even what I know of it I know for the most part in a thoroughly subjective way that I cannot express. When I consult a physician, I experience the difficulty of relating how I feel. Bodily feelings are vivid, yet vague and hard to put into words. I am the final judge of whether I really feel well. When no medical test reveals anything wrong with me, but I do not feel well, then I am not well.

Even if my sickness is imaginary, it is real at the psychological level and therefore is a psychological illness. At the higher ethical and spiritual levels, health also depends on an individual's own conscience, or spiritual discernment. Thus no one but the person ultimately can judge his or her own well-being.

Furthermore, this subjectivity is true not only of diagnosis, but also of treatment. The psychotherapist constantly has to remind the client: "No one, ultimately, can help you if you refuse to help yourself." Even the spiritual counselor must say, "God will help you by his grace, but you must let yourself be open to that grace."

Healing is a living process that must occur within the organism. It is true that near the end of life patients may be unconscious and completely passive about the surgery, medication, and injections thrust upon them, but these treatments seldom result in healing. Convalescence is an active process on the part of patients, and staying well is clearly something that they alone must do. No physician or nurse can make patients take pills, stick to a diet, or take necessary rest and exercise.

In a profound way, the will to life and health is the fundamental element in all healing, and this will to life must be intelligent, that is, a realistic search for the means to health. Most physicians and nurses seem to believe that the patient's courage is a critical factor in recovering health.

Therefore, whether in working to prevent sickness, to maintain optimal health, to assist recovery from disease, or to rehabilitate oneself after a crippling trauma, a person must make a commitment to life and health. It might seem that no special commitment needs to be made, because everyone has an instinct to live. No doubt the need to live, to grow, and to function well is innate; it is within the very design of any organism. But in persons who at their innermost depths are not instinctive but free, this commitment is not a given; rather, it must be freely made.

The commitment to life, which overcomes commitments to death, such as violence, pollution of the environment, drug and alcohol addiction, and treachery in human relations, is an affirmation of the value not only of pleasure, but also of freedom, intelligence, creativity, and love. As God says through Moses:

> I have set before you life and death, the blessing and the curse. Choose life, then, that you and your descendants may live, by loving the Lord, your God, heeding his voice, and holding fast to him. For that will mean life for you, a long life for you to live on the land which the Lord swore he would give to your fathers Abraham, Isaac, and Jacob. (Dt 30:19–20)

Such a commitment to life has to proceed from the spiritual level, although it is ordinarily manifested at lower levels as well. This deep commitment can be so blocked that persons profoundly dedicated to life in their spiritual center can yet suffer from an unconscious will to die at the psychological level. Some, of course, are so deceived by dualism that they do not realize that spiritual wholeness requires the integration of lower human functions. Thus, some pseudomystics have neglected ethical development, moral people have neglected psychological and physical health, and people concerned about psychological health have not always perceived its intimate connection with both ethical and biological health.

The Old Testament presents the Jewish view as profoundly life affirming. It constantly emphasizes the idea that God gives his friends health, security, children, and long life and that God has created men and women for life and wishes to prolong it for them. In consideration of the fact that the just often suffer persecution and martyrdom, the last books of the Old Testament affirm that God will raise his friends from the dead to everlasting life (cf. 2 Mc 7:22–23). Jesus approved of this teaching by saying, "God is God of the living, not of the dead" (Mk 12:27). Saint Paul also teaches (Rom 5:12ff.) that death (and by implication disease and aging) is somehow a consequence of sin (cf. Wis 1:13-15; see also chapter 11). Thus disease, aging, and death are not willed by God, but only permitted by him, as the inevitable consequence of the sin of the human race. Saint Paul joyfully affirms that in Christ all may be born again to everlasting life.

When Jesus prayed in the garden, "O Father, you have the power to do all things. Take this cup away from me. But let it be as you would have it, not as I" (Mk 14:36), he was affirming his own commitment to life, but expressing his willingness to endure death if the Father in his transcendent wisdom knew that only through death could doubting men and women be convinced that God and his Son truly love them for their own sake and not for the sake of honor or power.

Thus a sound theology teaches that the Father and Christ desire only life, a desire that is fulfilled in Christ's Resurrection. Following Jesus, Christians must always affirm life while being willing to endure the evil of death (1) as witnesses to others that faith, hope, and love cannot be overcome by the fear and despair of death; and (2) as sharers in Jesus's experience of death, by which we learn to be as unselfish, trustful, and hopeful as he was. The Christian, however, endures death serenely not because death is good, but because resurrection and eternal life are good and destroy death forever.

Thus it is essential to realize that Christian health care should never be directed to the passive acceptance of disease or death, as if they in themselves were somehow spiritual goods. In authentic Christian belief, every individual has a responsibility to choose life and to strive for it. Christians must strive for a full and abundant life and must accept disease and death only as inevitable incidents in the battle, but not as its final outcome.

Christian acceptance or resignation is not acquiescence, but rather a strategy by which good can be brought out of evil. Sometimes the enemy can be defeated only by patience, turning these evils into opportunities for growth and learning; but sickness and death should always be perceived as enemies. Christians should stand with Saint Paul in condemning death as the ultimate evil ("and the last enemy to be destroyed is death"; 1 Cor 15:26), especially if death is understood as the destruction of the human whole, that is, physical, psychological, moral, and above all spiritual death.

Our *first conclusion:* The person who has made a spiritual commitment to life will strive to achieve wholeness in every dimension of personality. A true understanding of the commitment to life leads to a balanced concern for the whole personality.

5.2 PREVENTIVE MEDICINE AND LIFESTYLE

Personal responsibility for health is often thought of as just going to a physician, but this is only a part of it. The famous dictum attributed to Hippocrates was that the physician should prescribe "regimen, medicine, and surgery" in that order, meaning by *regimen* the person's lifestyle of diet, rest, and exercise. Today, medical technology emphasizes the curative aspect of medicine more than the preventive aspect. In the future, perhaps, the center of medical care will shift from the hospital (curative) to a center for teaching people how to improve their lifestyles and maintain health.

Current lifestyles, in terms of physiological and psychological norms, seem to foster extremely unhealthy people. First of all, modern life often leaves insufficient time for rest, not merely in the sense of lack of sleep, but also in the sense of too much stress. It might seem that people have more leisure because machines have relieved them of much hard, servile labor. But this relief is more than offset by the routine of urban life that forces us, for example, to spend hours a day driving to and from work in the hazards of traffic. Clearly, as individuals, people are powerless to escape this system, but within it they do have some freedom to make choices that will gradually give their lives greater simplicity and a more natural rhythm, free from excessive competition and the drive for success.

Reduced stress also contributes to moral and spiritual health by making room for a contemplative atmosphere, for service rather than for ambition for power, for solitude and silence, as well as for more time to give to persons and less to things. In the past, men and women suffered from the burden of manual work, from fear of enemies, and from disease and hunger. Yet there was a natural rhythm of effort and of rest. Today, these natural rhythms are often broken up by artificial pressures and hectic overstimulation.

A stressful life can lead to addiction, the enslavement of human beings to the pursuit of intense pleasure or anesthesia as an escape from the pain of life. This addiction can be to hard drugs, smoking, alcohol, and tranquilizers; in a milder form, to the common addiction to overeating; and in a particularly corrosive way, to the anxious twentieth-century pursuit of sexual pleasure. In moderation, none of these things is unhealthy, but in addictive form they become obsessive and destructive to health.

Finally, modern people lack proper physical exercise. Although sports are highly cultivated, they are more watched than played by the average man and woman. Too many people do little manual work and seldom walk or engage in healthy exercise.

Assuming personal responsibility for health therefore requires a scientifically based knowledge of hygiene, good diet, rest, exercise, and moderation. These cannot be imposed from without. People need to design their lives to meet personal requirements, which differ greatly. To be healthy, people must express their personality in their lifestyle—not a false one, or a resignation to being half alive.

The problems of mental health are similar. People are overstimulated by sensation and passive imagination, but impoverished in active imagination, reflection, and meditation. They receive much input and information, but often little integration of symbols and feelings. They live at the top of their heads, out of touch with their feelings.

Concerning spiritual life, many persons live without clear commitments or goals and suffer from the emptiness, meaninglessness, and absurdity of life, and from loneliness, never seeking deep communication with others. Health therefore requires the courage to criticize the accepted norms of modern life and face the ethical dilemmas produced by modern technology. Perhaps it is futile to talk about a natural way of life, as counterculturists do. Has that point in human history arrived when nature must be replaced with a fabricated world, even with human beings, who have fabricated themselves?

Our *second conclusion:* Preventative medicine implies a need to recognize which goods of life are most important and to strive for those goods in an integrated manner.

5.3 CREATIVE STEWARDSHIP OF HEALTH

"The Lord God took the man and settled him into the Garden of Eden to cultivate and care for it" (Gn 2:15). Although humans are "masters" over lesser creatures, dominion over them and over themselves is only a stewardship for which human beings remain responsible to the one Lord.

Classical theology based Christian ethics on the conviction that God endowed all human beings with one common nature which remains essentially the same throughout all history from Adam and Eve to the Last Judgment. Human beings are stewards of this nature and of the world where God has placed them. By studying the God-given structure and dynamics of nature, it is possible, so theologians in the past thought, to formulate unchanging moral norms that are binding for every time and culture. Stewardship demanded that human beings abide by these norms, lest they destroy the garden of the world and the temple of their own bodies, which were given them to cultivate and care for.

Classical theology, in its account of human dominion, was too greatly influenced by the Old Testament image of the monarch God jealous of his supreme dignity and power. From the New Testament perspective, God is best revealed in Christ, who "though he was in the form of God, did not deem equality with God something to be grasped at, but rather he emptied himself and took the form of a servant" (Phil 2:6–7). Thus God is not jealous of his power but calls men and women to share in his work of making all things new (Rv 21:51). Such cooperation is not merely filling in details in a finished "plan of God." Rather, God has called human beings to use their own initiative and originality in completing his work. Thus the stewardship to which God calls us demands creativity on our part.

In creative activity, however, people have to respect their own limits and the limits of the materials with which they must work. The manipulation of stem cells and the Human Genome Project are excellent examples of the potential for human creativity but also of the need for careful control and planning. These limits of human nature are not set by God out of any concern for his own authority. God himself is "limited" by his own wisdom and love, which forbid him to do what is contradictory to his own nature. Human beings are far more limited by the fact that their share in God's knowledge and love is finite. No matter how they may progress in science, freedom, and power, they dare not contradict their own human nature without destroying themselves.

At any given moment in history, people's limits are set by their knowledge. Once they understand some aspect of nature well, they can freely choose to improve nature and surpass it. But when they lack that understanding, their efforts to improve on nature may prove disastrous. Our *third conclusion:* The evils of modern technology are not the result of creative use of knowledge, but of rash exploitation of a nature little understood. Above all, people have failed to understand themselves, their authentic needs, and their potentialities. Research and experimentation, with all the risks involved, are necessary, but we must proceed with reverence for the persons and the environment at risk.

5.4 DEVELOPING A WELL-FORMED CONSCIENCE

Given the limits just mentioned, the practice of modern medicine constantly involves both technological and ethical judgments. Practitioners must ask not only "Can it be done?" but also "Ought we do what can be done?" The claim by health care professionals that they can make autonomous decisions about medical therapy is invalid. That knowledge that makes these professionals experts in the techniques of medicine does not imply that they are experts in the use of these techniques, because use involves social, political, and moral values for which the patient retains decision-making responsibility.

Thus individuals who seek the services of a medical professional cannot simply delegate to that professional all decisions about their health on the grounds that the doctor knows best. Conversely, rarely is the individual competent to decide questions of medical therapy, unless he or she is given adequate information about the medical aspects of the decision. So there is a dilemma in medical decisions: Who has the knowledge both of the ethical norms and of the medical facts to make a responsible decision? And how are these norms and facts related to each other? This dilemma requires a discussion of the problem of developing a well-formed conscience.

Christian theology has always insisted that when it comes to concrete ethical decisions each normal individual has the capacity and the responsibility to judge and to act on his or her own judgment. This responsibility cannot be delegated to anyone else or to any institution; not to custom, to the law, or to advisers, and not even to civil or religious leaders. This is true in medical issues as well. The capacity to make practical judgment in matters involving ethical issues is called *conscience*. The Second Vatican Council, in the document *The Pastoral Constitution of the Church in the Modern World*, said of it:

> Conscience is the person's most secret core and sanctuary. There the person is alone with God whose voice echoes in the person's depths. By conscience, in a wonderful way, that law is made known which is fulfilled in the love of God and one's neighbor. Through loyalty to conscience, Christians are joined to others in the search for truth and for the right solution to so many moral problems which arise both in the life of individuals and from social relationships. Hence, the more a correct conscience prevails, the more do persons and groups turn aside from blind choice and try to be guided by the objective standards of moral conduct. (Flannery 1975b, n. 25)

Thus, when making personal decisions "guided by the objective standards of moral conduct" about health care, people have the responsibility to follow an informed conscience; that is, (1) to obtain as much relevant information as possible about a situation, both the facts and the objective moral standards (principles) that apply; and (2) to make and carry out a decision in accordance with this information. Sin is the failure either to inform one's conscience or to follow one's conscience after informing it.

Hence, in any question of health care, people have the responsibility (1) to learn the facts about the medical condition; (2) to determine in accord with an objective value system the needs and rights of the people involved; and (3) to come to a concrete, personal decision in spite of disagreement or pressures from others.

Does having all the information before making a decision definitely determine what the decision is to be? If it did, then there would be no such thing as freedom. Human beings are free not simply because they are relieved from any external forces coercing their decisions, but for two other reasons. First, usually there are many alternative means to a goal, some of which are clearly inappropriate, but often many of which are appropriate, each with its advantages and disadvantages. Hence some value choices will be between two or more good actions. Second, it is possible for people to reconsider their goals and to redefine or even alter them in view of some higher goal. Thus morality always involves a choice, and that choice is not always between a clear-cut good line of action and a clear-cut bad line. It may be between two or more good lines of action, and there may also be many wrong ways that involve different degrees of evil.

Because knowledge of the factors involved in any decision seldom results in a judgment that this or that action is best without qualification, it might seem that a rational decision is impossible. But knowledge or intellect is not the only factor involved in a decision of conscience; the will, supported by emotions, is also involved. Our decision is ethically good only if we have a good will (supported, if possible, by healthy emotions or virtues) that inclines us to follow our best information and ethical insight, even if they are not conclusive.

An informed conscience needs knowledge of the facts and of the law, but it also requires a disciplined or virtuous affection for what will truly satisfy our needs in an integral manner. The element of affection involved in ethical decision making is unappreciated by many contemporary ethicists, who seek to turn ethical decisions into rational balancing acts, without consideration of the virtues or character that make good ethical reasoning sure and easy.

If we are to follow our informed conscience, how does a Christian go about informing his or her conscience? Because Christians believe that the ultimate ethical principles are to be found in the life and teaching of Jesus Christ, this means going beyond merely philosophical ethics to the Bible, in which we have an inspired record of that life and teaching. Yet the Bible has been interpreted and applied in many different ways. How are we to know which is right? Catholics believe that Jesus himself provided an answer to this question by choosing twelve apostles to instruct the people and promising them the guidance of the Holy Spirit until the end of time (Jn 16:7–16).

Moreover, Jesus appointed Saint Peter as the head of this college of the apostles to maintain the unity of their teaching (Mt 16:17–19; Lk 22:30–34; Jn 21:15–19). This teaching authority (technically called the magisterium) continues in the bishops and the pope. Although there are disagreements among Christians about how to interpret even these texts of the Bible, it is difficult to deny that in the course of history the Roman Catholic Church has been able to maintain a unity and consistency of teaching difficult to find in the many Protestant denominations or the many national Orthodox churches.

Consequently, the Second Vatican Council, in *The Pastoral Constitution of the Church in the Modern World*, declares:

> Loyal submission of the will and intellect must be given, in a special way, to the authentic teaching authority of the Bishop of Rome, even when he does not speak *ex cathedra* (with full authority), in such wise, indeed, that his supreme teaching authority be acknowledged with respect, and sincere assent be given to decisions made by him, conformably with his manifest mind and intention, which is made known principally either by the character of the documents in question, or by the frequency with which a certain doctrine is proposed, or by any manner in which the doctrine is formulated. (Flannery 1975b, n. 25)

Therefore, a Catholic seeking to inform his or her conscience about some ethical question will first of all inquire if there is a teaching of the church on the subject and then whether the local bishop, or that bishop along with the National Conference of Catholic Bishops has given instruction on the question, and what type of instruction this is. For the United States, the conference has issued the *Ethical and Religious Directives for Catholic Health Care Facilities* (2001; see appendix 1).

The need to discern the type of teaching offered by the church follows from the custom of bishops and bishops' conferences, which often state that they are offering pastoral teaching, as opposed to defined teaching. Pastoral teaching is an application of defined teaching to contemporary social issues. Because such issues are changeable, the teaching of pastoral statements is not absolute and needs to be applied prudently by the persons to whom it is directed. If a Catholic finds that an ecumenical council under the leadership of the pope, or the pope in his own right, has declared that a teaching is contained in the Word of God and is to be believed by all the faithful, then such a teaching is to be considered definitive and certain ("infallible") and not subject to revision. Such decisions by the magisterium leave no room for further discussion, except for explanation, clarification, or further detail. Because these definitions are rare, they are called the use of the *extraordinary* magisterium.

Many statements coming from the Vatican congregations or even from the pope himself are not statements of the definitive magisterium, but only of the authentic magisterium (*Ad Tuendam Fidem*, John Paul II 1998). Although statements of the authentic magisterium are intended to direct us toward behavior that is in accord with Christian values, they do not have the same force as definitive teaching. As the statement quoted above from the

Second Vatican Council indicated, they are to be accepted with "loyal submission of the intellect and will" but do not merit a response of divine faith. Consequently, it is erroneous to quote church documents to settle ethical questions without carefully examining their precise authority, even when these documents issue from the Vatican or are signed by the pope himself.

However, there is a serious error rampant among many Catholics; they disregard anything that is not an infallibly defined teaching and maintain that they may follow their own "conscience" in matters of authentic teaching. This is often called the right to dissent from noninfallible teaching of the church. In the process of forming their consciences, however, Catholics will receive the best moral guidance from the teaching of the church. But what are they to do if they find that theologians disagree about some point of morals, or even dissent from the magisterial teaching? The fact that most theologians agree on a point is a sign that this point is correct, but when theologians, no matter how numerous and distinguished, disagree with the magisterium of the church, it does not make their opinion of equal weight or safe to follow.

More often than not, people maintain that they dissent from a teaching of the church when they really mean that the teaching is difficult to follow. Thus, several people state that they dissent from the teaching of the church with regard to contraception when they are expressing difficulties in following this teaching. The only situation in which a Catholic might dissent from the magisterium of the church would be when a noninfallible teaching is involved (authentic teaching). In such a situation, after study and prayer, if it seems clear that there is inconsistency with more certain church teachings or with certainly known facts, then the official teaching may be in error.

The Holy Father has acknowledged, for example, that with regard to certain scientific facts in the Galileo case, the teaching of the church was in error. Moreover, the church stated in a recent document (*Ad Tuendam Fidem*, John Paul II 1998) that, when the original statement was based upon contingent facts which in time might be proven wrong, the original statement could be subject to error. Finally, many people who maintain that the teaching of the church is in error (with regard to contraception, adultery, or abortion) seem to proceed from a dualistic concept of the human person or a secular value system.

The *fourth conclusion:* When a Catholic considers the teaching of the church in medical matters, he or she should not seek to merely obey that teaching but also to understand it, and above all to assimilate the values that give rise to the teaching. With regard to abortion, for example, one must learn to distinguish between direct and indirect abortion, but also one must seek to assimilate the value that each person is sacred, no matter what qualities and characteristics the person possesses or does not possess.

5.5 CONCRETE APPLICATION OF MORAL NORMS

Catholic health care professionals need not feel that they are sinking into a theological morass when applying church teaching to medical issues. They need only keep in mind that there are two different levels of moral certitude: (1) the theoretical level of principles and value priorities and (2) the practical level of concrete application of these principles to particular moral decisions. At the theoretical level of principles and values, Jesus Christ has given Christians ample guidance on "the weightier matters of the law, justice and mercy, and good faith" (Mt 23:23); and they are clearly expressed in the ordinary teaching of the church.

The practical level of concrete application of ethical principles is an area where official church teaching can be of great help, but where perfect clarity or undebatable certitude is often lacking due to the nature of particular decision making. At this practical level, one can only say, "I am as sure of my decision as I can be, but I realize that I could be wrong" (moral certitude). Health care professionals are well aware that the clarity and high probability of scientific laws are not to be expected in the application of these laws to particular medical decisions.

For example, it often happens that continued dialysis treatment does not seem beneficial for a patient, yet families are reluctant to stop this treatment, knowing the consequences. It is painful to have to make a life-and-death medical decision without being sure how the principles in the medical textbook fit the particular case; yet such decisions have to be made every day. In the same way, moral decisions cannot be made simply by referring to theological textbooks or to official church documents.

The fact that the pastoral guidance of the church at the level of concrete application leaves considerable room for individual and institutional judgment makes it obvious that the effort of Christians to acquire and act on a well-formed conscience involves no little risk and conflict. Hence a vital factor in such efforts is self-criticism or maturity of moral judgment. People have to be aware of their own biases, narrowness of experience and outlook, and half-conscious motivation. Consciences have their own psychological and spiritual pathologies—as do emotions—and they have often been weakened or distorted by defective ethical education.

In light of the foregoing, the material on well-formed conscience may be summarized in this *fifth conclusion:* When making a decision about health care, each person has the responsibility:

1. to inform himself or herself as fully as practically possible on both the medical facts and the ethical norms, especially those norms contained in the teaching of the church;

2. to form a morally certain practical judgment of conscience on the basis of this information;

3. to act according to this well-formed conscience; and

4. to accept responsibility for their actions.

5.6 ELEMENTS OF INFORMED CONSENT

The basis for informed consent is the right and responsibility that each person has with regard to his or her own well-being and pursuit of happiness and eternal life. Although the responsibility for obtaining informed consent rests primarily upon the physician, the patient or proxy is not passive insofar as decision making is concerned. Physicians and other health care professionals must never perform procedures or therapy without first obtaining informed consent from the patient or from the proxy.

Informed consent is also a basic right and consideration of all secular ethical systems utilized in the United States. But the foundations of the Christian concept of informed consent are different from those of secular systems. In the secular concept, the person has unlimited right to opt for whatever might suit his or her desires, including, for example, abortion or medical assistance in committing suicide. This is called the right of "personal autonomy." It can be symbolized in the oft-quoted phrase, "persons have the right to do whatever they wish with their bodies, as long as no one else is harmed."

In the Christian concept of informed consent, one has the right to request and choose the medical care that will fulfill one's responsibility to God, self, and neighbor. Hence, the natural functions of the body may not be sacrificed to protect other functions of the body unless there is danger to the whole body, as the principle of totality of the human person (see chapter 2) maintains. The Christian concept of informed consent or autonomy also limits the choice of persons with regard to abortion or the deliberate killing of the aged or infirm.

If a person is not able to give informed consent, it must be obtained from the patient's proxy. The proxy should make decisions in accord with the medical advice of the attending physician. Proxies are selected from the patient's family or by means of an advanced directive. The basis for allowing a relative or loved one to make decisions for an incompetent person is based upon the supposition that the relative loves the patient and will make medical decisions in the patient's best interest. Insofar as advanced directives are concerned, the person previously appointed by the now incompetent patient should be allowed to make medical decisions for the patient, but the physician and proxies must realize that circumstances may not warrant application of the original requests stated in the advance directive.

Informed consent was treated in an influential document sponsored by the federal government, the *Belmont Report* (CPHS 1978). It is still the gold standard for informed and proxy consent and may be summarized in three words: information, comprehension, and freedom. First, the specific information that should be provided for the patient or proxy concerns the purpose of the procedure, the hoped for results, alternative therapies, and truthful answers to any questions that the patient or proxy might have. Information should never be withheld for the purpose of eliciting consent.

Second, comprehension of the conveyed knowledge is a requirement more complex than it might seem at first. Because of the potential to understand medical terms varies so greatly, the material must be adapted to the subject's capacities. Health care professionals are responsible for determining that the subject understands the information, especially if the risk to the patient is serious. If the patient cannot understand, then the matter must be explained clearly to the person making decisions on his or her behalf. Research has shown that even people unfamiliar with medical terms can understand them and retain knowledge about them if explanations are well planned and given in plain language.

Third, freedom implies that the person understands the situation clearly and that no coercion or undue influence is exercised by health care professionals. However, it is difficult to discern where coercion begins and justifiable persuasion ends. The problem occurs frequently when seriously ill patients refuse therapy that would prolong the life of the patient for at least a little while. It would be inaccurate to think that patients with serious maladies are completely free insofar as choosing therapy is concerned. Freedom and voluntariness do not imply that the patient is free from all persuasion, but they do require that no deception be used to obtain consent.

The *sixth conclusion:* Informed consent is one of the most important ethical responsibilities for health care professionals, patients, and proxies, and may be summarized in the three words: information, comprehension, and freedom.

5.7 CHOOSING A PHYSICIAN

Because each person has the primary obligation to care for his or her own health, each person also has the obligation to seek and choose professional people to help advise concerning health care. Yet this does not mean that persons can surrender to others the responsibility of making decisions about their health. Professionals are helpers, not surrogate parents.

No one is a good judge in his or her own case; precisely because health is so personal a value, it is something about which it is hard to be objective. People tend to delude themselves both as to how well they are and as to how sick they are. Thus to be whole and healthy, each person must be humble enough to seek help from others who are more expert, or at least more objective, about their problems.

Not only humility, but also courage and hope are required. Fear, apathy, shame, and self-punishment are debilitating psychological and moral factors that prevent people from getting the health care they need. The most dangerous aspect of any disease condition is that it may make the victim despair of health or be afraid to seek help to obtain health. At the psychological level, neurotics and alcoholics notoriously deny their problems and resist therapy. Physically sick people also seem to have an almost instinctive dread of recognizing their illness and facing the pain of its cure. Even hypochondriacs, who seem only too eager to claim sickness, use the illusion of one disease to hide from themselves some other sickness—perhaps at the psychological, ethical, or spiritual level—that would be even more painful to face.

Even when people have the humility and courage to seek a physician, they are faced with very serious ethical problems in choosing a good one. For example, their choice may be very much restricted by the complex organization of modern medical care and the maldistribution of its services. Or the patient may not be able to judge accurately the professional ability of the physician. Certainly, it is true that in every age many, perhaps most, people have been quite irresponsible in selecting their medical guides. The very fears that prevent people from seeking help also cause them often to prefer the quack (medical, psychological, ethical, or spiritual) to the competent guide, whom they suspect may make them face a painful reality.

To escape enslavement to the incompetent or exploitative professional, people need to be conscious of the rights that correlate to their responsibility to choose professional help prudently. The Congress of the United States has made efforts in the past few years to agree upon a bill of patients' rights. They have had trouble reaching a consensus, mainly on the difficult issue of the ability of patients to sue their health maintenance organization or their employer if they feel they have received substandard care. How this dispute will be reconciled is difficult to determine; however, any legal document to define patients' rights should be based upon the following ethical norms:

1. the right to the whole truth;
2. the right to privacy and personal dignity;
3. the right to refuse any test, procedure, or treatment; and
4. the right to read and copy medical records.

The rights proposed above all rest on the fundamental concept of informed consent, as was discussed in the previous section. If the patient is to give free and informed consent, then he or she must also be able to refuse any test, procedure, or treatment. The right to privacy and personal dignity implies the right of patients to refuse to be involved in any professional procedures that make them objects to be examined or discussed for the benefit or convenience of professionals or students rather than for their own therapy.

If this consent is to be not only free but also informed, then the patient has the right to the whole truth, including access to read and copy medical records. Many professionals deny these rights on the grounds that the patient is not able to understand the technical information known to the physician and may be harmed by it. Such difficulties do not disprove patients' rights to know so that their consent may be fully informed, but only establishes the professional's duty to communicate this information in ways that are helpful, not harmful, to patients.

Patients have an obligation toward their physicians as well. Therefore, people should not accept lightly the idea that personal responsibility for their own health is satisfied merely by assuming a critical attitude toward physicians and demanding their rights from them. Such a responsibility also includes willingness to trust physicians once they have been prudently chosen, to make good use of their advice, and to cooperate with their healing efforts. Although people should never be afraid to protect their rights and to insist that physicians give patients all the information they need to give informed consent to treatment, they should also give them a deserved respect. Trustworthy and competent health care professionals do people a very precious service, for which they deserve profound gratitude, a good reputation, and fair and prompt payment.

The matter of patients' rights may be stated in the *seventh conclusion:* Because each person has the primary obligation to care for his or her own health, each person has the responsibility to seek and choose health care professionals to help him or her make good decisions concerning the use of health care.

SUMMARY

The primary responsibility for a person's health care rests with the individual. Each in his or her commitment to life must practice a stewardship of the body and mind given by God by making ethical decisions with regard to the pursuit of health, on the basis of an informed conscience. To inform their conscience properly, people need to obtain the best medical advice available. This implies a careful choice of the health care professionals who serve them and an insistence on their rights as patients. Moreover, Catholics should be aware of the teaching of the church with regard to health care and make use of this teaching as they form their conscience.

QUESTIONS

1. The philosopher Friedrich Nietzsche contended that Christianity is a "life-negating" religion, because Jesus was a celibate who allowed himself to be crucified without defending himself and who proclaimed an otherworldly Kingdom of God instead of affirming the maximum enjoyment of this life. How would you evaluate this understanding of Christianity?

2. Suppose you were asked to design a life plan promoting optimal health for a man or woman whose life work is that of a clinical nurse or a business executive. What habits are to be avoided and what encouraged?

3. How could the physicians of a small city be involved in the city's problems of environmental pollution and stewardship of local resources of water, green space, fauna, and flora?

4. List and describe the resources available to Catholic medical professionals faced with making conscientious decisions about difficult ethical problems.

CASES

1. Bill, a thirty-five-year-old cocaine user, has a high-paying job and no family responsibilities. He is told by his physician that recent studies have shown that cocaine presents a serious cardiac risk to middle-age persons because it releases large amounts of adrenaline into the system. Bill, however, figures that he can afford financially to continue the habit and that "we all have to go some day." Hence, he is willing to take his chances and continue his present lifestyle. Does Bill have any moral responsibility to give up cocaine? Why?

2. In Henrik Ibsen's famous play *An Enemy of the People*, a physician attempts to awaken the townspeople to the danger arising from the pollution of the water system. They do not want to hear his warnings, because his information hurts some people's reputations and his proposals for a remedy tread on other people's toes. Can you think of current situations where there is resistance by vested interests or by the public to problems of stewardship and preventive medicine? What could medical professionals do to overcome this? Does the medical profession itself sometimes support such resistance?

3. A number of Catholics have supported the legal right to "freedom of choice of abortion" despite the declarations against abortion by the Vatican and the U.S. bishops. They have argued: (1) It is not always necessary or helpful to support morality by law; (2) there is not a national consensus on the question of abortion; (3) a law against abortion could not be enforced; (4) such a law might lead to an increase of illegal abortions; and (5) in some cases, such as rape or danger to the mother's health, abortion seems medically justified. When forming one's conscience, is there a difference between a moral teaching of the church and the manner in which this teaching would be expressed in U.S. public policy?

6

Responsibilities of Health Care Professionals

OVERVIEW: Although each person is primarily responsible for his or her own health and health care, the social nature of the human personality makes it clear that we need the help of others in our endeavors to maintain or restore health. Thus we need the help of health care professionals and society. In this chapter, we consider the responsibilities of health care professionals. In chapter 7, we shall consider the ethical responsibilities of persons and institutions in providing adequate access to health care. We base our considerations in chapter 6 on the nature of a profession, the ideals of the medical profession, and the particular needs of patients. We apply the principles of human dignity, professional communication, and legitimate cooperation.

6.1 WHAT IS A PROFESSION?

Because health care is only one among several professions basic to the culture of any advanced community, to delineate the ethical responsibilities of the health care profession it is first necessary to consider the nature of the professions in general, then to define the specific role of the health care profession, and finally to identify its relationships with other professions.

In the classical sense of the term, the professions were ministry (theology), physic (medicine), and law. They were "person professions" centered on a counselor–client relationship. They did not produce goods for sale or works of art for enjoyment, but worked to heal, guide, or protect persons in a life crisis. Industrial society has fostered the professions greatly, but it has also depersonalized them. No longer do they center on relationships of persons; instead, they center on the productivity of an impersonal system. They no longer deal with improving interpersonal communication; rather, they deal with the more efficient exchange of power.

This slow depersonalizing transformation of the professions is reaching its completion today just as industrial society itself seems about to yield to a new postindustrial society. In postindustrial society, the source of power will no longer be economic ownership but rather knowledge and its communication. Such power means a still greater role for the professions. This knowledge can be used to bring about greater social conformism and dependency on professionals, or it can be used to open the system to wider, more genuine social participation by all. In either case, the professions would be radically reconstructed.

Will professionals become technocrats whose technological mastery must extend itself to behavior control? Or will they become the persons who help others to transcend the depersonalization of technological systems? If professionals choose the latter alternative, then the professions must again be personalized. They must be reconstructed so as to eliminate the threefold depersonalization that they have suffered in the epoch of industrial society: that of the client, the profession, and the client–professional relationship.

In medicine, clients have been depersonalized by the proliferation of specialism. Human beings are no longer thought of as complex organisms, but rather as collections of organs. The parts are healed, not the person, such that the very meaning of healing—that is, to make whole—has been lost.

Professions themselves have been depersonalized by a loss of clear identity. This loss is notoriously true for the ministry and is now evident in law, teaching, and medicine. A recent study showed that psychiatrists, psychoanalysts, and psychiatric social workers all do much the same thing, yet are considered members of three different professions. What is even more confusing is that many ministers, lawyers, and physicians counsel clients in ways not easily distinguishable from those of psychotherapists.

Contributing to this confusion of identity today is the tension within each profession between the goals of research and the goals of practice. How, then, can a professional make that kind of personal commitment always regarded as a mark of a profession if what he or she professes is not clear?

Moreover, the validity of the professional–client relationship is being questioned. Professionalism seems to imply an elitism that separates professional and patient and is ultimately socially destructive. The industrial model for organizing the professions has progressively restricted access to knowledge and skill, placing them in the hands of the elite, on whom the public is more and more dependent, but from whom the public receives less and less adequate service.

Today, the term *profession* is used for almost any prestigious occupation because it has the aura of an ideal. It is a symbol rather than a reality. Nevertheless, sociologists have devoted much time to developing a good empirical definition of a profession. Their role can be summarized as follows.

Professionals place value, first of all, upon systematic knowledge and intellect: knowing. Second, they value technical skill and trained capacity: doing. Third, they value putting this conjoint knowledge and skill to work in the service of others: helping.

Some sociologists use a scale to define professionalism. Professionals must rate high on the following six operational attributes:

1. They practice full-time occupations.
2. They are committed to a calling, that is, they treat their occupation "as an enduring set of normative and behavioral expectations."
3. They are distinguished from the laity by various signs and symbols and identified with their peers—often in formalized organizations.
4. They gain esoteric but useful knowledge and skills through specialized education, which is lengthy and difficult.
5. They are expected to have a service orientation so as to perceive the needs of clients that are relevant to their competency.
6. They have autonomy of judgment and authority restrained by their responsibility to use their knowledge and skill.

The problem with contemporary definitions of a profession (which fundamentally come down to "knowing–doing–helping") is that they fail to distinguish clearly the original group of person professions from other highly developed occupations to which the term has been extended but that do not deal directly with persons. Today, accounting, engineering, architecture and the other arts, and business are considered professions, because they also involve knowing, doing, and helping. Yet their immediate objective is not personal but productive. Obliterating the distinction between the person professions and productive occupations is characteristic of industrial society and its depersonalization of the professions. If professions are to be re-personalized, the distinction between profession and productive occupation must be drawn once more.

To call technological pursuits and the arts professions is confusing and dangerous because this designation disguises the fact that they produce things and do not directly help persons. Certainly, technological occupations should educate their practitioners to be more sensitive to the human uses to which their product will be put, but this humanization of technology will be hindered if industrial society continues the old tendency of lumping technological occupations and person professions together under one name and judging them all in terms of productivity.

A true profession, therefore, is rooted in theory but aimed at practice—a practice that does not produce things external to persons, but rather a service directly to persons themselves. Furthermore, this service is not applied to persons who receive it passively but facilitates those persons' own activity. It aims at healing them, at making them whole, at freeing them to act on their own. Person professionals should not act on clients or dominate them, but instead enable them to become fully, autonomously themselves. Thus a true profession cannot properly be elitist. It communicates power rather than enforces dependency.

Finally, professional help in the classical sense is concerned precisely with those problems that are deeply personal or are matters of life and death. Such help engages both professional and client in a profound responsibility both to each other and to the larger community. This personalistic concept of a profession can help in reconstructing the professions and professional education for the future.

The proper task of the medical professional is to deal with problems at the biological and psychological levels of human functioning. Obviously, at the psychological level counseling of a certain type plays a major therapeutic role. At the biological level, however, it is not so obvious that the health care professional's role is still primarily that of a counselor. Yet if the thesis put forth in chapter 5 is correct—that all persons have primary responsibility for their own health—then the physician's primary responsibility is to help patients make good health decisions (not make such decisions for them), which requires a counseling process. People cannot make a good decision about how to care for their health unless they have the required information.

Thus, the *first conclusion:* Physicians and other health care professionals are true professionals and serve their patients mainly as counselors helping them make the right decisions about health care. To some extent, the health care professional plays the role of a teacher in giving this information. But more is involved than that, because the information required is not abstract biological truth but a concrete assessment of personal health and the possible ways of dealing with the problems it presents.

6.2 IDEALS OF THE MEDICAL PROFESSION

To make sure that the personalistic concept of the health care professions is not a mere ideal but rather is fully explained so that it can be put into practice, we must take a brief look at the crosscurrents of purpose at work in the historical development of the medical professions. The health care profession includes others besides physicians. But physicians are the leaders of the health care team, and we can only understand the other health care professions if we grasp the history and ideals of the medical profession. For this reason, we concentrate on physicians in the rest of this section; much of the content, however, applies to other health care professionals as well.

The history of medicine shows that physicians have been considered both priests and scientists. This duality, upon closer examination, reflects the mind–body or psychosomatic duality of the human being who is sick. In Greece (where modern Western medicine originated), the first father of medicine was Asclepius, the "mild god." His priests presided over shrines (the first clinics), where the sick came to worship, sleep, and have their dreams interpreted. The symbol of the medical profession today is still a staff with entwined serpents, because the serpent—the symbol of wisdom and the healing power of Mother Earth (i.e., nature)—was the cult animal at these shrines.

This Greek myth of the god of healing manifests a basic truth about the medical profession: To this day, the physician retains something of a priestly ministry in the service of the healing forces of nature. Something similar is true of every person profession, because each one deals with the sacred dignity of the human person and rests on the sacred covenant of trust between client and professional.

This priestly ministry is especially true of the medical profession, because its direct relation to life and death gives it a sacred character. A person's trust in the physician is almost like trust in one's mother, a primordial confidence in life support. Although this trust can be abused and exploited, it is valuable when it is authentic. No one can be healed without trust. Thus the most significant distinction in explaining the history of medicine is not between scientific and nonscientific medicine, but rather between authentic medicine and quackery. Authentic medicine has both priestly and scientific dimensions.

The current debates about the humanization of medicine reflect the resurgence of the priestly aspect of the medical tradition, which never died and will always be part of medicine. Therefore the charismatic character of the physician—which arises from the priestly side of medicine but is also enhanced by the miraculous powers of scientific technology—should be respected. The charismatic atmosphere is an important element of the professional relationship and is essential to the healing process.

This atmosphere makes it possible for the patient, who is often distrustful, to place the necessary trust in professional help. It also gives medical professionals a sense of personal dignity, dedication, and responsibility that contributes immeasurably to their satisfaction and persistence in a difficult vocation. Moreover, self-respect guards other ethical values. Nothing is so likely to keep medical professionals from abusing their position for financial or other gains as this sense of self-respect. The increasing commercialization of medicine will be disastrous, and the medical professional will become an anonymous functionary in an industrial or a government bureaucracy, unless this self-respect prevails.

Our *second conclusion:* The physician who wants to develop sound ethical judgment must (1) have a profound respect for the medical profession as a vocation that has both scientific and priestly aspects and (2) have a clear understanding of the limits of this profession and of its interrelation with and dependence on other professions that also deal with the human person.

6.3 THE CHRISTIAN HEALTH CARE PROFESSIONAL

Christian health care professionals are called by their faith to understand this vocation in a special way, as are professionals of other religions or philosophies of life. Christians think of life as a gift from God and of the body as a marvelous work of divine creation to be reverenced as a temple of God (1 Cor 6:19; 2 Cor 6:16). They also think of the human person not only as a living body, but also as a body animated with a spiritual life that is open to a share in the eternal life of God. Consequently, the Christian health care professional thinks of sickness as an evil desecrating the temple. Even when sickness cannot be overcome, the struggle against it can be lived through as an experience that can further moral and spiritual growth. Thus the Christian physician or nurse is truly a minister of God, cooperating with him in helping suffering human beings overcome their suffering to live more fully. The Christian medical professional finds a model in Jesus Christ, the Healer. Although physicians do not have supernatural or miraculous powers, they do have medical skill, which is also a gift from God, and can imitate Jesus's compassion for the patient and his reaching out to the most neglected, even lepers. This Christian attitude cannot be a matter of mere pious words; rather it is a profound dependence on God, who gives the physician and nurse the inspiration, insight, and courage to carry out their work as professionally and as skillfully as possible.

Moreover, one should not make the mistake of thinking that the ethical aspect of medicine pertains only to its personal, priestly side, because it also penetrates its scientific aspect. The scientific approach to disease is built on a devotion to objective truth and on a courageous, persevering effort to advance this truth through research and criticism. Dedication to objective truth and scientific integrity is an ethical value of the highest order. Nothing is gained if the effort to humanize or personalize medicine interjects an unhealthy sentimentalism or occultism into its practice. Sound ethical judgment can be based only on critical scientific knowledge.

On the negative side, however, the scientific method as now understood and practiced often tends toward reductionism, that is, the assertion that the scientific method is the exclusive road to truth. Because the scientific method deals only with the limited aspects of reality that can be measured and experimented on, such a reductionist attitude can compel physicians to ignore and deny facts and experiences outside these rather narrow limits.

When reductionism is rigidly applied, the patient is treated as a soulless machine. In the history of medicine, this mechanistic approach has been profitable to the degree that it has allowed the intensive use of the scientific method, but it has ultimately limited the advance of medicine. Again and again, biologists and physicians sensitive to the holistic character of living organisms and the human person have revolted against reductionism and opened new, broader, and more fruitful lines of research.

The *third conclusion:* Sound ethical judgment must completely respect scientifically established medical facts, but it cannot rest on these facts alone. It must be open to all humanistic and spiritual approaches to understanding and evaluating the human condition.

6.4 PERSONALIZING THE HEALTH CARE PROFESSION

At the heart of every profession, there is a counseling relationship between persons, and this relationship takes on a special importance in health care. Although many models of counseling relationships may be applied to the professional–patient interaction, the most significant models from an ethical perspective are the psychoanalytical model and the medical model, because these are the models of relationship most prevalent in health care. We consider each model in order to indicate the ethical responsibilities of both patient and physician.

The Psychoanalytic Model

In the psychoanalytical model, the client comes to the therapist because of painful anxieties that make normal life difficult or impossible, with the goal of trying to resolve emotional conflicts whose unconscious origin is unknown to the client. The therapist's responsibility is not to diagnose the illness by labeling it, but rather to help the client understand the causes of his or her problems and cope with them more effectively. To achieve this, the therapist must gradually win the client's trust and help the client step by step to interpret the symbolism of the symptoms.

The therapist must grant the client the right to have his or her behavior interpreted as symbolic rather than judged morally and to have the client's sufferings counted worthy of sympathy. The therapist must help the client not to act out symptoms, but rather to discover their underlying meaning and thus to come to a deep, realistic self-understanding. Finally, the therapist must help the client acquire new skills to cope with the problems of life and eventually terminate his or her dependence on the therapist. To do this, the therapist must personally arrive at self-understanding through the same process.

The client must come to trust the therapist, speaking more and more freely, and cooperating by undertaking the task of working through symptoms. This process depends on an intense one-to-one relationship, in which the patient withdraws from the familial and social situation in which he or she became ill.

It also demands toleration by family and society of the patient's temporary withdrawal from ordinary relationships and responsibilities.

The dependence of the client on the therapist is essentially a recapitulation of the parental relationship, but a healthy one rather than the unhealthy one from which the client has suffered. Metaphorically, the therapist is a good mother in taking on the attitude of what Carl Rogers called "unconditional benign acceptance" and also a good father in the increasing role of interpretation and confrontation with reality. The libidinal, erotic elements of the transference of the client to the therapist are gradually turned toward the real love objects of the client's independent life. By no means is it easy for clients to come to such total trust in their therapists, because they have learned to distrust any mother or father. Clients must accept the tasks (1) of trusting the therapist and (2) of trying to recover health and normal independence.

For their part, therapists undertake the moral burden of being faithful to this trust given to them by their clients. They must approve and reinforce the client's progressive achievement of insight and gradually confront them more and more with the demands of reality. For therapists to be ethically true to this trust, they must be personally aware of any tendency toward countertransference (i.e., the development of a relationship in which the therapist begins to use the patient to meet the therapist's own emotional needs) and must strive to keep this human tendency within limits.

Today, these mutual duties are often formalized in a contract made at the beginning of therapy. Therapists are unethical when they fail to make such a clear contract (which is an aspect of informed consent) or fail to adhere strictly to it. Therapists should not assume moral obligations beyond the limits of this contract. The *fourth conclusion:* Psychoanalytic counseling aims at a relationship of trust between counselor and client, so that the client will be able to cope with reality and not be overburdened by emotional fear and depression.

The Medical Model

In strong contrast to the psychoanalytical model is the medical model. Yet it also gives rise to many ethical obligations. In the medical model, the professional goal is to treat a physical illness so as to restore normal physical functioning to the degree possible. The physician first seeks to diagnose the disease, then to prescribe a course of treatment (in which the physician is assisted by nurses and others) through medicine, surgery, nursing, or change of regimen. The physician must also make a prognosis and if possible offer the patient hope. The patient, conversely, is relieved from blame for his or her condition and from ordinary responsibilities to work and family, but is expected to be cooperative with the professional staff. Families and society are expected to support the patient psychologically and to contribute to the expenses.

Patient passivity raises the main ethical issue characteristic of this model. If the health care profession is only a servant to the patient because the primary responsibility for the patient's health remains the patient's, then it follows that the professional has no rights over the patient, except those given with the patient's informed consent. Hence, ethically speaking, an implicit or explicit contract must regulate all that goes on in the medical model.

What are the essential features of this medical contract? First, the contract limits the obligations assumed. In the medical model, a physician does not assume the role of a psychotherapist or of an ethical or spiritual counselor. Efforts to re-personalize medicine should not demand that the medical doctor assume all the roles proper to a complete health team. Of course, the physician needs to be aware of nonphysical factors that may be affecting the patient's health so that he or she can seek the help of other members of the health team in dealing with such factors. A well-known study of hospital care showed that a high percentage of patients were incorrectly diagnosed because of the failure of physicians to listen carefully to patients' complaints or to recognize nonmedical factors in their conditions.

The second essential feature of the medical model, as of other professional relationships, is trust. To develop a trusting relationship, the physician must seek to develop three personal attributes. The first is *concern*. Fundamental to the relationship is the physician's concern for the patient's well-being. Trust will never exist if the patient believes that the physician is concerned only about the fee or is acting out of mere routine like a machine or a bureaucratic functionary. This is the difficulty involved in setting time limits for treating patients, as is the practice in several contemporary health maintenance organizations. The physician must communicate interest in the patient as a person, not as a kidney or a heart, and a willingness to do for the patient whatever is professionally possible, without being limited by mere self-interested motives. For this reason, a well known theologian has rightly emphasized that the professional contract is something more than a contract; it is a covenant in the theological sense. Thus the professional contract also implies the promise to continue the care of the patient even when the patient is no longer able to insist on its fulfillment.

The second attribute is *knowledge and skill in medicine*. Health care professionals have the fundamental responsibility, within their specialties, to be experts in both the science and the art of health care, up-to-date in knowledge, experienced, of good judgment, and skilled in procedures. Personal warmth does not substitute for medical expertise. In times past, professionals communicated such expertise to patients with evidence of their education and licensing, by their reputation, and by the care and thoroughness with which they dealt with patients. With the advent of for-profit medicine, however, physician are often called upon to advocate the methods they use.

In this new atmosphere, honesty is the most important quality, lest people be led astray by the claims of aggressive health care suppliers.

The third attribute is *communication*. Because patients retain fundamental rights over their own bodies, and the knowledge of how they feel not only at this minute, but also throughout the day and in varied situations, physicians cannot hope to make a proper diagnosis, carry on successful treatment, or make an accurate prognosis without adequately communicating with their patients.

Health Care Fees

To these basic ethical obligations of the medical doctor, a fourth can be added that applies also to both the psychotherapeutic and medical models: to set or refuse an appropriate fee. In a capitalist society, it is assumed that a professional should be paid as any other worker is paid according to the laws of supply and demand. It is assumed that a service is just as much a commodity for exchange, with a value measured in monetary terms, as is any other product. Consequently, some persons argue that there is nothing ethically wrong with organizing the medical profession on the basis of profit like any other industry; they actually speak of the "health industry!" They believe that the stimulus of the profit motive has been the chief cause of the rapid technological development of U.S. medicine.

Yet the question can also be raised as to whether this capitalistic assumption is a realistic and practical fact. At no time in the history of medicine has the market system operated fully, because there have always been people who desperately needed professional help but could not pay for it. Either the professional had to provide free services or payment had to be made by a third party. In fact, since the rise of health insurance, Medicare, and Medicaid, most health care *is* paid for by a third party, the insurer or the government, which determines standard fees.

If our account of the nature of a profession is correct, it should be clear why profit cannot be the primary basis of any profession, but must be considered a secondary and highly variable feature. The medical profession, like any true profession, must rest not on bargaining but on trust; and it provides a service that is concerned with life and death, matters so precious as to be priceless. No monetary value can be put on the spiritual light given by a priest, the defense of human rights provided by a lawyer, the risk of his or her own life provided by a soldier, or the search for truth shared by a teacher. Nor is there any price for the service of a physician in the battle against disease and illness.

Hence professional fees are not payments measured by the value of the service provided (which is truly priceless), but a *stipend* to be measured only by what professionals need to live and work without distraction. The ability-to-pay principle is not unjust as long as it remains within the bounds of the more fundamental principle that professionals are public servants who have no right to expect in return for services anything more than a standard of living that will make it possible for them to perform those services with liberty of mind and health of body and to fulfill family and social obligations adequately.

Accordingly, the *fifth conclusion:* Christian health care professionals will pursue a lifestyle that is essentially modest and in which simplicity and freedom to be available to serve others is the only honorable measure of remuneration. Nor can the popular argument be accepted that physicians, because they spend years in difficult study, work long hours, and assume great responsibility, deserve to make money. The rewards of any profession are to be found not in some extraneous gain, but in the satisfactions of knowledge and of interesting, satisfying, and absorbing work. Such an ideal is not easy to realize, nor is it often realized in its purest form; but even when imperfectly realized it is what has given the medical profession its own vitality and health.

6.5 PROFESSIONAL COMMUNICATION

In health care, as in all professional relationships, adequate communication between professional and client is a fundamental ethical requirement. In the medical model, opportunities for such communication may be restricted rather sharply, but they are still crucial. Within the limits of the medical model, what are the duties of health care professionals?

The first obligation of the health care professional is to listen to the patient. The health care professional needs to remember that "the medium is the message"; that is, the way patients are (or are not) communicating may be the most significant symptom.

Therefore, no matter how busy they may be, health care professionals have the responsibility to acquire the art of medical dialogue, through which they can help patients say what needs to be said. The first rule of this art is for the professional to repeat back to the patient what the professional has heard that seems significant and to ask whether it is what the patient meant. A second rule is to obtain the patient's cooperation by explaining the purpose of questions, because unexpected and cryptic questions are often threatening and confusing.

Of course, professionals also have the right to require honesty and frankness from clients. When they suspect deliberate deceit, they should deal with the situation explicitly and directly as a breach of the patient's contract with the professional. In most illnesses, however, psychological factors may cause communication to be distorted by unconscious elements of denial, confusion, or panic. Psychotherapists, in particular, must deal with this perplexing inability of some patients to communicate openly. But other health care professionals also experience something of the same ambiguity.

Health care professionals cannot expect truth from their patients unless they are equally truthful with them. A lack of frankness by professionals is usually excused as concern to spare the patient, but is just as often the result of unconscious fear on the part of the professional. Chapter 12 discusses the problem of telling the truth to an incurably ill or dying patient. Here, it suffices to say that the fundamental principle in all such situations is that the patient has the right to the truth, however difficult it may be for the professional to communicate it.

In both the psychoanalytic model and in the medical model, the need for health care professionals to respect the dignity of their patients by observing confidentiality is most important. Patients have the right to the truth about their health because they have the primary responsibility for their health. They also have the right to privacy about those aspects of life that do not affect others directly. Human community is based on communication, which is impossible if confidences are not shared. But confidences will not be shared if the vulnerable party believes his or her privacy will be violated. Hence health care professionals have a serious obligation to maintain those confidences that would injure the patient's reputation if they were revealed.

How is a professional to act when questioned by others about a patient's condition? All Catholic moralists agree that it is always wrong to lie, even to protect confidentiality, but not all agree on how to define lying. The meaning of any human statement must always be determined from the context in which communication occurs. Consequently, when persons ask questions that they have no right to ask, the context renders any answer given essentially meaningless, so that it is ethically inconsequential whether that answer in a normal context would be true or false.

Therefore, health care professionals who are questioned about confidential matters may without lying or even falsehood reply in any way that protects confidentiality. This fact, however, cannot excuse a physician from answering frankly questions put by a patient or the patient's guardians, because these persons have the right to know the things that the physician knows about the patient. Whether one has the obligation to reply to a question with unambiguous and accurate information thus depends on the questioner's right to such information.

Hence, generally speaking, health care professionals have not only the right but also the duty to communicate information necessary to prevent serious harm to the patient or to others, even when it is given to them in confidence, to those who may be able to prevent this injury. When what is revealed is an intention to commit a crime (including suicide), the professional has the legal and ethical obligation to reveal to appropriate persons whatever information is necessary to prevent such a crime. When no crime is contemplated, but there is probably a danger of harm that can be prevented, the professional should do what is likely to be helpful in preventing such harm in a discreet way. Ordinarily, this should not be done without first warning the patient of exposure if the patient refuses to desist.

In recent times, the spread of acquired immune deficiency syndrome (AIDS) has reminded health care workers of the serious responsibility of confidentiality. Mainly because of the manner in which AIDS is acquired (people infected with the HIV virus often are homosexual, bisexual, or intravenous drug users), severe discrimination is exercised against AIDS patients. Thus, their privacy should be protected. People seem to forget that many people with AIDS have acquired the disease through blood transfusions or were born with it. Moreover, Christian compassion demands that respect be shown for those who acquire the disease through aberrant behavior, even though the activity that brings about the disease is not valued. Jesus never asked those he healed how they became ill.

The *sixth conclusion:* Health care professionals have the responsibility

1. to strive to establish and preserve trust at both emotional and rational levels;
2. to share the information they possess with those who legitimately need it in order to have an informed conscience;
3. to refrain from lying or giving misinformation; and
4. to keep secret information that is not legitimately needed by others, but that if revealed might either harm the patient or others or destroy trust.

6.6 PEER RELATIONSHIPS AND PROFESSIONAL DISCIPLINE

Health care professionals need good personal relationships not only with those they serve, but also with their colleagues on the health team. Problems of leadership and accountability, of common decision making and cooperation in carrying out decisions, and of adequate communication and mutual support not only have psychological importance, but also are profoundly ethical.

The need for improved peer relationships and professional communication is evidenced in medical malpractice suits. A federal commission concluded that malpractice suits frequently result (1) from poor communication between physicians and patients, and hence from inadequately informed consent on the patient's part; (2) from patients' frustration with physicians who seem unresponsive to their complaints; (3) from patients' misinformed, unrealistic expectations about the benefits of treatment; and (4) from growing public conviction that consumers need to defend themselves against arrogant, self-serving professionals. It is noteworthy that the first three of these factors (and perhaps in large part the fourth) can be reduced to a failure in communication, a skill in which physicians are often not well trained.

Two opposite remedies have been proposed for the malpractice problem. One answer is *peer review*. It is argued, plausibly enough, that in a field so highly technical as medicine no one is competent to evaluate professional performance except peers in the profession or even in the same medical specialty. Conversely, some observers argue that *peer discipline* has never been successful in protecting the patient or even in maintaining high standards of medical competence. A profession, they contend, is too concerned with its own autonomy to be very diligent in disciplining its members.

Consequently, these critics believe that disciplining a profession must first of all concern those who suffer from malpractice or neglect. Health care consumers must know and defend their own rights by all available economic, legal, and political means. Because the primary responsibility for health must remain with each person to whom the professional is only a servant, the ultimate right to call the medical profession to account must be in the hands of those the profession exists to serve. This is why the users of health services have the fundamental right to the final word in regulating the profession through public law.

The medical profession and every learned profession must have a genuine but limited autonomy. As health care users become more knowledgeable about what is and what is not good medical care, they will become more and more able to detect serious incompetence or negligence in the service they receive. But at last, this awareness will only raise questions; it will not be sufficient in most cases to pass judgment. People may have doubts that an operation recommended by their surgeons is really necessary, but all they can do to find out is either to ask for more convincing answers to their questions or to consult another professional.

It would seem, therefore, that a satisfactory system of discipline for the medical profession must be a combination of both peer discipline and consumer discipline. A medical review board must include both professional peers with requisite technical knowledge and experience and also health care users (along with legal advisers) to ensure that the medical professionals are more concerned for those served than for their own self-interest as the servants. Yet it is also essential that medical information be made more easily available to all users so that each can know and defend his or her own rights and interests.

Recently, government agencies and professional societies have called attention to the frequency of medical error, and the harm and expense inflicted upon patients as a result of medical error. (*To Err Is Human*, 2000, and *Crossing the Quality Chasm*, 2001; both National Institute of Medicine). Comparisons are drawn in these studies to practices that avoid error in the airline and nuclear power industries. In both of these industries, errors have been reduced by the practice of self-revelation. One problem of applying this method to medical error is that procedures and practices are not easily divided into right and wrong. True, some mistakes are egregious and deserve adequate redress. But others are a matter of more or less, not good and bad. To date, the medical societies and professional groups have not taken these studies seriously, and it seems that mistakes will be made in health care without serious efforts to correct the situation.

Although the above-mentioned studies would not seem to agree, we believe the real remedy for malpractice and unjustified malpractice litigation is a more personalized practice of medicine that will reduce misunderstanding between professional and patient and will correct human failure by professionals through mutual cooperation and discipline within the health team itself. The notion of fraternal correction is part of the Christian ethos (Mt 18:15B18). Applied to a profession, it means that the members do not simply ignore or hide the defects of colleagues out of indifference or self-interest, but instead are seriously concerned to help them overcome these defects and repair the consequences. It also implies that even workers in subordinate positions have a right and an obligation to correct superiors and that the superiors have an obligation to listen to such corrections.

The *seventh conclusion:* For a health team to develop mutual support and discipline, it must build up profound mutual trust and respect, which can only be achieved through persistent effort. One of the marks of a Christian health care facility, therefore, should be this striving to establish the personal relationships among the staff and administration that will be the basis for such professional cooperation.

SUMMARY

The many ethical responsibilities delineated and studied in this chapter are all derived from the concept of medicine as a profession. The professional relationship has no traces of debilitating paternalism, but it recognizes the need for health care professionals to offer their accurate evaluation of the patient's condition so that a collaborative decision will result. Moreover, fostering productive relationships between peers and coworkers in health care facilities is a serious matter. Recent studies indicate that medical care is not "problem free" and that more stringent efforts are needed to protect the well-being of patients.

QUESTIONS

1. What distinguishes the classical professions from other useful occupations? Why is the maintenance of high ethical standards in professions so important for society as a whole?
2. Are there any situations in which a medical professional is justified in revealing embarrassing or damaging information about a patient to a third party? Name and explain.
3. If you were a physician who wanted to set up a team approach to care for patients in an intensive care unit, what possible difficulties would

you anticipate? How would you avoid them? Do these factors involve questions of fairness (justice)?

CASES

1. Two physicians, Dr. A and Dr. B, were medical school classmates. Ten years later, however, they have developed very different "professional manners." Dr. A dresses very conservatively, always wears his white coat in his office, impresses his patients with a very crisp, authoritative manner, and always appears to be very busy. Conversely, Dr. B dresses informally, does not "look like a doctor," and cultivates a rather folksy manner with his patients. Dr. A's patients are afraid to ask him questions but have great confidence in his skill. Dr. B, who does not have as great a reputation, wonders if he ought to imitate Dr. A. Is Dr. B making a mistake? If so, what should he do about it? Or is Dr. A mistaken? How could he improve communication with his patients without losing their confidence?

2. Jane is fourteen years old and has become pregnant as a result of incest with her father. On a routine visit to the family physician, Dr. Y, she explains what has happened, and he confirms the pregnancy. She begs him not to tell her parents, because then her mother will discover what has happened. She is convinced that her mother will blame her, rather than her husband, because her relations with her mother are very bad. Dr. Y, a Catholic, tells her he never performs abortions, so Jane asks him to refer her to a physician who does. Dr. Y wonders whether professional confidentiality and perhaps even legal complications forbid him from informing the mother and trying to stop the abortion and the continuation of the incestuous relationship. But he is also worried that Jane will go to a disreputable and unsafe abortionist. What principles will help him solve his problem?

3. Nurse R has a low opinion of the professional conduct of Dr. Q. The latest example involved a comatose patient. She agreed with Dr. Q that the patient's family should be encouraged to give consent to disconnecting the respirator. After several days of discussion, the family called Dr. Q and gave their consent. That evening, he phoned Nurse R and ordered her to remove the respirator as soon as the family got there to be with the dying patient. She did not protest that this unpleasant task had been delegated to her, because she knew any protest would anger Dr. Q. With the family at the bedside, she removed the respirator, and to her and their horror the patient went into convulsions before dying. The family now blames her. What can Nurse R do to prevent such situations in the future?

7

Social Responsibility for Health Care

OVERVIEW: Individuals are mainly responsible for their own health, and the health care profession has a responsibility to be of service in this pursuit of health. But society also has a responsibility to individuals and the health care profession insofar as the pursuit of health is concerned. What are the ethical responsibilities of local, state, and federal governments? American culture and political thought are paradoxical in their prevailing attitude toward these questions. Although the principle was accepted long ago that government should promote and regulate free primary and secondary education for all children, for some reason Americans have hesitated to accept wholeheartedly the principle that government should promote and regulate universal free basic health care.

Although local, state, and federal governments have made efforts to extend health care to the elderly and poor through programs such as Medicare and Medicaid, we believe that these programs are part of a model of providing health care that is seriously flawed. This model does not recognize that health care is a right that should be allocated according to need, not ability to pay.

This chapter describes the models of health care used in the United States and offers an alternative model founded on Catholic social teaching. At present, health care reform is a topic on the minds of the U.S. public. Rather than discuss the details of the various reform programs that are being discussed, we offer a radical system for reform founded upon the teaching of Jesus in the Gospels, which will help to evaluate the various plans being proposed by the federal government. The principles applied in this chapter are the common good and subsidiarity, professional communication, and legitimate cooperation.

7.1 MODELS OF HEALTH CARE

Among citizens of the United States, and among health care professionals, there has been a tendency to discuss all social issues in terms of two opposing models: free enterprise versus socialism. Actually, three models of the social organization of health care are being debated in the United States: the *pluralist* model, the *centralized* model, and the *participatory* model.

The Pluralist Model

At this time, the pluralist model predominates in the United States. It is a blend of private and public health care facilities, of health care professionals working on either a fee-for-service basis or for a basic salary, and of various public and private financing agencies. The regulatory principle of this pluralist system is the market in which persons with health needs compete for the services of health care professionals, principally on a fee-for-service basis, and professionals compete to sell their services. Today, however, these professional health care providers no longer act merely as individuals, but are organized in a spectrum of health care institutions, of which the hospital is chief. In theory, the pluralist models favor competition to control costs. But in practice, because health care is not a commodity and because people are not free to select their health care as they are to select other goods, competition does not exist in health care.

Furthermore, an increasing number of physicians are organized in group practices of various types, such as health maintenance organizations and preferred provider organizations. In some of these organizations, physicians are prepaid by patients a fixed salary or a fee based on the number of patients served (capitation). Thus, in a pluralist system there is no single organizational structure but a plurality of providers, some acting individually, but most acting through some institutional group.

The difficulties with this present system have become very apparent in recent years. It is an inefficient system because it does not provide for long-range planning and it wastes resources in overlapping services and duplication of expensive plants and equipment. There are no national priorities for health care, so there are inconsistent actions: The federal government limits funds for Medicare and neonatal care programs while funding kidney transplants from living or cadaver donors. More serious still, the present system has not provided access to adequate medical care for many socially and geographically disadvantaged groups. Nor has it demonstrably raised the general level of health in recent years. Finally, it seems to be subject to ever-mounting costs, which now absorb about 15 percent of the gross domestic product.

Some economists who defend pluralism look for ways to bring free-market mechanisms into play to afford better cost control and greater effectiveness in meeting real rather than artificial needs. Although some doubt that professional monopoly is really the major factor in raising health costs, others assert this and call for restrictions on the monopolistic practices of medical societies, such as the use of ethics codes to prevent advertising and limit access to information by which consumers might be able to make competitive choices. Other economists believe some degree of government regulation is inevitable, but advise that it should not emphasize planning so much as provide economic motivation for hospitals to control costs (e.g., with budgetary measures, limits on new hospital construction, and encouragement to shift to more outpatient care).

One popular solution to the ills of our health care system is called *managed competition* or *managed care*. Although this system might bring about some economies insofar as record keeping and the use of clinical tests are concerned, managed care retains the same priorities as our present health care system. Thus, the health care of all the people is not a priority for this new system; rather, technology, aggressive acute care, and profit remain the priorities of managed care.

The Centralized Model

Because of such difficulties with the present pluralist model, a second centralized (or regional) model has been widely proposed and defended. In this model, the United States would be divided into regions, each having all health care organized in a unified three-layer pyramidal system. At the bottom of the pyramid would be a large number of primary care physicians and their auxiliaries, who would care for the great majority of health problems that require only a minimum of specialized knowledge and equipment. For cases exceeding such care, the second level would include hospitals or other facilities with complete staffs of specialists and advanced equipment. For cases of still greater difficulty, the third (and perhaps even fourth) level of institutions would be equipped to give the most advanced care; these institutions also would house medical education and research. In such a system, because long-range planning would be possible, the focus of health care could move away from curing disease and toward prevention, and each region more or less would become a health maintenance organization.

To think of the pluralist model as free enterprise and the centralized model as socialism is a serious mistake. Because of the monopolistic control by the medical profession, the pluralist model is in fact a free-enterprise system only in a very limited degree. In such a model, health consumers are seldom in a position to make intelligent choices between competitive alternatives, either because they lack information or because these alternatives are very limited.

Conversely, the centralized model is by no means incompatible with a free-enterprise system as it now operates in the United States. The American way of life has moved toward a high degree of rationalization and monopoly in industry, as well as in government. Such centralization has not changed the class structure of American society in any radical way. It would be perfectly possible to set up a centralized model in such a way as to leave a considerable choice to both the consumer and the provider. It could even include voluntary health insurance and fee-for-service features. What is essential to such a system is that it be centralized on a regional basis and open to strategic planning.

The Participatory Model

The participatory model is based on the view that there must be planning (as in the centralized model), but this is not the same as advocating a planned society. In a planned society, whether it be governed by a democratic bureaucratic elite or by a socialistic bureaucratic elite, individuals have their health cared for but lose any real control over how it is to be done. In a market system, individuals have scarcely more control because they lack the information or alternatives to choose from. What is needed, therefore, according to those who seek a third model, is a system in which consumers play a real role in the planning process. The great problem in adopting the participatory model is the resistance of health care professionals. They have been educated to believe that the maintenance of high-quality health care demands professional autonomy and forbids interference by laypersons.

The essential steps to developing a participatory model are (1) assumption of responsibility by each person for his or her own health, (2) restoration of a sound professional–client relationship, and (3) education of medical professionals to be able to work within this relationship.

Christian Social Thought

For Christian health care professionals, the first step in seeking a better organization of health care in the United States and in the world must be to free themselves from the ideology that leads Americans to analyze every social issue in terms of the American free-enterprise system versus socialism. Such identification of any human culture with the Gospel is certain to be misleading, because the Gospel stands as a prophetic criticism of every culture, approving some of its features but correcting others.

The authentic social teaching of the Catholic Church, for example, contains some strong criticisms of Marxist socialism and communism, chiefly on three grounds: (1) its atheistic materialism, (2) its denial of the right of private property, and (3) its tendency to totalitarian government. But this teaching also contains a vigorous criticism of capitalism on the grounds of (1) its deterministic reliance on economic laws, the so-called magic of the market; (2) its advocacy of unregulated competition and the profit motive; and (3) its neglect of Christian advocacy of the poor. Christian health care professionals, therefore, should base their thinking about the social organization of health care on the principles of the Gospel and not on the principles of the free-enterprise system, any more than on those of socialism.

No one economic system—any more than any one political system—is simply natural, right, or Christian. Such systems are human inventions, each with some advantages and some disadvantages, to be selected according to particular historical circumstances. These merits need to be evaluated both from a theoretical point of view and from a practical, experiential point of view. In judging them ethically, we must consider both their congruity with fundamental moral and Gospel principles and their pragmatic results in a given situation.

The *first conclusion:* Designing a fundamental revision for providing health requires radical thinking, and it is here that Catholic social thought can make an important contribution to finding new solutions. These solutions must rest on three principles, which have been previously expounded on in this book: (1) Every human being has a fundamental right to health, as acknowledged in the *Universal Declaration of Human Rights of the United Nations* (United Nations 1948; see appendix 2), Article 25, because human rights are based on essential human needs; (2) individual persons have the primary responsibility to promote their own health; and (3) as social beings, people also have the right to seek the help of others when necessary to fulfill this responsibility and reciprocally have the duty to give the same help to others as far as they are able. These concepts can be better understood in the context of analyzing the concepts of common good and subsidiarity.

7.2 GOSPEL PRINCIPLES OF SOCIAL ORGANIZATION

Common Good

The common good may be defined as the sum total of those conditions of social living whereby citizens are enabled more fully and more readily to achieve their own perfection. Most social evils and injustices are the result of the exclusion of some persons from the common good in which they have a right to share. The ancient evil of slavery was precisely such an unjust institution, wherein the slaves contributed to the common good but were not permitted to share fully in it—not only with regard to economic goods, but also with regard to such spiritual goods as education, freedom, political participation, respect, and even the right to worship the gods of the city. Thus the distribution of the common good is a fundamental demand of social justice.

Jesus, moreover, taught an ethics that clearly went beyond even this demand for distributive justice based on merit (i.e., each receives in proportion as he or she contributes). Jesus proclaimed the coming of the Kingdom of God

(Mk 1:15), which was not merely a heavenly kingdom but was also the fulfillment of the Old Testament prophecies of the Reign of God on the earth. When Jesus said to Pilate, "My kingship is not of this world" (Jn 18:36), in effect he was saying to Pilate, "I am not competing with you power brokers. I am building a kingdom built on a different principle; on service, not on dominion." He taught his followers to pray, "Your Kingdom come, your will be done, on earth as it is in heaven" (Mt 6:10).

The Beatitudes (Lk 6:20–22; Mt 5:3–11) are the joyful announcement to the poor (i.e., those excluded from the common good) that at last they are to be included in this common good, not only economically, but also spiritually ("the poor have the good news preached to them"; Lk 7:22). Consequently, the principle of the early church was "from each according to his [or her] ability, to each according to his [or her] needs," a principle Karl Marx borrowed from the Acts of the Apostles (32:35). Thus the common good requires love and mercy and the distribution of possessions according to need. The mark of all Jesus's work was his concern for the neglected, the outcast, the leper, the prostitute, the Samaritan heretic, and the pagan unbeliever.

A Christian ethics of health care allocation must be based not on merit, and certainly not on the ability to pay, but on need, because the needy are the most neglected. In this sense, health care is a right. Moreover, social oppression is the chief cause of illness. Hence those who are helpless by reason of poverty, disease, defect, or age (the unborn or the senile) should be the first to be considered under any health plan.

Yet all persons should contribute to the plan according to their ability. Thus the social responsibility for health care falls first on those who have the ability to heal, the health care professionals, and second on those who have the ability to pay, that is, those who have profited the most financially from society. For such affluent individuals to claim that they have made their wealth simply by their own efforts is an absurdity. They may have worked hard, but their wealth would not have been possible without the existence of the society of which they are a part. Consequently, their debt to the common good is in proportion to the wealth they have received from it.

Subsidiarity

From this notion of the common good, the notion of subsidiarity follows logically. Subsidiarity implies that the first responsibility to meet human needs rests with the free and competent individual, then with the local group. Higher and higher levels of the community must assume this responsibility (1) when the lower unit cannot assume it and (2) when the lower unit neglects to assume it. The higher level should never be content merely to take over responsibility, but it must work to return responsibility to a lower level. The main objection to many social reforms has been that they have not provided for this progressive decentralization. For example, the U.S. welfare system has perpetuated poverty rather than helped the poor and disadvantaged to become independent.

Before secular humanism became the dominant philosophy of modern society, Christian thinking was able to advance the notion that a society is not simply a two-level structure of government and citizenry, but an organic community containing many mutually interdependent functions. Hence the power to make social decisions ought to be kept as close as possible to those who experience those problems and are most strongly affected by the decisions concerning them. Only in this way can the dignity of the least members of a community be acknowledged and their interests served effectively by the greater members. A paternalism that decides everything for those it claims to serve is really nothing but a form of domination and tends to become self-serving.

Subsidiarity requires us to share decision-making power not only at various vertical levels of local, state, and federal government, but also among horizontal sectors representing various functional bodies. Each person in a society is related to as many such functional bodies as he or she has basic needs. The role of government is to coordinate and encourage the full development of these different organs of society, not to deprive them of their decision-making capacity.

The *second conclusion:* The kind of health care program that Christians can support consistently must aim at preventive medicine, at achieving a healthier people who can care for themselves, rather than an ever-increasing dependence on technical medical care and professional help. As Plato observed in the *Republic*, "A society that is always going to the doctor is a sick society" (1955, III, 405A). To achieve this fundamental objective, society must seek the sound political and economic organization of society.

7.3 FUNCTIONALISM

The application of subsidiarity to the organization of society on the basis of social functions—rather than on the basis of a struggle between isolated individuals defending their rights and a centralized government having all the powers of social decision—we call *functionalism*. Functionalism is opposed, on the one hand, to communism and socialism because they are totalitarian, concentrating all decision-making power in the hands of the state and the military. On the other hand, it is opposed to the competitive individualism of unregulated capitalism or free enterprise, with its hidden tendency to monopoly resulting in concentration of decision-making power in the hands of an interlocking power elite. Functionalism is not a mere theory, because it has been a powerful influence, through Catholic statesmen and stateswomen, on the formation of the European Union and of codetermination by management and labor in Germany, Japan, Yugoslavia, and other countries.

Politically, functionalism might seem to have little chance in the United States. Certain features of several institutions, however, are in fact functionalist. For example, higher education in the United States, in contrast to the statism of the lower school system, remains largely functionalist. Decisions about educational policies in our colleges and universities are for the most part still made independently of government by trustees, faculties, and accrediting agencies and by students exercising their right to choose their own schools. However, the increasing control of the government over schools by reason of their economic dependency is working strongly to destroy their functionalist character.

Similarly, the growth of labor unions in the United States once seemed to promise the eventual development of functionalism in the economic sphere. Unfortunately, the unions have largely neglected the social aspects of their original purpose and have been co-opted by the capitalist market system, in which they are becoming just another monopoly. Fortunately, this trend toward monopoly shows some signs of a reversal in the growth of consumerism, participatory democracy, and ecology, as well as in the increasing dissatisfaction with poorly designed liberal reforms, so many of which have served only to enlarge the power of government bureaucracy. Health care reformers need to take advantage of this growing criticism of the bureaucratic control of life to propose a more personalistic, functionalist conception of society.

In view of Christian goals, we should be aware of lessons learned by the United States with regard to health care. The first of these is that the pluralist system did not adequately care for the poor, nor did it do much about positive health improvement. It tended to pursue an exaggerated professional elitism, to place strong emphasis on monopolization and the profit motive, and it never produced a system of medical education that was personalistic. Yet the pluralist system should be credited with promoting very rapid technological and scientific progress and with developing a great number of health care facilities equipped to give high-quality care. It must be noted, however, that this progress has led rather to greater expenditure of resources on the sophisticated treatment of relatively rare ailments than to better care for the health of the majority.

The contemporary trend is to create a "market-oriented," centralized system aimed at correcting some of the defects of the former system, although not in a very radical manner. Such a new system will greatly increase the bureaucratization that—as evidenced by the welfare system, diagnosis related groups and other federal controls—can cost a great deal and accomplish very little. A centralized system will provide more health care, but there is no certainty that it will promote better health. Nor is a bureaucracy likely to personalize the health care it gives.

It seems, therefore, that although some form of national health care program is the only practical way available to extend care to the neglected of society, Christians should not have any illusions about the adequacy of such a program, but should critically support the new schemes for national comprehensive health care, stressing the need to incorporate into these plans as many functionalist features as possible. For example:

1. Comprehensive health care should aim primarily at the promotion of positive health, not merely at the curing of acute disease or the prolongation of life through sophisticated techniques. Therefore, it should work for the removal of the environmental and social causes of ill health, including the commercial exploitation of unhealthy patterns of living; and for the provision of preventive health education, which will give persons control over their own health.

2. Priority should be given to the problems of the most powerless, poorly informed, and least able to pay. These persons should not be cared for paternalistically, but should be admitted at once to participate in decision making about their own health needs.

3. Decision-making power should not be confined to a government bureaucracy or to autonomous professionals, but should be shared by all concerned in mutual interdependence.

4. Planning should proceed in such a way as to avoid tendencies to increase dependence on higher levels and to promote a gradually increasing decentralization, both in control and funding. This decentralization, however, should not be used as an excuse for the government to neglect the monitoring of health care and the supplementation and correction of defects at lower levels of organization.

5. Planning must be a continuous process of decision making that adapts to experience and new needs, rather than a fixed plan based on projections that may be mistaken.

The concepts underlying all such efforts to organize society, including its health care institutions, in such a way as to counteract tendencies to bureaucratism on the one hand, and competitive individualism on the other, can be summarily formulated.

The *third conclusion:* Human communities exist only to promote and share the common good among all their members "from each according to ability, to each according to need" in such a way that (1) decision making rests vertically first with the person, then with the lower social levels, and horizontally with functional social units; and (2) the higher social units intervene only to supply the lower units with what they cannot achieve by themselves, while working to make it easier in the future for lower units and individuals to satisfy these needs by their own efforts.

7.4 THE HEALTH CARE TEAM

Because of the highly specialized character of modern medicine, health seekers must entrust themselves not to a single physician but to a *health care team*. This section discusses those members of the health care team with whom the patient must deal directly—the physician, the nurse, and the social worker—to determine what reciprocal ethical obligations exist between the patient and these three kinds of professionals. To fulfill these ethical obligations, we suggest a new version of the relationship among team members.

Traditionally, the chief decision maker in any health care team is the licensed physician. Consequently, no serious step toward treating the patient can be taken without a physician's permission.

Today, the concept of the licensed medical doctor as a general practitioner has been vastly altered by the growth of medical specialization. In 1950, only about 36 percent of physicians in private practice were specialists, while in 2000 about 80 percent were specialists. This rapid decline of the general practitioner as the primary care professional has deprived patients of the advantages of having their health problems evaluated by someone who knows the patient in his or her family context during a long period and who thinks of the patient as a whole person with a continuous life history.

Perhaps the key to this difficulty of knowing the patient personally is to be found in a better understanding of the nurse's proper role. Originally, the nurse was the person most concerned with caring for the patient and in continuous contact with the patient. Therefore, patient-centered health care, which this book is advocating, would dictate that the nurse is the central professional figure, not the physician.

Today, however, nurses have been burdened with other tasks. For too long they spent much of their energy in housekeeping chores—making beds, carrying trays, and so forth. Now they have been largely relieved of these tasks by auxiliaries, but they are still much occupied with technical tasks, such as record keeping.

Under present circumstances, as nursing education has advanced, able nurses have sought administrative and teaching posts as the only way of advancement open to them. They would find nursing itself much more interesting, however, if it became the real focus of health care, so that the role of the nurse (female or male) in direct contact with the patient is seen as primary care and as the real source of the health team's unity. Then the nurse assigned to a given patient would become the authority with the responsibility for the patient as a person and would help the patient make use of all the resources furnished by the health team.

This personalistic, mediating function today is often performed by the medical or psychiatric social worker. Sociological study of the medical profession has led to the acknowledgment of the great importance of the social dimension in treating disease. Hence, persons trained in social process have been added to healing teams. The social worker interviews patients to discover possible social factors of ethnic culture, economic status, and family structure that may have caused the disease, may hinder treatment, or may prevent rehabilitation. Commonly, such workers help patients secure both their legal rights and their opportunities for public financial assistance and other matters connected with illness. They also act as liaisons with the patient's family and help find ways to assure family stability during the patient's absence from the home. Finally, social workers undertake the patient's reentry into society.

The social worker is chiefly concerned with patients in their normal life patterns, and the nurse with patients undergoing the actual experience of sickness and healing. Consequently, these two roles are very closely connected and together constitute primary care in the strict sense of direct concern with the patient as a person. The physician's role, however, is more specialized because it is focused precisely on the diagnosis and treatment of a pathological condition or its future prevention. If this analysis is correct, the physician cannot be the sole decision maker on the health team. Rather, the patient has the ultimate decision. The patient is helped in making this decision in the first place by the nurse and social worker, who are acquainted with patients in their total personalities and life situations; in the second place by the primary care physician; and in the third place by various specialist physicians.

Recently, some hospitals have begun to recognize the need for pastoral care—not as an occasional intervention of religious ministry from outside the institution by a visiting clergyman, or only as a convenience for patients who wish religious ministration by a resident chaplain, but as a regular part of patient care—because all patients, whether religious or secular, have problems of ultimate concern that affect the success of their healing process.

Physicians will not find it easy to reconcile their proper professional autonomy with the requirements of teamwork or to relinquish the idea that they have sole decision-making power in health care while all others are merely their executive assistants. If the health team concept is to have real significance, physicians must come to acknowledge that they need the help of others not only in carrying out decisions, but also in making them—if the people entrusted to their care are to be served well.

Commonly, when continuing education programs in ethics are offered to the professional staff of a hospital, nurses participate in them, but physicians are notable by their absence. Because physicians occupy a leadership role on a health care team, they must be as well acquainted with the ethical policies of the institution as are other members of the staff; yet they often excuse themselves because of their heavy workload, as if the nurses had it easy!

It would be entirely reasonable for Catholic institutions to specify as a condition of granting hospital privileges to physicians, or for medical staff and residents, that they must take a certain number of hours of continuing education in the ethical policies of the institution. A hospital administration that puts this issue on a professional, rather than informal, level will find that physicians will accept this responsibility as they do so many others and will soon come to view it as a reasonable, necessary part of the continuing education that today is demanded of all health care professionals.

The *fourth conclusion:* To recognize the personal and professional competence of health care personnel and the ethical needs of patients, we recommend a new relationship among health team members. This new relationship would be based upon a personalized concept of health care, as is explained above.

7.5   HEALTH CARE ETHICS AND PUBLIC POLICY

The federal government has made some attempt to give ethical guidelines for public policy with regard to health care. In the late 1960s and early 1970s, Congress became uneasy—in fact, disturbed—about the impact of scientific progress upon the rights of individuals and society. Revolutionary advances in science and technology were predicted (e.g., genetic engineering and DNA splicing), and it was feared that these advances might have damaging effects. At the same time, public outrage arose over some scientific research projects that had violated the human rights of individuals. For example, a study was made public in which aborted fetuses were decapitated so that they could be used for pharmaceutical tests. Moreover, the press exposed the Tuskegee syphilis study, in which the cure for syphilis was withheld from poor African American men afflicted with the disease in order to prolong the research.

Because of general apprehension about revolutionary scientific developments and the sharp public reaction to specific abuses in the area of research, Congress established the National Commission for the Protection of Human Subjects of Biomedical and Behavioral Research (CPHS) in July 1974. As its name indicates, the mandate for this commission was to set ethical guidelines for research projects involving human beings, especially those whose rights might be violated.

When the term of this commission ended, the secretary of the then–Department of Health, Education, and Welfare appointed an Ethics Advisory Board (EAB) in the spring of 1978 to continue the study of ethical issues and public policy. This board was superseded a few months later by another group created by Congress, the President's Commission for the Study of Ethical Problems in Medicine and Biomedical and Behavioral Research (PCEMR).

The productivity of these three federal commissions was impressive. The CPHS published more than ten studies in its four-year life on subjects such as research on fetuses, children, prisoners, and the mentally infirm. It also studied psychosurgery, put forth ethical guidelines for the delivery of health care by government agencies, and set standards for institutional review boards. In the *Belmont Report* (CPHS 1978), the CPHS sought to synthesize the ethical principles pertaining to informed consent, which it had used in its studies.

The EAB, because of its short existence, studied only one ethical problem at length, that of in vitro fertilization, and prohibited the creation of fetuses for research purposes. The PCEMR was commissioned by Congress to consider many ethical issues, such as brain death, access to health services, withdrawal of life-support systems, and testing in regard to genetic disease. During its existence, the PCEMR published ten studies on these and other topics.

As 2000 approached, President Clinton appointed a Presidential Ethical Commission to consider some of the more difficult ethical issues arising in research. This commission considered such issues as stem cell research, with cells derived from abortions, and the creation of fetuses for research purposes. For the most part, the commission's findings were not greeted with satisfaction by those who maintain that life begins at conception, and thus Congress did not approve their conclusions. As even neutral observers have indicated, the commission really did not proceed in accord with any ethical theory, but only seems to have concluded in favor of more research, no matter whose rights could be violated. President George Bush has also been involved in ethical issues resulting from human research, especially insofar as the use of embryonic stem cells is concerned. We shall discuss this issue at greater length in chapter 10.

Although we shall not attempt to evaluate in detail any of the documents emanating from these federal commissions, we offer five general comments. First, it is a step forward that the president of the United States and Congress recognize that there is a need for ethical norms for research and therapy carried out with government funds. For the most part, the norms set forth by the commissions are useful and protect the rights of scientists and physicians as well as subjects and patients.

Second, the norms formulated by the commissions are designed with our pluralistic society in mind. Thus, they seek to enunciate what most scientists, politicians, and religious thinkers can all agree on. Although they do not state it explicitly, it is clear that they avoid controversy, so some of the more difficult and important ethical issues are not considered, such as the value of fetal life, the moment at which human life begins, the meaning of health, and the value of prolonging life versus the value of a good moral life.

Third, although some of the more important norms concerning physician–patient relationships are considered (e.g., informed consent and justice in selection of research subjects), there is little detailed consideration of the pressing ethical questions concerning the society–physician–patient relationship, such as: Is there a right to equal health care for all? Should all feasible care be financed publicly? What are the goals for our national health programs?

Fourth, the basis on which these ethical statements are formulated is not the nature of the human person, the covenant between physician and patient, the just society, or religious teaching. Rather, the basis is what is culturally acceptable, that is, those norms that seem acceptable to the U.S. public. Deciding ethical responsibilities in this manner is dangerous because it justifies whatever is popular. The ethicist should continually question and evaluate what is culturally acceptable, judging it on more fundamental values.

Fifth, the motivation for observing the norms of the federal commissions is mainly monetary. If a person or institution does not observe these norms, the person or institution will not receive federal funding for research or therapy and might be subject to malpractice litigation. Thus, in a certain sense, these "ethical statements" emanating from the federal commissions are legal norms insofar as the motivation to observe them is concerned. Although ethicists may differ in detail as to the proper motivation for ethical activity, avoiding legal sanctions is not considered by any ethicist to be the ultimate justification for ethical action.

In the late 1980s, Congress once again sought to establish a national ethics commission. But the country was so polarized at that time, and probably still is, that a representative commission could not be agreed upon. Various pressure groups in society insisted that members representing their interests alone had to be appointed to the commission. As a result of this pressure, although federal funds were allocated to create the commission, the effort was abandoned.

The *fifth conclusion:* The deliberations of federal commissions have been worthwhile in that they have brought to our attention the need for ethical norms in the field of research and therapy. Yet because the commissions have avoided some of the more important questions while concentrating on expressing consensus and because the norms are based on a weak foundation, more rigorous thinking must be applied to the modern ethical issues in medicine, research, and health care.

7.6 THE CATHOLIC HEALTH CARE FACILITY

Originally, Catholic health care facilities were founded principally by religious orders of sisters and brothers to give health care to the neglected and, especially in areas where Catholicism was not the chief religion, as a means of witnessing to the ethical and spiritual aspects of health care in accordance with Catholic values. Today in the United States, the dominance of secular humanism as a philosophy of life has so influenced and pressured the operation of Catholic health care facilities that many wonder whether these institutions are any longer Catholic in any significant respect.

What qualities should characterize a Catholic health care facility? In the United States, such a facility has several obvious characteristics. The Catholic Health Association recently has published some excellent studies on Catholic Identity for its member facilities. We briefly describe five of the more prominent elements outlined in these studies. First, Catholic health care facilities seek to carry on the healing ministry of Jesus Christ. This ministry receives apostolic direction from the bishop of the diocese. Under his guidance and interpretation, it follows the *Ethical and Religious Directives for Catholic Health Care Services*, promulgated by the National Conference of Catholic Bishops (2001), which outline the proper spiritual care patients should receive, the duties of the hospital as a representative of the Catholic Church, and the medical procedures prohibited in Catholic health care facilities. Many of the ethical problems presented in this book are treated in the *Directives*.

Second, a Catholic hospital is usually sponsored by a religious community of sisters or brothers who have basic financial ownership and responsibility for policy. But more and more, Catholic hospitals are sponsored or governed by members of the laity, or at least board members of these corporations are often laity. The lay form of sponsorship will probably become more prevalent in the future. It is not a revision of the concept of health care as the apostolic work of the church, but rather an expression of the laity's call to the apostolic life resulting from Baptisms and outlined in the *Decree on the Apostolate of Lay People* from the Second Vatican Council (Flannery 1975a).

Third, Catholic health care facilities are for the most part nonprofit institutions. Their principal goal is the service of the right to health of all persons, and especially the neglected. Thus, these facilities have chosen what Pope John Paul II and the U.S. bishops call "the option for the poor." Although investor-owned corporations are not evil in themselves, they are out of place in the health care setting, because their primary goal is making a profit for investors, not assuring the health of people in need.

Fourth, Catholic health care facilities offer a pastoral care program that involves sacramental as well as a counseling ministry staffed by priests, religious, and laypersons. In larger health care facilities, there may be full-time ministers representing religious communities other than the Catholic Church.

Fifth, such institutions usually are marked by various Catholic symbols, such as statues, religious pictures, and crucifixes in the rooms. Moreover, there are usually chapels in Catholic hospitals where daily Mass is often available.

All of these characteristics (even the last) are more than superficial. They express the character of the hospital as a ministry of the Catholic Church, which is based on the interrelations of the whole person in all the biological, psychological, ethical, and spiritual dimensions dealt with in this book.

At the deepest level of Catholic identity is the proclamation that the health care facility is as an extension of the ministry of Jesus Christ. In his earthly ministry, Jesus was prophet and teacher, king and shepherd, and priest and sanctifier. The Second Vatican Council has taught that his three-fold ministry should be reflected in all the works of the church and in every member. Healing is integral to the shepherding function of the Christian community, because building this community entails concern for each weak member who needs restoration to vital life and participation.

Jesus healed people radically by penetrating to the spiritual core of the human personality and liberating the person from original or social sin and also from individual, personal sin. A Christian hospital, therefore, also seeks the radical healing of those for whom it cares. The experience of sickness and healing in such a hospital should be also an experience of personal spiritual growth through suffering and redemption.

What should make a Catholic hospital a special kind of community and a model for other healing communities is that its members, both professionals and patients, are clearly aware of the presence of Christ the Healer in the midst of the community making use of his ministers—physicians, nurses, techni-cians, administrators, and patients in relation to each other—in his work of healing. This presence of Christ should also be celebrated ritually through the sacraments and proclaimed through the word of Scripture and of preaching, with Christ's promise of renewed life more powerful than death.

A significant development in Catholic health care is the recent formation of health care corporations, in which a number of hospitals under the spon-sorship of the same religious order or several religious orders are united in a single corporation. This enables the corporation to provide the individual hospitals with much needed research and education and a more effective public voice to influence public health care policy. It is essential that such large corporations give as much attention to the Christian values to which they are dedicated as to economic and administrative problems. Otherwise, they become a business and do not promote the values that should charac-terize health care.

Our *sixth conclusion:* A religious conception of a health care institution should enhance its competence in all the arts and sciences of modern medi-cine. Unless a Catholic health care facility gets its vitality from its own reli-gious faith and system of values, it will become more hurtful than healing, a scandal rather than a witness to Christ's presence in a suffering world.

SUMMARY

Perhaps the greatest ethical issue in health care in the United States is social responsibility. The U.S. health care system is advanced and sophisticated insofar as research, knowledge, and therapy are concerned, but it is poorly designed to provide care. Too many people, especially those without health care insurance or without adequate coverage, are unable to receive the care they need; the poor and frail elderly are especially deprived.

There are no easy answers to the problem of providing adequate access to health care for all. But some solution to the problem must be found in the immediate future. The federal government must cooperate with the health care community to overcome the injustices that are present in our provision of care. Neither the federal government nor health care professionals and corporations will act, however, unless private citizens express their displeasure with the shocking lack of care for many people.

As part of a national effort to provide health care, Catholic health care facilities and professionals have definite social responsibilities that may be summarized in the phrase: They are to continue the healing mission of Christ.

QUESTIONS

1. If a national or even a regional system of universal health care is developed in this country, what policies should be built into it that will maintain subsidiarity and limit the growth of a cumbersome and oppressive bureaucracy?

2. According to the concept of functionalism, health care is an autonomous sector of our national society whose concerns should have easy access to government power without resorting to covert lobbying. In what respect is this now the case in the United States, and in what respect is it not?

3. Many television dramas have hospitals as their settings and health care professionals as their characters. In what ways do they and do they not realistically portray health care facilities as human communities?

4. What changes would you make in the Catholic health care facility best known to you to make it more authentically Catholic?

CASES

1. In a city of 75,000 population, there are two nonprofit hospitals, one Catholic and one nondenomintional, which compete with each other. Neither is usually filled to capacity. A group of physicians builds a for-profit hospital in the city that competes with both nonprofit hospitals. The doctors' hospital has a financial advantage in that it refuses charity patients beyond the minimal percentage required by government regulations. The Catholic hospital has always gone beyond this minimum, and the nondenominational institution has followed the

same practice so as not to fall behind the Catholic institution in public support. The for-profit hospital intends to bring advanced equipment into the city and thus attract those able to pay. What are the legal and ethical aspects of this situation?

2. Dr. N moves from Canada to the United States because he resents the government regulation involved in Canada's national health care system. He says that, in his experience, these regulations make it more difficult for a conscientious physician to follow his own best judgment in fulfilling his obligation to his patients. In the United States, however, he finds that Medicare requires a great deal of paperwork, and so he decides to refuse Medicare patients. He then finds that his income falls. To increase it, he is tempted to recommend more surgery than he might otherwise have done. What are the ethical questions that Dr. N must ask himself?

3. In a city public hospital, tax revenues set severe budgetary limits. This hospital is the recipient of many minority patients with low incomes, who are rejected by other local hospitals because they lack insurance. It is proposed that heart transplants begin at this hospital because Dr. M of the staff, an excellent cardiac surgeon, is very interested in the procedure. Objections are raised that becoming involved in something so sophisticated and expensive in this type of hospital is a poor use of resources. Dr. M points out that charity patients have even more heart disease than the average population. Do they not have a right to full care at community expense? What would be your position?

4. Saint Ann's General Hospital is sponsored by a congregation of Catholic sisters. Because of declining vocations, they have only a few sisters on the staff, none of whom is actually engaged in nursing. The medical staff is only about 30 percent Catholic, and the nurses are of many religious affiliations or none. The sisters' congregation, however, retains ownership of the corporation and influential positions on the board. What should be their objectives in policy decisions if the hospital is to remain Catholic in more than name? What relation should the hospital have to the local Catholic bishop?

8

Human Research and the Allocation of Resources

OVERVIEW: In this and the remaining chapters, we apply the twelve principles of ethical decisions explained in chapter 2 to the chief ethical issues debated today in health care. First, we consider issues involved in medical research and in the allocation of scarce medical resources (triage) because these are general issues affecting all aspects of health care. Research is a concern of contemporary health care ethics because history indicates how easy it is for research to be utilized for goals that endanger the well-being of the persons enrolled in the research programs. Allocation of health care resources is also a continuing ethical concern. If we strive for justice in our society, a fair distribution of health care resources will be a prominent concern because health is such an important human good, and many other human goods depend on a person's health. In this chapter, we apply the principles of stewardship and creativity, totality of the person, informed consent, and double effect. When discussing the allocation of scarce resources, the principle of common good or participation in community is also applicable.

8.1 HUMAN RESEARCH

Research can be defined as a deliberate change of conditions without foreknowledge of the results but with observation of the results. Research designates an activity designed to test a hypothesis, permits conclusions to be drawn, and thereby develops or contributes to generalizable knowledge. Research is usually described in a formal protocol that sets forth an objective and a set of procedures designed to reach that objective. In human research, several categories of subjects may be involved: (1) normal healthy adults, including the investigator and elderly persons; (2) sick adults, including the acutely and terminally ill; (3) people living in highly controlled situations, such as prisoners, soldiers, and students; (4) children, both healthy and ill;

(5) mentally incompetent persons, whether adults or children; and (6) unborn fetuses or still-living aborted fetuses. Each of these categories presents special ethical problems. A comprehensive and significant study (Katz, Capron, and Swift-Glass 1972) pinpoints the source of ethical problems in research upon human subjects when it states:

> When science takes man as its subject, tensions arise between two values basic to Western society: freedom of scientific inquiry and protection of individuals inviolability. (p. 1)

It is undeniable that research on human beings is often useful and necessary for the health of society and for the good of individuals. Many beneficial vaccines and other therapies, such as open heart surgery and successful treatment of certain birth defects, have required human research. But research has often been abused. The world will never forget the horrors of the experiments carried out on innocent human beings in the name of scientific progress in the Nazi concentration camps. Other egregious violations of human rights have occurred during research projects in the United States, such as the withholding of newly discovered penicillin from patients in the Tuskegee syphilis study; the Willowbrook experiments, which used retarded children as subjects; and the injection of live cancer cells into unknowing subjects in the Chronic Disease Hospital case. Psychological research has also given rise to serious debate about behavior control. Such abuses often are not the product of demented or perverted minds but rather result from a lack of care and ethical sensitivity on the part of well-motivated researchers who overlook the rights of human beings in an effort to ensure scientific progress.

A modern form of abuse of human subjects occurs in the use of human embryos for research purposes with the loss of life for these incipient persons. Many study groups throughout the world have examined the ethical issues associated with research on embryos, usually considering embryos that are generated by means of in vitro fertilization. The Warnock Commission in the United Kingdom tried to avoid the ethical issues by coining the term *pre-embryo* and declaring that every blastocyst should be considered a pre-embryo up to fourteen days, thus, denying the newly formed entity the rights of personhood.

The reports on fetal research produced by study groups in the United States, commissioned either by the president or Congress, have used a utilitarian approach, emphasizing the valuable knowledge that would be derived from research on human embryos and being silent concerning the rights of the newly conceived. However, Congress has prohibited the use of federal funds for research that destroys fetal life. The Australian Research Committee studying the issue stated that the respect due the embryo from the process of fertilization onward requires its protection from destructive "non-therapeutic experimentation." The Australian committee reached this conclusion because it could find no marker after fertilization that would serve to separate the embryo from its identity as a human entity with rights. Pope John Paul II puts the argument against research upon human embryos in theological language when he states:

> Genetic manipulation [research] becomes arbitrary and unjust when it reduces life to an object, when it forgets that it has to do with a human subject capable of intelligence and liberty and worthy of respect. (John Paul II 1983, n. 6)

Research with fetal tissue, especially with stem cells, also causes ethical concern. In this form of research, the issue is not the use of stem cells for therapy or research, but rather the fact that many stem cells are derived from fetuses destroyed in elective abortions, or from embryos that have been frozen and later thawed to extract stem cells. But human stem cells may be obtained from adult tissue. Thus the ethical issue arises from the manner in which the stem cells are obtained. The scientists who isolate these cells from frozen or aborted fetuses maintain that they have nothing to do with abortion, and that the material is already there and will go to waste if they do not use it. The ethical evaluation then involves the principle of cooperation.

Given the fact that the research or therapy in question is a good action, is the researcher or therapist who isolates stem cells involved in the unethical act of abortion or in support of that unethical action? It would seem that the scientists harvesting the stem cells from frozen embryos or dead fetuses resulting from elective abortions do indeed agree with the destruction of the fetuses. But what about scientists who use cells lines developed or cultured from the original stem cells? In some cases, it seems this form of cooperation would not be formal, but rather mediate material cooperation. Thus, a hard and fast disapproval of research with stem cell tissue cultured from stem cells that are far removed from the original source of tissue is difficult to posit at this time.

The president of the United States has stated that no federal funds may be used to destroy fetuses in order to obtain stem cells, but he has allowed the use of federal funds for research and therapy using cell lines developed from the original stem cells. In making these announcements, he also stated that adult stem cells are a promising source for research and therapy, and that the optimistic statements about the potential therapeutic value of stem cell research should be tempered with the realization that about ten years ago scientists were optimistic about the therapeutic value of fetal tissue resulting from abortions but that the results of this form of research and therapy were negative.

Today, in an effort to obviate excesses and facilitate progress, the federal government requires that every institution that carries on research projects with public funds establish an institutional review board (IRB). An IRB monitors the research protocols mainly by analyzing the risk–benefit ratio for the patient, by evaluating the informed consent process, and by examining the procedures required by the research protocol insofar as they might affect the safety of the human subject.

Because there is risk to the human subject involved does not mean that a research protocol would be rejected by the IRB, but the IRB requires that the risk be proportionate to patient benefit, that free and informed consent on the part of the subject be assured, and that the protocol of the scientific investigation be as safe as possible. If not, the research project must be rejected by the IRB. In the United States, most research is carried on in medical schools with funds from the National Institutes of Health. However private corporations, using private or federal funds, are becoming more and more involved in research projects. Many complain that research by private corporations becomes very difficult to control.

Research on human subjects should be distinguished sharply from therapy for human subjects. The primary purpose of therapy is to heal the person receiving the therapy. Research, however, proposes to provide new knowledge that will benefit society as a whole. But because research and therapy are often combined in one protocol, it is helpful and valid to classify human research as either therapeutic or nontherapeutic. This distinction surfaces immediately when the ethics of research is discussed. Therapeutic research allows one to accept greater risk of harm than nontherapeutic research. Therapeutic research studies the effects of using diagnostic, prophylactic, or therapeutic methods that depart from standard medical practice but hold out a reasonable expectation of success for improving the condition of the subject. Nontherapeutic research, conversely, is not designed to improve the health of the research subjects; rather, it seeks to gain knowledge or develop techniques that may benefit people other than the subject. For example, when the vaccine for poliomyelitis was developed, the goal of the protocol was to obtain knowledge that would protect society now and in the future.

The *first conclusion:* Research protocols that involve human beings are necessary but must be carefully monitored by institutional review boards, whether the research is combined with therapy or is only pure research.

8.2 NORMS FOR RESEARCH ON HUMAN SUBJECTS

The proper manner of conducting research on human subjects has become one of the most discussed bioethical questions of recent years. Through seminars and studies sponsored by the federal government on the subject, several ethical principles have been developed to serve as a guide for researchers and for those who support research. As a result of studies by legal, medical, and ethical groups throughout the world, especially in the generation immediately after World War II, some principles for human research have become widely accepted, even though there may be disagreement concerning their applications in particular cases.

These norms produced by medical and legal experts, such as the Nuremberg and Geneva statements on research with human subjects (World Health Organization 1946, 1967), are largely in harmony with Christian teaching on human dignity. Here we give nine norms for ethical research that involves human subjects. Some of these norms are pertinent to psychological research; some to medical research. Some of the norms are self-evident, but some need explanation for their ethical implications to be clear.

Norm 1. The knowledge sought through research must be important and obtainable by no other means, and the research must be carried out by qualified people.

Norm 2. Appropriate experimentation on animals and cadavers must precede human experimentation.

In recent years, research upon animals has become an ethical as well as a political issue, with some people claiming that animals have rights and that all animal experimentation is unethical. As a result of protests and organized objections, research with animals has been curtailed. Given the responsibility of humans to respect animals as an important part of creation and the universe, the more cautious approach to animal experimentation is to be encouraged.

The extreme rejection of research upon animals must be resisted, however. It is a perversion of the term to maintain that animals have rights. Only beings able to choose between right and wrong actions have rights. Moreover, the effect of some pharmaceutical and surgical procedures cannot be developed without research upon animals. Computer models for research upon living tissue are simply not efficient. Finally, in any analysis of evolution or creation, animals contribute to and are significant for the well-being of humans. This relationship between humans and animals allows for and requires the prudent use of animals for research purposes.

Norm 3. The risk of suffering or injury must be proportionate to the good to be gained.

Because the principle of double effect is used to justify the possible ill effects of human experimentation, the proportion between risk and potential benefit is an essential criterion, the benefit being the good effect and the risk being the foreseen but undesired bad effect. Of course, predicting the degree of risk with certitude is seldom possible. Sometimes—as in the case of the poliomyelitis inoculation in 1954, when the use of some poorly prepared live vaccine resulted in the death of children; or in the 1980 swine flu inoculation disaster, when many elderly became very ill and some even died—the risks may be greater than predicted.

Hence, absolute certainty concerning the nature and degree of the risk cannot be required. To demand such certitude would paralyze all scientific research and would very often be detrimental to the patient. Care must be taken, however, to predict as accurately as possible the nature and magnitude of risk from any particular human experiment, and the bias of enthusiastic researchers in favor of the promise of some new procedure must be subject to review by an IRB. When discussing risk, it is important to distinguish between the frequency and the gravity of a risk. Thus a researcher may state that a risk is light if it happens in only 3 or 4 percent of cases. But if the risk in question is death or serious impairment, then it is a very grave risk for which there may be no proportionate benefit.

When determining the degree of risk that a person might undergo, one must always bear in mind this difference between therapeutic and nontherapeutic research. If the research project is therapeutic, then persons may undergo greater risk because they are seeking to avoid serious illness or death. The principle of totality is thus involved in therapeutic research. Hence, a person may endanger or even sacrifice an organ or function to avoid death.

The same principle of totality cannot be invoked in the case of nontherapeutic research, however, because one person is not related to another person or to a group of persons (the society) as part of the whole. Although a relationship of extrinsic finality exists among different people, a relationship of intrinsic finality or form does not. One person does not exist for the other, nor is one person ordered to another person as a means to an end. Each individual person is an end or being in himself or herself and cannot be sacrificed for another. This is the basic reason that the public authority has no right to sacrifice individuals for the interest of the state or for scientific progress.

Experiments carried out for the good of the state or for scientific progress may provide new knowledge or medical techniques and thus seem beneficial, but if they do so at the expense of human rights and human dignity they are immoral. In research directed to the common good and not to the individual good of the research subject, the matter of free and informed consent becomes paramount. One may risk one's life for others, but the level of risk must be assessed and the action must be freely performed for it to be ethical.

Norm 4. Subjects should be selected so that risks and benefits will not fall unequally on one group in society.

Justice demands that the burdens associated with human progress be shared equitably. In recent years the poor of the world, especially in the United States, have borne an unequal burden insofar as medical research is concerned. Although they have been involved in the experimental studies that develop the new drugs, the price of the new drugs when approved is often beyond their reach. Research protocols must be designed to offset this imbalance and to ensure that when the poor take part in an experiment their human rights are respected and they are given the freedom their human dignity demands.

Norm 5. To protect personal integrity, free and informed (voluntary) consent must be obtained.

Requiring informed consent is perhaps the most important and the most debated of the principles involved in human experimentation. All agree that the requirements for informed consent may be summed up in three words: information, understanding, and freedom (see chapters 5 and 6). Thus, the subject must not only know the process or procedure in question, but he or she also should be able to comprehend it because it is explained in understandable language. Freedom does not imply that one is free from the natural coercion of the need for therapy that might accompany an illness, but it does mean that there is no deception or external coercion involved. However, consent should be obtained, and how knowledge must be communicated to subjects should be debated extensively. Moreover, the debate must increase as impaired or imprisoned human subjects or children are considered for research protocols.

The most puzzling problems in research occur when one person gives consent for another person who is unable to consent for himself or herself. Such consent is commonly called proxy consent. As such, proxy consent simply means that one person represents the interests of another and by some legitimate title gives consent for the experiment in place of the subject because that subject is unable to do so. Decisions of proxy consent must be made in view of the good of individual person, not for society's good, a class good, or the good of another person. Otherwise, the person is being manipulated and treated as a thing. If the research is therapeutic, there is a reason for the proxy to allow risk in proportion to the good that might accrue to the incompetent individual in question, because that would be acting in the person's best interest. If nontherapeutic experimentation is involved, however, then the risk allowed to the subject is limited.

Proxy Consent for Nontherapeutic Therapy

As has been stated, nontherapeutic research results in knowledge that will be beneficial to others but does not benefit directly the subject of the research. Children, the retarded, the dying, fetuses, and newborns are considered by some to be fitting subjects for nontherapeutic research. These proponents argue that this research is ethical because it gives subjects an opportunity to contribute to the common good, something they should desire. Others maintain, however, that a guardian has no right to expose a ward to any risk. The justification for this position is that a proxy should make a decision in accord with the subject's best interests. But because it is not evident how nontherapeutic experimentation is in the subject's interests, and, because the subject does not have the capacity to make a free choice about a free matter, the proxy (guardian) has no right to presume or say anything on the ward's behalf.

Others would allow exposing children and others who cannot consent for themselves to "minimal risk." They maintain that there are some things a child as a human being should do for others, for example, take part in experiments where there is hope of general benefit and only minimal risk. The U.S. Commission for the Protection of Human Subjects, when determining the norms for fetal experimentation and for children, followed the minimal risk theory when considering nonbeneficial research. Indeed, the commission would even allow more serious risk of harm if a national committee recommended it.

We follow the more protective opinion, maintaining that proxy consent is not licit in nontherapeutic experimentation, even when the risk is minimal. Two considerations convince us of this. First, because of the principle of human dignity, guardians have responsibility for wards who cannot care for themselves. This principle affirms that no person can achieve fulfillment without sharing in the common good and contributing to it. Hence, when a guardian or proxy consents to subjecting a ward to research, the proxy has the right to do so not on the basis of the presumed consent of the ward, which is merely hypothetical, but on the basis of the ward's actual need for care. Thus theories of presumed consent based on what the ward should do if the ward could consent are weak.

Second, granting permission to expose incapacitated people to minimal risk would open the way for an extensive interpretation. Risks that are objectively serious may be called minimal if the guardian is not aware. Thus, a guardian should be an advocate, jealous of the ward's rights, not ready to yield these rights for the sake of others who cannot act for themselves or for the hypothetical rights of future generations of other children.

Double-Blind Protocols

A special ethical issue arises in double-blind research. The objectivity of scientific research depends largely on the use of controlled experimentation, in which a group of subjects is divided into two subgroups. One group receives the experimental therapy while the other group, the control group, receives the standard therapy or a placebo. Sometimes three groups are used, one group receiving the experimental therapy, one receiving a placebo, and one receiving standard therapy or no treatment at all.

This method of research sometimes is called a randomized clinical trial. To ensure even greater objectivity, a double-blind control may be used. Not only are subjects not informed as to which kind of treatment they are receiving, but even those researchers who evaluate the effects of the treatments do not know which subjects have received which therapy. Only the double-blind technique can eliminate the placebo effect, that is, the improvement frequently experienced by patients who expect it and the effect of bias on the part of scientists. This raises ethical questions, however, because it seems (1) that those patients who do not receive the new therapy are at a therapeutic disadvantage and (2) that none of the patients in the double-blind experiment could have given informed consent to a specific treatment.

This form of research has been criticized by acquired immune deficiency syndrome (AIDS) patients. They maintain that it is unfair to give a patient a placebo or ineffective therapy when some patients will receive a therapeutic agent. AIDS patients often have the substance they are receiving tested, and if the substance is not the new therapeutic agent, they will drop out of the study. Certainly, the nature of informed consent has been rightfully questioned by AIDS patients.

In double-blind experiments, therefore, the subjects should be informed that if they consent to the experiment some will receive the new treatment and others will not, but that none of the subjects will know. The potential subjects will then be free to consent to these experimental conditions or to refuse to participate. If the clinical trial involves a placebo for the control group and the project aims at finding an agent that will mitigate or cure a lethal or disabling disease, then a special ethical issue arises, because the control group may not be receiving adequate therapy for their illness or disease. This is especially true if there is some justification for thinking that the new therapy might be much more effective than older ones.

Thus the same protocol may be therapeutic for some and nontherapeutic for others. IRBs and researchers then must be doubly cautious when a double-blind placebo protocol is being designed or reviewed. If the new therapy proves to be effective, then the protocol must be interpreted and the new therapy made available to all. Of course, a rush to judgment concerning the efficacy of a new therapy must be avoided.

Norm 6. At any time during the course of research, the subject (or the guardian who has given proxy consent) must be free to terminate the subject's participation in the experiment.

The reason for this norm is that the consenting subject or proxy may not have been able to anticipate correctly the subjective factors involved—the amount of suffering, anxiety, or depression—until they begin to be actually experienced. Moreover, the subject or proxy may even discover that the information given was inadequate, deceptive, or imperfectly communicated, or the subject or proxy may have second thoughts about his or her own understanding or freedom when the consent was given.

Psychological Research

Special problems are involved in psychological experiments. To discuss these problems more fully, we defer the consideration of ethical issues in psychotherapy to chapter 11, where they are explained thoroughly. At this point, however, we consider issues that might arise in any psychological research. In such research, all the precautions necessary in medical experiments must be preserved, especially informed consent, careful calculation of risks and benefits, and precautions against the bias of researchers in favor of their own freedom. We must also add the following special rules.

Norm 7. In psychological experimentations that shade imperceptibly into social research, the researcher should work with rather than on the human subject.

That is, the researcher must gain the subject's cooperation in the experiment so that the subject will participate with the purpose of gaining greater insight into himself or herself as a person to become freer and more realistic in coping with life's problems and also with the purpose of sharing this knowledge and freedom with others.

This norm is based on the fact that psychological experiments with a human subject are also psychological experiences for the subject, which can be healthy and psychologically therapeutic or traumatizing. Only in very few cases will such experiences be neutral. Even the experience of filling out a questionnaire can be educational or terrifying. Any experience in which the patient is treated as a passive object rather than as a person cannot be beneficial.

Norm 8. The researcher must avoid breaking down human trust by lying or manipulation, although subjects can give free and informed consent to experiments in which they must learn to interpret ambiguous communications or meet puzzling situations.

In many psychological experiments, the researcher does not seem to have any qualms about lying to subjects. Not only is lying intrinsically wrong and contrary to professional ethics, it is also psychologically harmful to the subject because it breaks down the social trust on which human relations are built. Commonsense proof of this is supplied by the fact that those who have been subjected to such manipulation often react indignantly when they discover the deception and feel they have been treated unfairly. This is especially true when dealing with mentally disturbed patients, because elements of distrust, withdrawal, and paranoia present in most forms of emotional disturbance can only be reinforced by deception on the part of professionals who claim to be especially trustworthy and authoritative.

This rule against lying, however, does not prohibit experiments in which previous warning is given that the experiment may involve games in which ambiguous clues are given and embarrassment and defeat may possibly experienced. These are risks of the experiment, to which the subject must have a chance to give free and informed consent or refusal. Deception in such a case is not a lie, because traditional moral theology has always insisted that it is permissible to use ambiguous clues or language in situations where others are forewarned either explicitly or by the very nature of the situation.

Such games do not usually break down trust if the researcher sticks to the rules. Moreover, they may be highly educational for the participant, because through them the subject gains insight as to how important it is to base one's interpretation of reality on solid evidence rather than on ambiguous evidence or subjective feelings.

Norm 9. Researchers must not take serious risks of reducing the subjects' abilities to perceive reality as it is or to make free choices, except as a temporary experience through which the subjects can learn to cope with distortions of truth and attacks on their freedom.

This norm states more exactly the special risks involved in psychological experimentation. It excludes permission for any more than temporary damage to patients' ability to remain or become free in managing their own lives. Thus, an experiment would be forbidden if it might cause organic brain damage or induce drug addiction. Similarly, experiments must be avoided that might make the subject unduly liable to hypnotic control or to compulsive patterns of behavior (as might take place in some forms of behavior modification) or that create recurrent hallucinations. A special case of psychological research that may involve risks to freedom is research in dealing with human sexuality. This issue is discussed in chapter 9 in connection with therapy of inadequate or perverted sexual behavior.

The *second conclusion:* Research upon humans must be conducted in accord with the aforementioned norms, and the researcher has a personal responsibility to follow these norms.

8.3 ALLOCATING RESOURCES: MICRO AND MACRO ISSUES

Allocating resources for health care occurs at two levels: first, at the micro level, that is, at the level of individuals; second, at the macro level, that is, at the level of various groups within a national society or at the international level. In chapter 7, we discussed Christian principles for allocating health care resources within our national economy. In this section, we shall consider the principles concerned with micro allocation and with macro allocation at the international level.

Allocating resources between individuals is called allocation at the micro level or *triage,* a French word meaning to pick or sort according to quality. According to Stewart Hinds, this term came into medical usage as a result of wartime experiences and was first explained by Jean Larrey, chief surgeon of Napoleon, in his *Memoirs:*

> Those who are dangerously wounded must be tended first, entirely without regard to rank or distinction. Those less severely injured must wait until the gravely wounded have been operated upon and dressed. The slightly wounded may go to the hospital in the first or second line; especially the officers, since they have horses and therefore have transport. (Hinds 1975, 6)

Recently, however, triage has come to have a wider significance, pertaining to any situation where individuals must be selected for immediate treatment because limited resources dictate that not all can be given equal care.

Ethicists generally agree that triage does not violate justice if it respects the rights of patients as completely as possible in an emergency situation. In applying the principle of triage in emergency situations, two questions must be asked: Who is in greatest need of treatment? Who will benefit most from treatment? In the classic cases of wartime or disaster emergencies, as Larrey noted, these two questions yield a threefold division of victims: (1) the dying, whose need is great, but who will benefit least from treatment and who should be made comfortable and left to die; (2) the wounded who will survive without treatment because their need is little and who can be left to care for themselves; and (3) the wounded who will die unless treated, but who will probably survive if treated. Because these last have both the greatest need and can benefit most, they deserve most attention.

Today, triage problems arise not only in emergency situations but also in situations where no real emergency exists. For example, it may be necessary to select which patients are to be given a new vaccine or drug when a sufficient supply for all is not yet available. The recipients of scarce organs for transplantation are also subject to a form of triage. According to recent federal legislation, they are classified by need, and regional centers distribute available organs. Again, in supportive health facilities, where patients require almost unlimited attention for chronic, debilitating diseases, similar selective problems are common if the supply of life-support devices is limited.

Sometimes, to apply triage, it may also be necessary to use a random principle of selection not based on need or benefit, such as a lottery or the rule of first come, first served. Such procedures are not unfair if the need and benefit are approximately the same for all, or if there is no way of discriminating on a need and benefit basis.

The principle of subsidiarity provides that charity begins at home; that is, those closest to us and whose need is best known to us should be cared for first. Thus it is not unjust for a family to seek the best obtainable care for its members, or for physicians to give special attention to their regular patients with whom a special relationship of trust has been built, as long as no one else is treated unjustly. The same principle, however, requires that those responsible for a larger group (e.g., any health care facility open to the public, even if privately owned) should attempt to distribute resources to protect the basic rights of all but to give the greatest care to those who have most need and will benefit most.

One of the most difficult problems in applying this kind of justice arises when a choice must be made between supplying a few patients with expensive and lengthy treatment that may only keep them living for a while in very restricted activity (e.g., kidney dialysis or heart transplantation) and supplying a larger number of persons with simple treatments (e.g., a vaccine or dietary supplement) that may keep them normally active for many years. On the one hand, in the second case the benefit for the many is great, whereas in the first case the benefit for the few is small. On the other hand, for each of the few the need is very great indeed, and the benefit (from their point of view) is very real.

Nevertheless, it seems that in the social distribution of health care, priority should be given to that kind of preventive medicine or treatment of acute disease that will raise the general standards of health, especially for the young, over elaborate modes of treatment for the aged or seriously handicapped, because the first kind of care will help more people and enable them to lead a more beneficial life. The problem with our national health care program today is that there are no priorities for the expenditure of funds. Thus the more dramatic and colorful programs, such as transplant and dialysis, receive ample funds, while the more basic preventive programs, such as prenatal care and vaccinations, receive insufficient support. Although public health departments offer free vaccinations, because of restricted funds they are often unable to implement programs that would effectively contact poor children, who consequently go unprotected.

Even more difficult questions arise when the triage principle is extended to problems of health care distribution on the international level. An adequate discussion of this topic exceeds the scope of this book, but we believe that U.S. health care professionals must think about health in global terms. This problem of social triage was dramatized by Garrett Hardin (1974) in his proposal for a "lifeboat ethics." He argued that because of the crisis of the population explosion and world hunger, industrial countries are faced with a hard choice. To continue to send medical aid and food to developing countries will only increase their overpopulation, with the result that even more people will starve than are starving now. Consequently, Hardin advocates that food be given only with the condition that these countries institute very stringent (even compulsory) population controls, or all foreign aid be terminated.

Hardin further argues that industrial countries would be foolish to lower their own standards of living and health for the sake of poor countries, because they need all they have to raise healthy, well-educated children, who are the only hope of the human race for the future. No matter how much is given to poor countries, they can never produce such children.

If Hardin is right in believing that the crisis is so close that only short-run solutions are possible, then it is doubtful that anything at all can be done about the situation, because social policy seldom can move so rapidly. However, most experts believe that, in the long run, various possibilities still exist to bring world population and food resources into balance. The present situation has come about because industrial countries have introduced modern medical technology into developing countries, not merely for humanitarian reasons, but to further their policies of political and economic colonialism. Unwittingly, industrial countries, by introducing modern medicine, also upset the ecological balance and produced rapid population growth, without producing the standard of living that in industrial countries motivates and facilitates responsible parenthood. Thus, justice demands that industrial countries help restore the balance that they themselves destroyed.

The United States and other wealthy industrial countries need to undertake such a restoration of justice—not only for their own sake, but also for the sake of self-preservation. It is quite unrealistic for wealthy nations to suppose, as Hardin does, that they can sail away in their lifeboat and leave the rest of the world to sink. There is no place to sail to and no ocean to absorb the millions who look enviously at the wealth we hoard. Nor is it true that poor countries are without power, because the ultimate weapon may turn out to be not the atom bomb, but sheer numbers.

Thus, in the social triage situation, the fundamental principle must be equal justice for all members of the world community, even the least privileged. If resources are scarce, then these resources must be assigned first to those members of the community who can use them best and most justly for the good of all. But whoever makes this selection must avoid the danger of being judges in their own case. Even according to Hardin's argument, would it not be wiser to attempt to select from *all* countries those citizens on whom the future of the race can most securely depend, rather than waste resources on so many in the United States who consume much and contribute little?

The *third conclusion:* Allocation of scarce resources, or triage, must be done in an ethical manner. The criteria for allocation must be made known to all, and the needs of the poor and powerless must be respected.

SUMMARY

Research and the allocation of scarce medical resources are prominent ethical issues in health care because they affect or influence all aspects of care. The ethical difficulties concerned with research usually result from neglecting subjects' rights to informed consent. For this reason, people who are more easily manipulated, such as children, prisoners, and the elderly, require special protection under the law and in the ethical norms recognized by legitimate researchers.

The United States has been ambivalent with regard to the allocation of scarce resources, seeking whenever possible to avoid the ethical challenge of making difficult choices. Thus, for example, when it became obvious that some people might not receive treatment for end-stage renal disease, the federal government decided to fund a transplant and dialysis program for anyone needing treatment. No norms to evaluate the program were ever offered. The same situation seems to be developing with regard to organ transplants; who has a right to receive the scarce organs? There is public pressure to try to supply organs for all, even when the chances of success are slim and the costs are exorbitant. Is it time to set some ethical standards for allocating scarce resources?

QUESTIONS

1. What practical difficulties might arise when researchers seek informed consent or proxy consent for therapeutic or nontherapeutic research?

2. What are placebos? Under what conditions may they be used in experimentation with human subjects? When should researchers interrupt the protocol to discontinue the use of placebos?

3. If each human being has an equal right to health care, when a disaster occurs (e.g., a plane crash or train wreck), why may greater medical attention be given to some less seriously injured victims than to others who are more seriously injured? Could triage be applied to individual nations with regard to the world food supply?

4. What responsibilities does the U.S. government have with regard to helping developing countries improve their health care systems?

CASES

1. In June 1992, a thirty-five-year-old man with endstage renal disease due to hepatitis B infection received a transplanted baboon liver in an experimental procedure. In addition, the transplant physicians employed experimental antirejection drugs to try to prevent xenograft rejection. Patients with hepatitis B infection do not do well with human liver transplants, because the virus tends to destroy the new organ in the same way it did the original organ. "The baboon liver," stated the transplant physicians, "is less susceptible to the hepatitis." The patient encountered many complications after the transplant surgery. He never left the hospital, dying a few weeks after the transplant surgery. Comment on this surgery, using the principles of ethical research and the principles for the ethical use of scarce resources.

2. You are a researcher seeking a cure for acquired immune deficiency syndrome (AIDS). Desiring to test a vaccine that you and your colleagues have developed, you seek to infect yourself with the AIDS virus. Discuss this action from an ethical perspective.

3. The neonatal care unit at Children's Memorial Hospital has six respirators available and eight newborn infants in need of pulmonary assistance. What ethical norms would you use to determine which infants will be able to utilize the respirator?

9

Sexuality and Reproduction

OVERVIEW: The topics of sexuality and reproduction give rise to several different ethical issues. Before seeking to solve the many issues that are associated with these topics, we begin this chapter by considering the meaning of human sexuality, and how it influences our personal and social lives. Then we consider a question: When does human life begin? The answer to this question will control how many of the other questions that arise in the study of human conception and development will be answered. After considering this pivotal question, we consider the questions of artificial reproduction, abortion, ectopic pregnancy, contraception, sterilization, and treatment for rape. The many principles used in this section are a well-formed conscience, human dignity, totality and integrity, stewardship and creativity, inner freedom, and personalized sexuality.

9.1 THE MEANING OF SEXUALITY

When discussing human sexuality, it is important to realize that *sexuality* is an ambiguous term. First of all, it is used to denote the capacity of persons to love other persons and be united with them in friendship and community. In this sense of the term, every human being is a sexual person. In his "Instruction on the Human Family," Pope John Paul II (1981) emphasizes that in our totality as persons that we are male or female, and thus sexuality is the source of our relationship as human persons. Personhood transcends sexuality, so that purely spiritual beings such as the angels can love and communicate without being sexual; but human persons are embodied spirits. Hence "sexuality" in this broad sense grounds human "relationality." Persons are born from the sexual relations of their parents and achieve their fulfillment through relations with other sexual persons, even if they remain celibate. Our capacity for affection, communication, and sympathy in all relationships is rooted in our physical and psychic sexuality. Through sexuality, men and women are called by God to either marriage or the single state.

When discussing the human family, Pope John Paul II writes (in "Instruction on the Human Family"):

> God inscribed in the humanity of man and woman the vocation and thus the capacity and responsibility of love and human union. Love is therefore the fundamental and innate vocation of every human being. Christian revelation recognizes two specific ways of realizing the vocation to love, marriage and virginity (the single state). (John Paul II 1981, n. 2)

The second way the term sexuality is used refers to actions that are *genital* and seek orgasmic satisfaction. Here and in subsequent sections, we are principally concerned with ethical questions about genital activity within marriage. Therefore, we consider autoerotic or extramarital sexual activities only as they help us understand the relations of married couples. Human sexuality, in this second sense of the word, is a complex of many values that are generally recognized in every culture and ethical theory. However, their interrelationship is a subject of disagreement. These generally recognized values of marital sexual activity can be reduced to five major categories. As we discuss these five major values, it will become clear that some of them are acquired, at least particularly, through sexual activity in the first sense of the term:

1. Sexual activity is a search for sensual pleasure and satisfaction, releasing physical and psychic tensions.
2. More profoundly and personally, sexual activity is a search for the completion of the human person through an intimate and personal union of love, expressed in and through the mutual gift of the lovers' bodies. It is also the mutual complementing of the male and female so that each achieves a more integral humanity.
3. More broadly, sexual activity is a social necessity for the procreation of children and their education in a stable family so as to expand the human community and guarantee its future beyond the death of individual members.
4. Still more broadly, our sexuality opens us up, married or single, to all the human relationships of friendship, sympathy, cooperation, compassion, and reconciliation that constitute the network of human society.
5. Symbolically, sexual activity is a sacramental mystery, somehow revealing the cosmic order and our human destiny, because it stands for the creative love of God for his creatures and their loving response to him.

Because of this cosmic symbolism, these values are celebrated as sacred gifts in all the great religions and philosophies of life and are protected and developed in every viable human culture. The five values of human sexuality that we have identified, all of them not limited to genital activity, are affirmed in natural law and Christian ethics. The Catholic Church, often influenced by the culture or philosophy of the times, has emphasized various aspects of these five values at different times. When agricultural production required more human labor than it does today, the church emphasized the need for large families.

In contemporary times, to respond to our culture's great concern for the subjective factors in human development, the church looks to human sexuality from a new perspective. Through the thought of the Second Vatican Council and the writings of Pope Paul VI and Pope John Paul II, the church has proposed a new formulation of the values of marriage that better balances its social and personal meanings. The earlier language that spoke of the value of procreation as the "primary end of marriage" has been clarified by stating as the basic principle of the theology of sexuality "the inseparability of the unitive and procreative meaning of marriage." Marriage is also no longer called a "contract" but more specifically a "covenant of love."

This new formulation has caused confusion in the minds of some theologians, who seem to think that the church makes love between the spouses as the primary end of marriage and procreation merely an optional consequence. However, the real aim of the new formula is not to rank the unitive and procreative values of marriage or to subordinate one to the other, but to make clear that they are inseparably connected so that one value cannot define the marital relationship in isolation from the other. Taking into account the church's reformulation of its teaching on marriage, how are the facts of biology, psychology, anthropology, and sociology to be interpreted? Genesis 1:27 teaches that God created human beings as male and female and blessed our sexuality as his great and good gift. Jesus confirmed this teaching and perfected it by demanding men to be as faithful in marriage as the Scriptures required women to be faithful (Mt 19:3–12). He also emphasized the dignity and worth of the child as a fully human person (Mt 19:13–15).

What, then, is the meaning of sexuality for married people who have no children because they are infertile? Childless couples may love each other no less, but through no fault of their own cannot enjoy the full generative expression of their love in a family. Yet they can still exercise this generatively by extending their love to the service of others in need. Adopting children, for example, is one way for infertile couples to fulfill their generativity. Hence, the bond that holds man and woman together is not just a bond of self-interest and need, but above all, a bond of self-giving love. This is a special kind of love, specified by human sexuality. Single persons also can express their generativity by concern for child welfare or for general social justice, and they often do so even more effectively than some parents.

Jesus also taught that although married sexuality is a great gift, its use is only a relative value and can be freely surrendered for the "sake of the Kingdom" (Mt 19–12). Thus, for the Christian, the celibate or single life, with its freedom from domestic cares, can be of service to others and can be personally maturing and fulfilling. Saint Paul praised the holiness of married love as symbolic of Christ's love for the church, yet gave preference to the freedom enjoyed by celibates who devote all their energies to the service of God and human community (1 Cor 7:25; Eph 5:22). Like Jesus, Saint Paul and countless other Christians have chosen the single life to devote themselves in the name of God to the service of others.

Hence, the Catholic Church has maintained the institutions of sacramental marriage and consecrated virginity or celibacy as complimentary to one another. Jesus said: "At the resurrection they neither marry nor are given in marriage" (Mt 22:30), indicating that the married state will be transcended, although the bond of love that marriage fostered will endure forever. Hence, the *first conclusion*: Sexuality, a term used in two different ways, is the function of the human person by which we form friendships, create community, and ensure through the marital act the continuation of human race and the bond of unity between husband and wife.

9.2 HUMAN SEXUALITY

When Does Human Life Begin?

Because many of the medical problems associated with sexuality are connected with its reproductive aspect and depend upon answering the question of when human life begins, we will deal with this question before considering the ethical aspects of this human function. Embryologists who are asked this question in a purely scientific context usually answer without hesitation: "A human organism, a member of the human species, comes into existence when a human ovum is fertilized by a human spermatozoa and a one-celled zygote is produced."

Nevertheless, the abortion controversy has led many people, even embryologists, to question the acceptability of this answer or at least its ethical significance, especially when the term concept that "a human person is the subject of human rights" is introduced into the discussion. When the ethical implications of these words become evident, many people opt for a theory of "delayed hominization," thus maintaining that human personhood, if not human life, does not begin until sometime after conception. Some people even wish to redefine conception, maintaining that it occurs only after implantation of a fertilized ovum in the wall of the uterus. This is contrary to biological fact, because the embryo actively implants itself, which it could not do unless it was already an integrated organism.

Our definition of a person relies upon structure and function; a person is a living animal with the radical capacity to think intelligently and to make free decisions. Thus, a definition of human personhood begins with the notion of the person as conscious, intelligent, free adult, but it must include the entire life story of the unique organism whose personhood is fully self-conscious and fully evident in structure and function only at certain periods of the story. Thus, not only the actual here and now performance must be considered but also the potential capacity for other activities. The life cycle of any human person includes remarkable morphological and functional changes. At any stage in the cycle, a person has the active potential to develop different structures and thus different functions; this is especially true of a young person.

The term *potentiality* has many meanings in current usage. Some confused uses of the term are very evident in current arguments about the origin of the human person. First, any kind of stuff or material has the potentiality to be made or formed into an unlimited number of very different kinds of things. In this sense, the subatomic particles that formed from the Big Bang were potentially the human race. Potentiality in this sense of mere stuff is something passive, like clay in the hands of a potter. But there are other senses in which potentiality is conceived actively as the power to modify and develop passively potential material. Thus the potter has the active potentiality (capability) to form clay into a variety of vessels.

This active sense of potentiality is especially useful in understanding living organisms. At any given moment of its life, an organism has both a structure and a variety of functions. These functions are active potentialities that depend upon the existence of a structure as an actuality; for example, a bird has the power to fly only when its wing structure has been actively developed. But what is more important is its potentiality for self-development, that is, to elaborate its own structures and thus to acquire more diversified function. This capacity for self-development is the function that gives unity to all the others and guarantees the particular identity of each organism.

Delayed Humanization

An argument that some offer for delayed humanization stems from Aristotle's obsolete biological theory, which influenced Catholic thought because of it acceptance by Albert the Great and Thomas Aquinas. Aristotle argued that until an organism has developed to the point that it has a central organ with the minimal structure required for psychological function it should be considered a vegetative rather than an animal organism. For Aristotle, this primary organ was the heart. According to modern biology, the primary organ is the central nervous system and the cerebrum. Because the cerebrum is observable only toward the end of the third month of gestation, this would mean that before this stage the embryo or fetus is not even an animal organism and therefore not human.

The weakness of this argument is that it defines incorrectly the minimal structure necessary for the organism to be a human person in the sense it has the active potentiality to develop into a human adult, capable of intelligent and free activity. We now know, as Aristotle and Thomas Aquinas did not know, that before the appearance of the brain as the primary organ of the fetus a sequence of primordial centers of development goes back to the nucleus of the zygote. This nucleus has contained, from the beginning, all the information and active potentiality necessary to eventually develop the brain and bring it to the stage of adult functioning. Thus, although it is true that the developing fetus at first exhibits only vegetative and animal functions and only later and long after birth specifically human functions, it possesses, from conception, the active potentiality to develop all these functional abilities. The minimal structure necessary for this active potentiality of self-development and necessary or adult psychological activities is present in the one-celled zygote.

Officially, the Catholic Church has never based its position against direct abortion on the claim that the human soul is created at conception. The "Declaration on Procured Abortion" (Congregation for the Doctrine of the Faith 1974), while affirming that from the time of conception direct abortion is always a grave sin, appended a note saying: "This declaration leaves aside the question of the moment when the spiritual soul is infused" (n. 11). The advances in embryology however, have made the church more confident that the theories of delayed humanization are scientifically obsolete, so that a more recent instruction, *On Respect for Human Life* (Congregation for the Doctrine of the Faith 1987) states:

> Certainly, no experimental datum can be in itself sufficient to bring us to the recognition of a spiritual soul. Nevertheless, the conclusions of science regarding the human embryo provide a valuable indication for discerning by the use of reason a personal presence at the moment of first appearance of human life . . . Thus the fruit of human generation from the first moment of its existence, that is, from the first moment the zygote has formed, demands unconditional respect, that is morally due to the human being in his bodily and spiritual totality. (I, 1)

Some question about exactly how to pinpoint the time of conception remains because the fertilization process from the penetration of the sperm to syngamy (i.e., the fusion of the ovum and sperm into the single nucleus of the zygote) is not instantaneous, and the chromosomes and their maternal or paternal origins remain identifiable. More probably, the new organism comes into existence at syngamy rather than at penetration by the sperm, because only then does a new, single nucleus with its complete set of chromosomes exist to unify the new organism and direct its orderly development. However, the time between penetration and syngamy is much too brief to be a practical significance from an ethical perspective.

Another common argument for delayed humanization is based upon the fact that identical twins originate from the division of a single embryo in the period (not more than two weeks) before implantation. This has led some embryologists to speak of the *conceptus* at the pre-implantation phase as the *pre-embryo*. The potential for identical twinning is interpreted by some to mean that the pre-embryo is not a single individuated organism but simply a collection of cells. But given the self-actuated activity of the embryo even at this stage of its existence, the term pre-embryo is simply meaningless.

The exact cause or causes of identical twinning are still not certain, but there are two possibilities: (1) Due to an anomaly in the process of fertilization, not one but two zygotes may have been produced from the beginning, in which case the argument against each zygote being a person has no validity, especially when each twin has its own amniotic sac. (2) Due to a developmental accident during the incipient state of development, a cell or group of cells becomes detached from the original organism, and because those cells are still totipotential, they are able to develop into a second individual (for a discussion of the concept of totipotentiality, see chapter 10). The fact that one person is produced from the other is no proof that the first person was not an individual organism, any more than the possibility of cloning human persons denies the existence of the original organism from which the clone was derived. This second explanation is favored when the twins have a single amniotic sac. Moreover, it is simply not true that the pre-embryo is every simply a loose collection of cells. From the first cell division, cytology shows that a very definite pattern of development and differentiation is taking place in a carefully synchronized sequence determined by the genetic code. This would be impossible if the cells were not in constant communication.

A final argument for delayed humanization is based on distinguishing between genetic and developmental individuation. It is asserted that although the zygote is genetically individuated, its developmental individuation takes place only gradually. Furthermore, even its genetic individuation is questioned on the grounds that the development of the embryo is determined not only by the nuclear genes, but also by cytoplasm factors contributed by the mother after implantation, and perhaps by other maternal influences.

This argument rejects the fact that the normal development of the human organism is a unified process of self-development, and thus from the very beginning that process must be guided principally by the genetic information present in the zygote. The development also requires the appropriate environment provided by the mother. Yet all that is known of embryology shows that the organism is not formed by its maternal host, but develops from within itself, implants itself in her womb, and triggers her body to expel it at the proper time. An ethically adequate definition of human personhood must consider not only the person as a conscious, intelligent, free adult; it must also consider the entire life cycle of the unique organism, whose personhood is fully self-conscious and full evident in morphology and behavior only at certain points during that life.

As embryological research advances, the evidence that life begins at fertilization becomes overwhelming. The medical profession therefore, needs to work toward a consensus on this issue of who is a person with human rights on the basis of what is best known, namely biology and psychology. The definition of what it is to be a human person with human rights must not contradict biological facts or depend simply upon pragmatic consideration. To do so is to become open to racism and all kinds of discrimination. Thus, our *second conclusion:* From biological evidence, it is clear that human life begins at conception and the various arguments for delayed hominization lack credibility.

Artificial Reproduction

Artificial reproduction is any process by which a human sperm fertilizes a human ovum in a manner that takes place not as the result of sexual intercourse. Although there are many different methods of bringing about conception outside of human intercourse, the current more common methods are in vitro fertilization (IVF) and artificial insemination by a husband or donor (AIH or AID).

IVF involves collecting sperm and ova from the couple who will generate the child and starting the process of human generation in a petri dish and then transferring two or three (or more) fertilized ova to the womb of the prospective mother. This process is performed in private clinics and is very expensive, especially if success is not obtained in the first attempt. Live births resulting this form of artificial generation occur about 20 percent of the time. Excess embryos resulting from this process are often destroyed or frozen with the possibility of revivifying them should the initial process fail. In artificial insemination, whether AIH or AID, sperm is introduced into the woman's vagina artificially. Judging from the number of scientific and popular articles written about these two forms of artificial reproduction during the past twenty-five years, many thousands of children have been conceived in this manner, but it is difficult to obtain accurate statistics.

Although the church has spoken often against the generation of children outside of the marital act, the most complete explanation of church teaching is contained in the instruction *On Respect for Human Life* (Congregation for the Doctrine of the Faith 1987). The teaching of the church in this document can be summarized as follows:

1. Human procreation must take place in marriage. The procreation of a new person, whereby the man and the woman collaborate with the

power of the Creator, must be the fruit and the sign of the mutual self-giving, love, and fidelity of the spouses.

2. Using the sperm or ovum of a third party is not acceptable, because it constitutes a violation of the reciprocal commitment of the spouses. Moreover, this form of generation violates the rights of the child to a filial relationship to its parents.

3. The generation of the new person should occur only through an act of intercourse performed between the husband and wife, in an act that is per se suitable for the generation of children, to which marriage is ordered by its very nature.

4. The fertilization of the new human person must not occur as the result of a technical process that substitutes for the marital act because it separates the proceative and unitive aspects of marriage.

Unfortunately, in our opinion, the directive pertaining to this topic in the *Ethical and Religious Directives for the Catholic Faith* (hereafter, the *Directives*; see appendix 1) is not precisely stated:

> Those techniques of assisted conception that respect the unitive and procreative meanings of sexual intercourse and do not involve the destruction of human embryos or their deliberate generation in such numbers that it is clearly envisaged that all cannot implant and some of them are simply being used to maximize the chances of others implanting, may be used as therapies for infertility. (directive 39)

This directive seems to imply that there are such methods of fertilization. In reality, none have been developed. Some Catholic physicians and theologians have advocated the gamete interfallopian transfer (GIFT) method of reproduction as ethical if masturbation is not employed to obtain semen. But it seems, in the GIFT process, that even if fertilization is not extracorporeal, it is not the result of the marital act but rather of a technician's manipulation. Hence the *third conclusion:* Methods of human generation that occur outside the marital act are unethical because they result in the destruction of fertilized ova, and because they bring about the generation outside the method in accord with the natural law and the design of the Creator.

9.3 ABORTION

Technically, the term *abortion* includes spontaneous (miscarriage) and deliberately procured (or induced) termination of pregnancy with the resulting death of the human being at any stage of its development. Usually the term abortion is used in regard to the latter. A direct abortion is one that is induced with the immediate purpose of destroying the human fetus at any stage after conception. An indirect abortion is one in which the direct, moral object of the action (immediate intrinsic purpose of the procedure) is therapy for the mother, but in which the death of the fetus is a side effect that cannot be avoided; for example, the removal of a pathological tube containing a fertilized ovum in an ectopic pregnancy or the removal of a cancerous gravid uterus. Such indirect abortions are justified by the principle of double effect since (1) the act itself is directly aimed at treating a pathology in the mother and hence ethical; (2) the mother and physician would save the child if that were possible; (3) the death of the child is not a means to treat the mother, but only a side effect of the procedure; and (4) the proportionate reason for the procedure is to save the mother's life.

The prohibition of direct abortion has always been consistent with church teaching. Jesus preached the good news of God's love for the "little ones," the outcasts rejected by secular and religious authorities, including powerless little children, whom he declared should be given special respect in the Kingdom of God (Mk 9:33). The sacredness of human life is so fundamental to the teaching of Jesus and to the New Testament's moral exhortation that it does not even mention abortion.

The *Didache*, however, a catechetical instruction for baptism contemporary with the later books of the New Testament, shows that early Christians were forbidden to have abortions. In the times following the early church, abortion and infanticide were widespread in Greek and Roman culture, but the church continued to condemn the practices. The church continued its condemnations until modern times. The Second Vatican Council, for example, condemned abortion and infanticide as "unspeakable crimes." In 1995, John Paul II in the encyclical *The Gospel of Life* declared unequivocally that abortion and euthanasia cannot be reconciled with the church's constant teaching:

> Therefore by the authority which Christ conferred upon Peter and his successors, in communion with the bishops who have condemned abortion and who in the aforementioned consultation albeit dispersed through the world, have shown unanimous agreement concerning this doctrine. I declare that direct abortion, that is abortion willed an end or a means, always constitutes a grave moral disorder since it is the deliberate killing of an innocent human being. (John Paul II 1995, n. 62)

Hence, acceptance of this teaching is required of all Catholics. If they are true to their beliefs in the advocacy of the helpless, Catholics need to work for practical legislation defining the subject of human rights, but at least for positive efforts to reduce the number of abortions. Undoubtedly, the task for Catholics as a community should first and last be educational rather than merely political. Jesus taught us to trust in the power of truth, love, and forgiveness rather than in the power of law or law enforcement. Political action cannot be neglected, but it must be supported by a transformative educational effort. The Catholic health care professional and Catholic health care institutions have crucial roles to play in this educational effort regarding all medical-ethical issues and their social impact. The *fourth conclusion:* Direct abortion is intrinsically evil, and the church—following the teaching of Jesus—has affirmed this truth from its beginning.

9.4 DISPUTED CASES: ECTOPIC PREGNANCY AND ANENCEPHALIC INFANTS

Over the years, the ethical treatment of ectopic pregnancies and anencephalic infants have been controverted. An ectopic pregnancy occurs when a fertilized ovum attaches itself to the wall of the fallopian tube instead of passing through the tube to the uterus and attaching itself to the wall of the uterus, as normally happens. This results in a pathological condition, which may lead to death or serious morbidity for the woman if the fallopian tube should rupture. The *Directives* state that in treating a woman with this condition, "no intervention is morally licit which constitutes a direct abortion" (directive 48).

But physicians and moral theologians do not agree upon which procedures to remove the fertilized ovum would be direct abortions and which would be indirect abortions. All agree that it would be licit to remove the portion of the fallopian tube that is pathological (salpingectomy), even though the fertilized ovum would also be removed, by reason of the principle of double effect. But there is dispute in regard to performing a linear salpingostomy (merely splitting the tube and removing the fertilized ovum), which allows the tube to heal and perhaps be useful for future pregnancies. In contemporary medicine, methotrexate is often used to cause the separation of a fertilized ovum from the wall of the uterus.

Although it would be wrong to detach a child from its normal site of implantation, to detach it from an abnormal site that constitutes a pathology in the woman's body would seem to be licit. In this case, removing the fertilized ovum from the fallopian tube by means of salpingostomy or methotrexate does not have as its direct intrinsic intention (moral object) the death of the fetus; rather, its intention is to treat the pathological condition. For this reason, it is our opinion that salpingostomy and the use of methotrexate do not result in direct abortion.

The proper therapy for an anencephalic infant and other infants with severe genetic defects is also disputed. Anencephaly and some severe genetic defects can be diagnosed well before the normal time of birth. Would it constitute an abortion to deliver infants before viability if they will be allowed to die shortly after birth, knowing they will die when they are removed from the womb? Some moralists have maintained that early delivery before viability, or even after the time of viability, would be licit because it may help the mother avoid psychological suffering. Furthermore, some have maintained that anencephalic infants would be considered as organ donors even though they would die shortly after an early delivery.

However, these opinions seem to use the term viability in an equivocal manner. Viability is not a general characteristic that all infants acquire at the same time. Moreover, no aggressive care will be given to an anencephalic infant delivered early, whereas it will be given to a normal infant who is delivered early. Speaking about the viability of a fetus when the intrinsic intention of the procedure is to bring about the death of the fetus is at best a misnomer.

Hence, it seems that the proximate purpose of early delivery for an anencephalic or a genetically deprived infant is to hasten or cause the death of the infant. Thus it is our opinion that anencephalic and genetically deprived infants should be allowed to go to term, be baptized, and be allowed to die in their parents' arms. This opinion is in accord with norms published by the National Conference of Catholic Bishops (1996) in "Moral Principles Concerning Infants with Anencephaly." The *fifth conclusion:* The ethical issues concerning treatment for ectopic pregnancies and anencephalic infants depend upon the proper medical treatment of the pathologies involved. The implantation of the fetus in the fallopian tube is a medical pathology, which can be treated by surgery or pharmaceuticals, but the impaired physiological condition of an anencephalic infant is not a true pathological condition.

9.5 THE MORALITY OF CONTRACEPTION

Contraception is the performance of sexual intercourse with the deliberate intention of rendering infertile an act that could be fertile. The most common form of contraception practiced today is the hormonal pill (the pill), which is taken orally to prevent ovulation and thus separate by human endeavor the unitive and procreative effects of intercourse. Several other forms of contraception, such as an intrauterine device (IUD), condoms, and contraceptive jellies, are also used to prevent conception. These latter mentioned devices are questionable methods, because they are often ineffective. Moreover, IUDs have been found to make women permanently sterile or to cause other bodily harm.

The practice of contraception has become so common today that many Catholics practice it and do not understand why the church considers it to be sinful. They think it is an arbitrary rule made up by conservative clergy. In fact, however, this question, like that of abortion, has been present since the very beginning of Christianity and was opposed by Christians as a feature of a decadent paganism that had no regard for human dignity. Although its practice was less effective than modern methods, it was very common and often led, as it still does today, to abortion.

Throughout history, contraception has been condemned not only by the Catholic Church, but by all the other Christian churches, because they understand that it is contrary to the Creator's design for human sexuality and that it would be harmful to the human family and social welfare. Its acceptance by some Protestant churches in the last century has proved to be disastrous, because it is a principal factor in the so-called sexual revolution that, in the name of freedom, has in fact enslaved persons to depersonalized sex. In our culture—where sexual abuse, rape, the treatment of women and children as sex objects, teenage sexual activism, divorce and its harmful effects on children, and injustice to women have become common—the church's wisdom in preserving the true meaning of human sexuality as existing for the sake of human happiness has become very clear.

Contraception is intrinsically wrong, not because of any arbitrary rule of the church, but because it destroys the true meaning of sexual love and in the long run leads to serious personal and social evils. Although married couples who practice it may deny its harmfulness to their relationship, what has happened in our society to marriage proves the contrary. For a fuller discussion of how this tragic state of affairs has come about and why we need a deep cultural change in attitudes toward sex, see the fourth edition of our *Health Care Ethics*.

For our purposes in this volume, we will simply quote the teaching of recent popes, to indicate the reasons underlying the teaching and the fact that the teaching has not changed. Pope Paul VI, in the encyclical *On Human Life* stated:

> The Church's teaching on contraception, often set forth by the Magisterium, is founded upon the inseparable connection, willed by god and unable to be broken by human beings on their own initiative, between the two meanings of the conjugal act; the unitive meaning and the procreative meaning. (Paul VI 1968, n. 12)

Pope John Paul II added in *Reflections on the Encyclical "On Human Life" of Pope Paul VI*:

> The pertinent principle of conjugal morality is therefore, fidelity to the divine plan manifested in the "intimate structure" of the conjugal act. . . . and the inseparable connection of the two significances of the conjugal act . . . love and potential fecundity, which two aspects cannot be deprived of their full and adequate significance by artificial means. When couples, by means of contraception, separate these two meanings that God the Creator inscribed in beings of man and woman in the dynamism of the sexual communion, they act as arbiters of the divine plan and they manipulate and degrade sexuality

and themselves by manipulating the value of total self-giving. (John Paul II 1984, 23)

Various Conferences of Catholic bishops throughout the world have attested to the truth of this teaching, while recognizing the difficulties that married couples may have in following this teaching of the church. We shall have more to say about these difficulties when we consider the pastoral aspects of this teaching. The *sixth conclusion:* Contraception—the separation of the unitive and procreative aspects of the marital act by human means—is intrinsically evil.

9.6 NATURAL FAMILY PLANNING

In recent years, the church has emphasized that to be truly human, married couples must consider the intelligent planning of parenthood so as to provide for the proper care and education of their children. Catholics therefore cannot be indifferent to the growth of population and the ethical problems that it causes. In general, the church proposes natural family planning (NFP) as a means of limiting the number of children when there are reasonable and serious reasons for such limitation.

Some critics of church teaching have maintained that approving of family limitation is not consistent with the teaching on the natural inseparability of the unitive and procreative aspects of the conjugal act. But in the method of family limitation recommended by the church, the couple does not practice contraception (artificial interference with the two aspects of intercourse) but "uses an opportunity given them by nature." That is, infertile periods are recognized, and the couple has intercourse only during these periods. In "Instruction on the Human Family," Pope John Paul II observed: "It is a difference which is much wider and deeper than is usually thought, one which involves in final analysis two irreconcilable concepts of the human person and human sexuality. The choice of accepting the cycle of natural fertility-infertility of the woman thereby involves accepting dialogue, reciprocal respect, shared responsibility and self control" (John Paul II 1981, 38).

NFP is not based on calendar computations but rather upon a scientific study of human physiology. Two modern, well-tested methods of determining the time of ovulation and the periods of fertility and infertility are the sympto-thermal method and the ovulation method, often called the Billings Method after the physicians who developed it. Scientific studies conducted under the auspices of the World Health Organization show that the method effectiveness of NFP is as good as or better than any other method of family limitation, save surgical sterilization. The use effectiveness, however, is not as high, because of the failure of couples to abstain at a time when they knew they might be fertile. The proponents of NFP also point out that:

1. Such methods place responsibility on both partners, not merely on the woman, as do most methods of family limitation.

2. Many women who use NFP report an enhanced sense of personal dignity resulting from an awareness of their own body and its natural rhythms.

3. Abstinence from intercourse can help a couple to have confidence in the strength of their love and express it in other ways besides orgasm.

4. Periodic abstinence removes something of the sexual routine and enhances the experience when it is actually decided upon. The degree of abstinence it requires is not significantly greater than couples often accept today as a matter of course for reasons of occupations, travel, and health. Moreover, couples who practice NFP report that, overall, they engage in marital intercourse more often than couples using artificial methods to prevent conception.

Hence, the *seventh conclusion:* Natural family planning is an ethical, effective, and proven method of limiting the size of families.

9.7 SURGICAL STERILIZATION

If infertility is the result of a surgical procedure to counteract some pathology in the body (e.g., a hysterectomy), it is called an indirect sterilization. More frequent, however, are direct sterilizations to prevent potential fertility, accomplished either by a vasectomy for a man or a tubal ligation for a woman. Direct sterilization, which is a form of contraception, is intrinsically unethical because it not only separates by human endeavor the unitive and procreative aspects of the marital act, it also mutilates the human body in that it destroys a human function when there is no pathology that would justify it. Sterilization is less risky to health than oral contraceptive and intrauterine devices, but it is more final than temporary forms of contraception. Some success has been developed in recent years in reversing sterilizations, but doing so is far from a safe and sure practice.

Elective surgical sterilizations of women usually take place in acute care hospitals, especially at the time of cesarean section childbirth. Because the Catholic Church sponsors many acute care hospitals in the United States, the issue of performing sterilizations in Catholic hospitals has often been a point of contention. First, the distinction between a direct and indirect sterilization has not always been clearly defined. Second, given the popular acceptance of sterilization as a means of family limitation, many representatives of Catholic health care have urged a policy of toleration with regard to people and physicians who wish to practice this procedure in apparent good faith.

The teaching authority of the church has stood firm, however, in maintaining that unless there is a present pathology that needs to be corrected, sterilizations are intrinsically evil and may not be performed in Catholic hospitals nor in non-Catholic hospitals under the management of Catholic hospitals. Thus, the *Directives* state: "Direct sterilization of either men or women, whether permanent or temporary, is not permitted in a Catholic health care institution. Procedures that induce sterility are permitted when their direct effect is the cure or alleviation of a present and serious pathology and a simpler treatment is not available" (directive 53).

The *eighth conclusion:* Direct surgical sterilization of men or women is intrinsically evil, but a procedure to treat a present pathology that causes infertility as a side effect is not prohibited.

9.8 CARE OF RAPE VICTIMS

Rape is one of the most common social crimes. Because many rape victims hesitate to expose themselves to shame and notoriety, it is difficult to ascertain with any degree of accuracy the number of rapes committed in the United States each year. There is evidence that rape is motivated by hostile impulses—a desire to assert aggressive powers by the rapist and to humiliate the victim—more than a desire for sexual pleasure. Because it involves sexual acts, however, we consider it a violation of natural sexual activity, which should be an act of mutual love.

A victim of rape should be given the most sensitive and charitable care possible. Victims often complain justifiably that they are treated by police and medical personnel alike as though they were responsible for provoking the attack. Many cities have formed task forces to help educate police and medical personnel concerning the humane treatment of rape victims, and also to present the crime by alerting the public to the signs of possible attack. Because most victims of rape are treated in hospitals, health care personnel should attempt to accomplish the following:

1. offer psychological support and counseling that the woman needs to overcome the trauma of attack; often, this will require follow-up treatment;
2. provide medical care for injuries or abrasions that might have occurred;
3. gather evidence to be used if the rapist is apprehended; and
4. provide treatment to prevent venereal disease and pregnancy.

The fourth point, preventing pregnancy, raises special ethical problems. The victim of rape has a right to avoid pregnancy, which is a tragic violation of her human rights, but once she has conceived she must also respect the rights of the child within her, because both are equally human persons and have equal rights. A woman who has consented to intercourse takes the responsibility for this act as a free person, and thus she should use the act in accord with its intrinsic significance of love and procreation. A rape victim, however, has no such responsibility, because she has not consented to the sexual act and has no responsibility to fulfill its intrinsic meaning.

Therefore, Catholic moralists maintain today that even a woman who is in danger of sexual attack may take contraceptives to prevent conception. And it is a common teaching among Catholic moralists that a woman who has already been raped may take contraceptives to prevent ovulation or to render the sperm inoperative. Thus, the *Directives* state: "A female who has been raped should be able to defend herself against a potential conception from the sexual assault" (directive 36). Usually, contraceptives will be offered to rape victims by hospital personnel. From our discussion of abortion, it is clear that no action that would destroy or prevent the implantation of an already fertilized ovum should be performed.

Although a woman who has been raped has the right to protect herself from conception, she does not have the right to do so at the expense of another human being. A woman would not restore her personal dignity by destroying another person. Before using any method to limit ovulation that also might be cause an abortion, efforts must be made to determine whether or not ovulation has occurred in the current menstrual period. If ovulation has not occurred, contraceptives may be used to prevent ovulation. If ovulation has already occurred, then contraceptives may not be used because their only effect would be to cause an abortion. If the woman is not sure whether or not ovulation has occurred, a dilemma arises.

Joseph Piccione and Gerald McShane (1997) have designed an ovukit that determines with some degree of accuracy whether ovulation has occurred. This facilitates the treatment of rape victims in accord with Catholic teaching. Unfortunately, not all Catholic hospitals have the ovukit available, so therapy will often be utilized in presence of some doubt. The *ninth conclusion:* Methods of preventing ovulation may be utilized in Catholic hospitals, provided efforts are made to ensure that the woman has not already conceived as a result of the rape.

9.9 PASTORAL CONSIDERATIONS

The church has no desire to condemn people who abuse or contradict the natural good of human sexuality or reproduction. Rather, it recommends patience, sympathy, and time to help people realize the injury they inflict upon themselves and others by contradicting the values of virtuous human sexuality. Typical of this attitude are some recent statements of Pope John Paul II in the encyclical *The Gospel of Life*:

Decisions that go against life sometime arise from difficult or even tragic situations of profound suffering, loneliness, a total lack of economic prospects, depression and anxiety about the future. Such circumstances can mitigate even to a notable degree subjective responsibility and the consequent culpability of those who make these choices, which in themselves are evil.

I would like now to say a special word to women who have had an abortion. The Church is aware of the many factors which may have influenced your decision and it does not doubt that in many cases it was a painful and even shattering decision. . . . The Father of Mercies is ready to give you his forgiveness and peace. . . . You will come to understand that nothing is definitively lost and you will also be able to ask forgiveness from your child who is now living with the Lord. (John Paul II 1995, n. 18)

Moreover, in response to theologians who criticized the teaching of the church concerning human sexuality, the church has stated (in *The Moral Norms of Humanae Vitae*):

Christian moral tradition has always maintained the distinction—not the separation much less the contra position—between the objective order and subjective guilt. For this reason it becomes a matter judging subjective moral behavior within the norm which prohibits the intrinsic disorder. It is perfectly legitimate to give due consideration to actions of individuals not only to their intention and motivations but also to the various circumstances of their lives and above all to the causes that might impair their consciences and their free will. This subjective situation, which can never change into "order" what is intrinsically "disorder," can have some bearing of the responsibility of the individual's behavior. (Congregation for the Doctrine of the Faith 1989, n. 3)

This distinction between objective morality (i.e., what is helpful or harmful to the human person by reason of the moral object) and subjective culpability (i.e., a person's own understanding and responsibility for good or ill) is fundamental to pastoral care, which is directed toward helping people overcome the gap that often exists between moral truth and moral sensitivity. In 1980, the Synod Bishops said:

In no way do we ignore the very difficult and trying situations of many Christians who although they sincerely want to observe moral norms taught by the Church, find themselves unequal to the task because of weakness in the face of difficulties. (Congregation for the Doctrine of the Faith 1989, n. 20)

The wisdom of pastoral counseling recognizes that the acceptance of moral truth and the development of moral sensitivity are gradual processes. The reform and renewal of morality are not accomplished through condemnation, but through patience and compassion. Hence, the meaning of the distinction between objective and subjective morality does not imply that people have a right to form their own consciences without referring to church teaching. Rather, it implies that church teaching in some instances will be difficult to follow because of the many situations of contemporary society that impinge on moral decision making and behavior. Counselors of people who in good faith do not understand why the church condemns contraception and who think that they can disregard its teaching on this subject should patiently seek to help them achieve this understanding step by step and develop the courage to follow the church's guidance. The first step in such help is to begin not with the issue of contraception but with the person's better understanding of his or her sexuality and how the proper use of it is so important for their true and lasting happiness and the happiness of their marriage.

Health care professionals can sympathize with the pastoral dilemma of the Catholic Church from the analogy of their own dealings with patients. We live in an unhealthy society, which makes it difficult for people to understand healthy living or practice it. Often, they have also lost trust in their physicians because of what they have heard of malpractice and alternative medicine. Should a physician refuse care for such patients who do not cooperate? Surely, the right policy for physicians is to tell patients the truth about ways to strive for good health and to persuade and encourage them to live better.

Similarly, the church must be patient with people who have become confused about fundamental Christian values and about the trustworthy authority to guide them. Many see no other solution for their problems than in ways plausibly promoted in the secular milieu, which in fact are morally harmful. Conversely, the church must not lack the courage to keep trying to educate its members concerning what Christian morality and sound ethics tell us is good for the family and its members. Hence, the *tenth conclusion:* Pastoral considerations seek to help people follow the norms of sexual morality so that they will grow as persons and integrate their personalities. The distinction between objective and subjective morality does not result in a separation of mind and body, but rather in an effort to help people develop moral character.

SUMMARY

Catholic tradition with regard to the generation and birth of children is based upon the firm conviction, drawn from Sacred Scripture and reason, that the family is the God given entity for co-creating human life. Moreover, the acts of love and unity proper to married couples are the only human acts worthy of bringing new life into the world. The family is not only the proper source of life but also the proper setting for educating the young about virtue.

Closely allied with the teaching of the church with regard to family and reproduction is its teaching on the sanctity of each human person. Thus, the teaching of the church about abortion and fetal testing are of great importance in contemporary society. Unfortunately, however, contemporary society is blind to the sanctity of life—especially for the weak—and to the meaning of family as the only proper context for reproduction. In a word, the teachings of the church are countercultural. The task of Catholics is not only to live the teaching of the church, but also to defend and explain it, using the science and language of contemporary society.

QUESTIONS

1. Why does the church spend so much time and energy explaining the teaching of Christ and the natural law with regard to human sexuality?
2. How are the four values of marriage related to family health and why is it unethical to deliberately separate these values?
3. What values or ethical norms should be used in planning the size of one's family?
4. Why is NFP an ethical practice, if contraception and sterilization are not?

CASES

1. Anne went into septic shock in the seventh month of her pregnancy. It is virtually certain that she will die of this condition if the source of the infection is not removed. In removing the placenta, the source of the infection, her unborn child will also be removed and may die. Is this a direct or an indirect abortion?
2. In a mid-size Catholic hospital, the obstetrics-gynecological staff maintains that the *Guidelines* prohibit the practice of "good medicine." It is rather difficult to identify their specific complaints, but they are threatening to leave the hospital and start their own facility unless changes are made. As a board member, what process should you follow in considering their complaints?
3. One of the professors in your university maintains that "sex is for fun" and that the teaching of the Catholic Church inhibits having fun from sexual activity. Would you agree with him, or would you be able to defend the teaching of the church?
4. A few years ago, two young women who were six months pregnant were diagnosed as having cancer of the uterus. Both decided to delay surgery or chemotherapy until their infants could be delivered with a firm hope of viability. Both died shortly after their children were born. What were their ethical options? What were they saying by delaying therapy for their condition?

10

Reconstructing Human Beings

OVERVIEW: In recent years, medical technology has moved from the mere capability of repairing the human body to new capabilities of remodeling the body by surgical reconstruction (transplants and sexual reassignment) as well as by genetic reconstruction, which may alter not only an individual but also all his or her descendants. Some of these new capabilities are already practical; others are still futuristic. We discuss many of them in this chapter, applying the principles of stewardship, human dignity, and totality.

10.1 HUMAN DOMINION OVER NATURE

A basic axiom of medicine has always been the Greek dictum, *Art perfects nature*, which implies that a human person can be healed (or patched up) and develop to maturity but cannot be essentially remade. Today, however, we must face the questions, Is it right for persons to become their own creators? Can and should human nature be remade? Can genetic engineering or some type of surgery at a very early age hasten the processes of evolution by eliminating troublesome wisdom teeth or appendixes? Might the technology of the future greatly reduce the complexities of the digestive system, which so often becomes diseased, and can human beings be fed in some simpler way, perhaps by a more effective intravenous method? To avoid sexually transmitted diseases, might all human beings be sterilized and reproduce artificially, or even be neutered?

The basic ethical issue here seems to be the extent of human dominion over nature. This is the classical way of posing the issue, but theologians of the past seemed to be influenced too much by the Greek image of God as a jealous monarch who becomes angry when Prometheus infringes on his prerogatives. Thus, they limited the powers of human dominion over the human body significantly. Others see such attempts to improve on humankind as an insult to the work of the Creator, whose masterpiece is the human person, or at least as a fatal temptation to pride.

Today, however, in considering radical human redevelopment, two theological points must be stressed. (1) God is a generous Creator, who in creating human beings also called them by the gift of intelligence to share in his creative power. Consequently, God does not want humans to leave fallow the talents he has given them, but encourages them to improve on the universe he has made. (2) Such improvement is possible because theology can accept the idea that God has made an evolutionary universe in which humankind has been created through an evolutionary process that is not yet complete. Thus, God has called humankind to join with him in bringing the universe to its completion, and in doing this he has not made humans merely workers to execute his orders, or to add trifling original touches on their own, but has made them genuine coworkers and encourages them to exercise real originality.

It is important to remember, however, that human creativity depends on a human brain, and the activity of the brain depends upon the emotions and the biology of the body. Any alteration that would injure the brain and hence, a person's very creativity, would indeed be disastrous mutilation, especially if this were to be transmitted genetically, thus further polluting the gene pool with defects that might be hidden and incalculable.

It is generally admitted that knowledge of this wonderful brain, sometimes called the "two-pound miracle," is still in its beginnings. The complexity of the brain is beyond any other system imaginable, and this complexity is reduced to a relatively small organ capable of self-development from the embryo and of self-maintenance, but not of self-restoration. The human brain may be near the limit of complexity and integration possible in organic, living systems.

This is certainly not so true of other organ systems, and it is possible to imagine that someday in other environments it might become necessary, for example, to replace the human lungs with other ways of obtaining oxygen or adapt our digestion systems to new forms of nutrition. In principle, such changes would seem be ethical (1) if they gave support to human intelligence by helping the life of the brain and (2) if they did not suppress any of the fundamental human functions that integrate the human personality.

Thus, alterations that would make it impossible for a human being to directly sense the external world at least as effectively as it now does with five senses would be contrary to the principle of totality. So would alterations that would make it impossible for human beings to experience the basic emotions, because emotional life is closely related to human intelligence and creativity. Again, alterations that would make human beings sexless and incapable of parenthood would also be inhuman. Grave ethical difficulties arise when we consider whether society has the knowledge or virtue to modify the human body wisely. Attempts to improve the human body or any set of organs would undoubtedly affect negatively other functions of the human body or other organ systems.

With these thoughts in mind, the *first conclusion* with regard to restructuring the human body comprises three points. First, the use of surgery and genetic manipulation to improve human bodies is ethically good, provided that the people conducting this form of experimentation take full account of the risks and are not carried away by false ambition, without regard to the real meaning of being human. In particular, Christians should be concerned that such innovations do not weaken the human family or the realization that children are a unique gift from God, not something to be manufactured at will by other humans.

Second, genetic engineering of the present human body would be permissible if it improves rather than weakens basic human functions, especially as they refer to human creativity and intelligence. In this regard, we need not draw a line between somatic cell germ cell intervention and germ cell intervention, as long as such intervention is in accord with the ethical norms already mentioned.

Third, the principle of stewardship and creativity throws light on many of the possibilities for human reconstruction. Natural law should not be conceived as a fixed unchangeable pattern of human life to which human beings are forever confined. Rather, the Creator has made human beings free and intelligent, and precisely this intelligent freedom is human nature and the foundation of natural moral law. Human intelligence, however, is not disembodied; it depends upon a brain and a body that have specific structures and purposes.

Three levels of remaking the human body are possible: (1) surgical procedures; (2) manipulation of embryonic cells; and (3) genetic engineering, which introduces different genes into the already constituted human genome. We shall treat these possible levels of remaking separately.

10.2 SURGICAL PROCEDURES

Organ Transplants

Two types of transplants using human organs are possible, one involving an organ or tissue taken from a dead person and given to a living person, and the other involving an organ taken from one living person and given to another living person. Transplanting an organ or tissue from a dead person to a living person presents no ethical problem. With few exceptions, religious groups as well as humanistic ethicists have recognized the worth and ethical validity of such transplants. If a serious question arises concerning this type of transplant, it stems from factors other than the transplant itself.

For example, concern has been expressed about the worth of heart transplants—most of it arises either from the great expense of money and personnel involved in a medical procedure that brings very little substantive value to society or from fear that in some cases the organ donor had not actually died. But these concerns are not focused on the transplant as such, and they have been somewhat dispelled as a result of better survival rates in recipients of heart transplants and a greater ability to ascertain the criteria for total brain death. In *The Gospel of Life*, Pope John Paul II—echoing Pope Pius XII—summed up Catholic teaching on transplants involving human organs:

> The Gospel of Life is celebrated above all else in the daily living of life which should be filled with self giving for others. . . . A particular praiseworthy example of such gestures is the donation of organs performed in an ethically acceptable manner with a view toward offering health and even life itself to the sick who sometimes have no other hope. (John Paul II 1995, n. 86)

There are many more difficulties, however, and less consensus concerning an organ transplant between living persons. At first, some theologians sought to justify transplants between human beings by reason of the principle of totality. But close examination of this principle indicated that a person cannot endanger his or her own life to assist another by reason of this principle. Because the body and its organs exist principally for the good of the individual, the power to give organs to another living person is limited. The principle that justifies donors to sacrifice an organ for transplantation is not that of totality, because the actual donor is mutilated, but the principle of common good or charity, the supreme commandment of the love of neighbor.

Because, however, that command is "to love your neighbor *as yourself,*" donors cannot injure their own bodies or seriously risk their own lives for another when this risk may in fact do little good. Consequently, one can donate an organ only when it is probable that one's own health will be preserved and the recipient will receive a proportionate benefit. Yet because such a donation is not one of justice but a free act of charity, it is possible for donors to refuse to make such a free gift, nor should others pressure them into doing so or condemn them for not doing so.

It is also essential to distinguish between *anatomical integrity*, which can be sacrificed, and *functional integrity*, which cannot be sacrificed. Anatomical integrity refers to the material or physical integrity of the human body. Functional integrity refers to the systematic efficiency of the human body. For example, if one kidney were missing from a person's body, there would be a lack of anatomical integrity, but if one healthy kidney were present and working, there would be functional integrity because one healthy kidney is more than able to provide systemic efficiency.

This distinction between anatomical and functional integrity, which we have incorporated in our formulation of the principle of totality, explains why the church has approved blood transfusions and skin grafts and why theologians have approved elective appendectomy if the abdominal cavity is open for another legitimate reason. In these situations, loss of anatomical integrity may occur through loss of blood, skin tissue, or an internal organ, but no loss of functional integrity occurs.

Given the fact that the more successful transplants among the living are between members of the same family, familial or social pressure to offer one-self as a donor may at times be severe. But the courts (rightly, we believe) refuse to compel such donations. Pope John Paul II, as quoted in *Dolentium Hominum*, summed up the essence of being an organ donor in the following words:

> Transplantation presupposes a prior, explicit, free and conscious decision on the part of the donor or of someone who legitimately represents the donor, gen-erally the closest relatives. It is a decision to offer without monetary reward, a part of one's own body for the health and well-being of another person. In this sense, the medical action of transplantation makes possible the donor's act of self-giving, that sincere gift of self which expresses our constitutive calling to love and communion. (John Paul II 1992, n. 2)

Hence, organ transplants between two living persons are licit if the donor's functional integrity is maintained, but we would caution that great care be taken in weighing the merely potential benefit against the actual risks. Consent should not be given unless the prognosis is good, because some recipients of transplants die within a short time because of "rejection," even if the transplant is "successful." Therefore, it is necessary to weigh the value of such a brief prolongation of life against the lifelong risk to the donor.

Along with justifying the donation of an organ on the basis of the prin-ciple of the common good, some Catholic theologians go a step farther and seek to justify these procedures either by expanding the principle of totality or by treating the whole process as a curative action, even though two peo-ple are involved and one will be injured. In so doing, they destroy the limits that protect the integrity of donor. The human unity of body and soul is ignored by these theories, and the body is treated as merely something used by the person, the parts of which are at the disposal or "over against" the person and thus may be sacrificed by the person for any higher good. Falling heir to Cartesian dualism, which renders appreciation of the body–soul unity of human nature impossible, one author even concludes that both eyes may be donated "for the good of another person."

Finally, arguments for the gift of human body parts lose their force when it is a question of sale, even the sale of blood. Such a sale is ethically objec-tionable for two reasons: (1) It is contrary to the dignity of the human body and depersonalizing, and (2) all those who need such a gift should receive it, rather than only those who can pay. Recently, the U.S. Congress passed laws against selling organs when it passed a bill to establish better methods of collecting and distributing human organs.

Because so many different organs and tissues are now subject to trans-plant—not only the heart and kidneys, but also lungs, liver, parts of lungs and livers, pancreas, spleen, skin, and bone marrow—there is a continual shortage of suitable organs and tissue for transplant. Research is even under way to use organs from animals for human transplants, the problem of rejection being addressed by adding human genes to the animal organ. There is no ethical objection to using animal organs for human transplants. An exception must be made, however, for transplants of reproductive organs, if this would involve the possible conception of children who would not be genetically linked to their parents in the normal manner. Finally, the hope of supplying organs and tissue to replace dysfunctional material will be a reality if stem cell research, which we consider below, is successful.

At present, the system of obtaining organs and allotting them is not well defined. Regional transplant centers, which are funded in part by the federal government, publicize the need for organ donations; maintain waiting lists, including those who need transplants; and assist physicians in allotting the available organs. For the most part, when organs become available in a particular region, they are usually given to a person in the region. Recent legislation has set guidelines for the national sharing of available organs on the basis of genetic matching between donor and recipient. In general, the organs are allotted to those in gravest need who also have a chance of survival. The *second conclusion* may be formulated as follows:

1. The functional integrity of the donor as a human person should not be impaired, even though anatomical integrity may suffer.
2. The risk taken by the donor as an act of charity is proportionate to the good resulting for the recipient.
3. The donor's consent is free and informed.
4. The recipients for the scarce organs are selected justly.

Sexual Reassignment

A special type of reconstructive surgery is *transsexual surgery*, a procedure by which the sexual phenotype of a male is altered to resemble that of a female, or vice versa. Such surgery, along with hormonal treatment and psychotherapy, is called *sexual reassignment*. Some physicians believe it to be helpful in dealing with the puzzling and painful condition called *transsexualism* or, more accurately, *gender dysphoria syndrome*, which is characterized by great anxiety over one's phenotypic sex and socially imposed gender role.

Such procedures involve a radical mutilation, namely, castration and construction of a pseudo vagina for a male, or mastectomy and hysterectomy (sometimes also the construction of a nonfunctional pseudo-penis and testes) for the female, along with hormonal treatments with possible serious side effects. These obviously raise the ethical question of whether the attempt to change a person's biological sex is ever a legitimate aim of medical care.

Catholic moralists have always admitted that in cases where a child is born with ambiguous genitalia, the parents should raise the child as belonging to that sex in which it is most likely to be able to function best. Nor does there seem to be any objection to the use of surgery or hormones to improve the normal appearance or function of such a person in accordance with the sex in which he or she is to be or has been raised. The reasoning behind this position is that a person must "live according to nature," insofar as this is humanly knowable.

Recently, however, knowledge of sexual development has increased vastly, and sexual ambiguity in development is seen as far more complex and common than formerly thought. The biological determination of sex depends on the presence or absence of the Y chromosome in the one-cell zygote, which in the beginning constitutes the human person. When present, it produces the H-Y antigen as early as the eight-cell stage of development, and the person begins to move toward maleness; otherwise, all zygotes develop as females.

All embryos originally have undifferentiated gonads and two sets of sexual ducts, the Wolffian and the Mullerian. But at seven weeks, the male gonads differentiate and begin to produce hormones that destroy the Mullerian ducts and cause the development of the male genitalia; otherwise, the Wolffian ducts are absorbed and the gonads and the Mullerian ducts develop into the female sexual system. Yet the differing hormonal balance in the two sexes causes certain differences in the male and female brain, in particular, preparing the female brain to regulate the menstrual cycle. It seems that these neurological differences also result in behavioral differences in the two sexes.

All these biological determinations are at work before birth. After birth it is probable, but not yet proved, that biophysical events at the unconscious level, similar to the imprinting demonstrated in animals, also promote sexual differentiation, such as the way the mother cares differently for a female and male child. Finally, at the conscious environmental level, the person learns his or her own gender identity and assumes a gender role in society. In this long and complicated process, many things can go wrong at each stage, with the result that in the human population a whole spectrum of conditions exists between the normal masculine and feminine conditions, meaning by "normal" a condition determined by the intrinsic teleology of sex optimal for species survival.

Among these possible abnormalities *homosexuality* is a highly varied condition, probably having many etiological factors, in which a person who is phenotypically unambiguously male or female and in no doubt about his or her gender is conscious of greater sexual attraction to those of his or her own sex than to others, and who consequently is unable to enter into a satisfactory marriage. *Transvestism* is a condition in which a person, usually heterosexual in orientation, is more comfortable sexually while wearing clothing symbolic of the opposite sex; it is probably a form of fetishism. *Transsexuals* differs markedly from the foregoing by gender dysphoria syndrome (i.e., an anxiety, sometimes reaching suicidal depression, as the result of the obsessive feeling that one's "real" sex is the opposite of one's phenotypic sex).

Sexual reassignment would be acceptable ethically if it were possible to demonstrate that a transsexual is similar to a person born with ambiguous genitalia. At present, we do not believe that this can be shown to be the case, for several reasons. It has not been established that the cause of gender dysphoria syndrome is biological. No such cause is obvious at the level of either the genotype or phenotype, and as yet the evidence is tenuous that the reason transsexuals feel from early in their lives that they have a "soul different from my body" is due to some developmental accident in the central nervous or hormonal systems.

It remains more probable that the determining causes of transsexualism are at the psychological level of development. A renowned expert in the field stated: "I have seen any number of men who would like to live as females and vice versa; I have not seen one with a reversal of core gender identity." Consequently, the gender ambiguity in question appears to be primarily psychological and should thus be treated by psychotherapy, rather than surgically. Unfortunately, today the social construct that stereotypes some persons as "gay" or "lesbian" has discouraged adequate research on the causes of these developmental defects. Surgical efforts to accommodate them rather than prevent or remedy them are obviously not either medically or ethically the best approach to solving the tragic human difficulties they produce. As too often happens today, pragmatic solutions are accepted rather than fundamental ones.

From a theological point of view, it is clear that transsexual surgery does not really solve personal existential problem, because it does not enable patients to achieve sexual normality and enter into a valid Christian marriage or have children. Because many of these individuals are somewhat asexual, their problem is not primarily sexual satisfaction but the relief of the burden of anxiety, which can usually be at least considerably lightened by psychotherapy. The *third conclusion:* On the basis of the present state of knowledge, surgery for sexual reassignment is unethical. Certainly, compassion should be extended to this small but greatly suffering group of human beings, but it should take the practical form of psychotherapy and pastoral guidance.

10.3 MANIPULATION OF EMBRYONIC CELLS

Sex Selection

The issue of parents' need and right to have children or even to order the sort of child by manipulating the genetic makeup of the embryo gives rise to a host of ethical problems. This is an effort to control and produce at will new combinations of genetic traits in the offspring.

One of the simplest forms of this manipulation would be to determine at will the sex of the offspring by selecting sperm that do not or do have the Y chromosome that determines maleness and then using selected sperm for artificial insemination or in vitro fertilization and implantation. Even if a technique could be invented to promote or suppress the production of one or the other type of sperm in the father without interfering with the normal process of sexual intercourse, the social and ecological consequences of such intervention could be counterproductive.

Biologists are convinced that evolutionary selection has developed the process of sexual differentiation by a genetic mechanism of the sort we find in the human species, which produces an approximate 50–50 split among the sexes. Studies predict that if couples were able to choose the sex of their offspring, however, most couples would choose to have a boy first, and then a girl, and the eventual distribution of males and females would be near 50–50, as it is now.

It seems, therefore, that the promotion of sexual selection might not be seriously deleterious to society, although it certainly would have risks and would have few, if any, social advantages over leaving it to nature. Its only advantage would be that parents would have freedom to choose. Although this preference is probably cultural and subject to cultural modification, it possibly also has a sociobiological foundation in the greater mortality of males.

Ethically speaking, is the free choice whether to have a boy or a girl beneficial for the child? After all, parents should not let their subjective preference operate at the expense of the child. It would be unethical to convince a child to be a doctor or a lawyer if this were not in the best interest of the child. Christian teaching shows that it is important for children to be accepted as a divine gift—to be loved for what they uniquely are, and not merely because they conform to their parents' hopes or expectations. If society says "You are loved because you conform to your parents' preferences," this seems to be an injustice to the child and further reinforces the cultural message that children exist primarily to fulfill their parents' needs rather than for their own sake.

The fourth conclusion: The selection of the gender of the child is unethical if this would upset the 50–50 balance of males and females in the population, or if the method involves artificial reproduction. Moreover, it would tend to lessen the sense that every child is a gift to the parents, not their property.

Splitting Embryonic Cells

The human embryo, as we indicated in chapter 9, begins as a one-celled living being. It quickly grows into a two-celled, then four-celled and eight-celled entity. Any one of these eight cells can be isolated from the rest and begin the process of multiplication all over again. This may be what happens sometimes in the formation of an identical human twin who is really a "natural" (or rather an "accidental" but not artificial) clone. The second twin is a slightly younger clone of the first twin that already exists as an ensouled human person; yet the clone has a human, spiritual soul because God creates a soul for every truly human body.

Thus, each one of these cells is considered to be *totipotent* in its very early stages—that is, it may be removed from the others and allowed to develop into another human being on its own. Because not all eight cells have identical DNA, if a cell without a particular genetic abnormality can be discerned, it would be possible to develop a human being without a particular genetic weakness, which the other cells may have inherited from the parents whose germ cells contributed to the original zygote.

An example of this phenomenon occurred recently. Molly Nash, a six-year-old child, was diagnosed with Franconi anemia, a genetic disease that normally results in death at an early age. Her parents sought advice from medical scientists, who suggested that if the parents had a second child without the disease, the child's blood might be transfused into Molly and save her life. Because both parents had the Fanconi gene, their chance of producing a child without the disease were one in four.

But the scientists, by means of in vitro fertilization, were able to examine a newly conceived embryo in its earliest stages before implantation. Selecting one totipotent cell that did not have the defective gene, they implanted it in the womb of the mother, destroying the other totipotent cells that did have the defective gene. When Adam, the second child, was born, his blood was transfused into Molly. It is not clear as yet whether the total process, which cost hundreds of thousands of dollars, was successful. But it shows the potential for therapy using stem cells from embryos.

The *fifth conclusion:* Because this form of therapy requires the destruction of living embryos, and the generation of human embryos in an unnatural manner, it would be unethical.

Screening Embryonic Cells

The medical specialty of diagnosing inherited or genetic defects and their treatment, as well as the task of screening populations for these defects, and of counseling couples that are or may become parents of defective children is developing rapidly; special institutes dedicated to it are being founded throughout the United States. The need for testing for genetic defects is evident from the following statistical considerations.

There are more than 3,000 single-gene defects identified at present. Moreover, each of us carries between five and eight mutant lethal equivalents (genes), which we are all able to transmit to subsequent generations.

Thus, we are all mutants, in the strictest sense, although only about 5 to 8 percent of us actually manifest some form of genetic mutation. An estimated 0.5 percent of all live births are attended by chromosomal imbalances such as trisomies and chromosome maldistributions. Three-quarters of these, or 0.29 percent, are deleterious defects. (Also, an estimated 9 percent of all early embryos are chromosomally abnormal, most of them lethally so.)

Major single-gene mutations—homozygous and heterozygous—(e.g., autosomal dominants and recessives and X-linked disorders) occur in 1.8 percent of the general population. The polygenic conditions (e.g., diabetes mellitus, gout, and some allergies) occur in 1.7 to 2.6 percent of all live births. (These figures appear to remain fairly constant throughout the world.) Add the figures, and we have the 4.8 to 5 percent incidence of genetic defect in all live births.

Techniques of diagnosing genetic defects after conception at early stages of human development are being perfected (e.g., amniocentesis, by which some genetic defects can be determined by examining the amniotic fluid in which the fetus floats in the womb; and chorionic villi sampling, a procedure that is less invasive than amniocentesis but also enables genetic diagnosis before birth; chorionic villi are the waste matter of the chorion, which is the envelope containing the fetus).

Sonography is often used to "picture" the position of the infant and prepare for a safe delivery. The benefit of sonography is presently questioned by health care economists. Today, sonography is often combined with amniocentesis to ensure that the needle introduced through the abdomen of the pregnant woman to gather amniotic fluid does not injure the infant. When properly performed, amniocentesis and chorionic villi sampling are relatively safe procedures. However, many couples that would not have an abortion even if genetic screening revealed genetic anomalies thus choose to have only sonography. A woman would be well within her rights if she requested the prior record of success and failure of the hospital before submitting to prebirth genetic screening.

In the instruction *On Respect for Human Life*, the Congregation for the Doctrine of the Faith (1987, I, n. 2) treated the topic of prenatal diagnosis and stated: "If prenatal diagnosis respects the life and integrity of the embryo and the human fetus and is directed toward its safeguarding or healing as an individual, then the practice is allowed." In *The Gospel of Life*, Pope John Paul II (1995) also approved of prebirth genetic testing, provided that the testing is not used as an indication that an abortion should be performed.

The reason for justifying these procedures is that prenatal diagnosis makes it possible to anticipate earlier and more effectively the need for certain therapeutic medical or surgical procedures. Satisfying the curiosity of the parents with regard to the sex of the child does not justify amniocentesis or chorionic villi sampling, but it might justify sonography or other noninvasive procedures. Of course, the procedure would be immoral if it were done with the intention of having an abortion if the results were not acceptable to the parents. An unfavorable diagnosis should not be the equivalent of a death sentence for the infant in the womb. The *sixth conclusion:* Screening embryonic cells for genetic defects is an ethical procedure, provided it is performed for legitimate purposes.

Genetic Counseling

Genetic counseling may occur before conception or when the child is in the womb. Because many ethical issues are common to both types of counseling, we will consider them simultaneously. Genetic counseling may be characterized as a process of communication that attempts to deal with the human problems associated with the occurrence of a genetic disorder. This process helps an individual couple comprehend the medical facts, understand the ethical options for dealing with a positive diagnosis, choose the action that seems most appropriate, and act in accordance with that decision. The counselor should also help the couple make the best possible adjustment to help the affected member of the family.

Generating children is conditioned by the capability of parents to provide for them. Prospective parents therefore must consider these factors: (1) their own need to have children as the completion of their mutual love; (2) their own capacity to care for these children; and (3) the risks that each particular child may suffer from grave handicaps that require special care, including the possibility that this child will be faced in his or her turn with the question of whether he or she should pass on defective genes to the next generation. Some significant risks of defect exist for *every* child and could not be eliminated, no matter what means were utilized.

Thus, in all cases parents must decide whether they have the capacity to care for a potentially defective child. Furthermore, it is the duty of the genetics counselor and of society to assist the parents in accepting and meeting reasonable risks. For genetics counselors or society at large to encourage in parents the attitude that they should not have children unless the children are perfect and require the least care possible is as reprehensible as to encourage parents to reproduce fatalistically with no account of their genetic compatibility.

Studies demonstrate that many counselors are inclined to recommend abortion if the infant in the womb has a serious genetic defect. In accord with the Christian concept of human dignity, however, the counselor should never recommend abortion as a solution. If the parents declare a firm intention to abort, the counselors should present other options and avoid formal cooperation in an abortion, because the counselors should protect the infant's right to life as they would the right of a child already born. In sum, if abortion is in question, the counselor should respect the conscience of the parents while doing everything possible to protect the life of the child. Clearly, one of the prominent ethical issues in genetic counseling is the shortage of well-qualified counselors.

The possibility of cooperation in an abortion, however, should not prevent a Catholic health care facility from instituting a preconception or postconception screening program. Such programs must be conducted prudently, however, because serious questions may be raised. First, the research purposes of genetic screening must be regulated in the same way as any other kind of research on human subjects. Thus, it seems that because amniocentesis involves a risk to the fetus (usually less than 0.05 percent at more competent centers), it cannot be used for research purposes unless proportionate benefits exist for the fetus.

Therapy for infants still in the womb is a possibility; for example, a hydrocephalus fetus may be treated before birth. Therapy of this type justifies amniocentesis, and the potential for treating genetic anomalies before birth is increasing. Some ethicists maintain that the benefit that comes to the parents from amniocentesis—either knowing that the child is normal or being able to prepare themselves for the birth of a debilitated child—would justify the amniocentesis.

Hence, the use of preconception screening to promote responsible parenthood is in general a laudable purpose, because there can be no doubt that couples should not bring children into the world for whom (with the reasonable assistance of society) they cannot adequately care and that the care of defective children presents special burdens. Consequently, prospective parents have the duty to seek the scientific information useful to such decisions through preconception screening, and society has the duty to assist them in obtaining such information, if there is reasonable suspicion of genetic defect and this information is economically available to them.

But extreme caution is necessary if the program involves *negative eugenics*. Proponents of this type of screening argue that modern medicine has upset the ecological balance by saving the lives of more and more defective persons who would have died before they could reproduce. Negative eugenicists thus maintain that the load of defective genes in the gene pool is increasing and that a much higher level of genetic disease may soon occur in the population. But scientists also have stated that the consensus of the best medical and genetic opinion is that whatever genetic deterioration is occurring as a result of decreased natural selection is so slow as to be insignificant when contrasted with "environmental" changes, including those produced by medical innovation.

Hence, if only those persons who themselves suffer from a particular disease are prevented from reproducing, this would not eliminate heterozygous carriers, who would continue to transmit defects dependent on recessive genes. Moreover as defective genes are eliminated from the gene pool, they are constantly replaced by mutations caused by environmental factors.

Hence the *seventh conclusion:* The genetic counselor has the function of helping prospective parents prepare themselves for the possibility that a fetus will be defective and to plan ways to provide for this eventuality. The counselor also has the responsibility of helping parents care for children who have been born with birth defects.

10.4 GENETIC MANIPULATION

Efforts to use genetic manipulation or engineering to eliminate actual or potential disease or to improve the human genotype may be applied in one of three different ways: through splicing into human cells a healthy gene to displace a defective gene, by administering pharmaceuticals containing altered cells, or by stifling harmful genes by interfering with their protein production. The development of these methods will be dependent in the future upon the findings of the Human Genome Project (HGP).

Few scientific enterprises have been as grand as the HGP. According to its leaders, the project is "an ambitious effort to understand hereditary instructions that make each of us unique" (Collins 1995). It is intended to find the location of the 30,000 human genes and to read the entire genetic script, all three billion bits of information, by the year 2005. Researchers have announced that, although some chores remain, the task of identifying and sequencing the human genome is substantially complete. They hope that all this new knowledge will help scientists to identify defective genes and either neutralize their debilitating qualities or replace them entirely with "good genes." In time, science may be able to wipe out some diseases all together. Moreover, it is hoped that the new knowledge will change the delivery of health care. In the past, physicians diagnosed an illness as the result of a clinical examination, confirming it through biomedical testing. If the HGP is successful, these methods will become obsolete. In *Life Script*, Nicholas Wade describes the potential of medicine as follows: "Consider a new way of healing the body. Instead of cutting flesh with scalpels, poisoning it with chemical drugs, or burning in with radiation, the physician would gently treat the body with nothing but cells and proteins, seeking to mend like with like" (Wade 2001, 19).

Some of the efforts at molecular diagnosis or genetic engineering are already in use:

- Each year, clinical labs perform millions of tests aimed at detecting potential or actual diseases caused by genetic defects.
- Newborn infants are screened for sickle-cell anemia, a metabolic illness called phenylketonuria, and congenital thyroid defects.

- Other tests reveal whether people who are predisposed by family history to develop cancer have in fact inherited dangerous genetic mutations.

We know, however, that although genetic makeup determines human physiology, it contributes only a predisposition to human disease. Environment and behavior are also significant factors insofar as acquiring disease is concerned. A few years ago, some scientists were saying that they would soon find the genes that "cause cancer" and find a way to replace them. Today, however, scientists see the development of disease, especially an inherited one, as much more complex phenomena: Indeed, it seems that some diseases mainly are caused by environmental factors, whereas others have a mainly genetic origin.

Efforts to modify the activity of the human genes by eliminating genes or introducing new genes into the human genotype have not to date been successful. But indicators for future success in this effort should not be discounted. The efforts to eliminate defective genes through splicing new genes or by limiting the activity of defective genes are ethically acceptable. In a certain sense, they resemble the effort to use pharmaceuticals to sustain or improve health.

The use of stem cells to treat disease or improve health does cause ethical concern, however. Stem cells are best described in the context of normal human development. Human development begins when a sperm fertilizes an egg and creates a single cell that has the potential to form an entire organism. The fertilized egg is totipotent, meaning that the cells of this organism can develop into other cells, even into another distinct organism. In the first hours after fertilization, the cell divides into two totipotent cells. This means that either one of these cells, if placed in a woman's uterus, has the potential to develop into a human fetus. In fact, identical twins develop when two totipotent cells separate and develop into two genetically identical human beings.

Approximately four days after fertilization and several cycles of cell division, these totipotent cells begin to specialize, forming an outer cell mass called the blastocyst and an inner cell mass that will go on to form virtually all of the tissues of the human body. These inner-mass cells are *pluripotent*— they can give rise to many types of cells, but not all types of cells necessary for fetal development. Pluripotent stem cells are capable of developing into any one of the 220 types of cell that make up the human body. Researchers feel that pluripotent stem cells can be nudged down certain pathways and thus develop the material that will replace diseased parts of the body or overcome impaired functions.

Pluripotent cells offer the possibility of renewable sources of replacement cells and tissue to treat such genetic illnesses as Parkinson's and Alzheimer's diseases, to say nothing of spinal cord injury, and replacing degenerated heart muscles and the entire pancreas to cure diabetes. There is almost no realm of medicine that might not be touched by this innovation. Scientists believe that the challenges to this type of therapy are significant but not insurmountable.

The main ethical issue regarding research and development of stem cells arises from the source of these cells. To date, the source of most of these cells has been aborted fetuses or fetuses that have been frozen at the moment of conception and stored for future use. In either case, obtaining stem cells from embryos is contrary to the teaching of the Catholic Church because it involves the destruction of human beings, or close cooperation with those who are destroying human beings, even if the persons destroyed are in their first stages of existence.

Because cell lines have been developed from stem cells that were originally derived from aborted fetuses, several politicians and scientists maintain that using these cultured cells is far removed from actual participation in the destruction of human fetuses. We believe that the scandal arising from the use of these cells, even if they were cultured, would be so grave as to prohibit their use in a Catholic health care facility.

The ethical debate could be avoided because stem cells may also be obtained from adults, as well as from fetuses. In fact, some scientists maintain that this source of stem cells is so promising that the use of embryonic stem cells will be irrelevant in the future. Clearly, adult stem cells seem more adapted to overcoming rejection because they may be taken from the very persons who need genetic therapy in the form of new tissue or organs. The U.S. Congress has prohibited funding for nontherapeutic research, but some ethicists, scientists, and politicians seek to reverse this prohibition.

As we consider genetic reconstruction, it will be wise to remember four points. First, it is more feasible, technically and ethically, to improve the human condition by improving the environment and development of the individual (i.e., the phenotype) than by modifying genetic endowment (i.e., the genotype). Therefore, priority in research and investment of medical resources should be given to the former effort. Genetic research is extremely important, however, to explain the interactions of genotype and phenotype.

Second, presently proposed methods of genetic reconstruction of human beings involve in vitro fertilization and other procedures that are ethically objectionable because they separate reproduction from its parental context and involve the production of human beings, of whom some will be defective because of experimental failure and thus will probably be destroyed. This contravenes the basic principles of ethical experimentation with human subjects.

Third, proposals to improve the human race by sex selection, cloning, or genetic reconstruction are ethically unacceptable in the present state of knowledge. Unless limited to very modest interventions, they would restrict the genetic variability important to human survival, and they would separate reproduction from its parental context.

Fourth, the principle of stewardship throws light on many of the problems of human reconstruction. Natural law should not be conceived of as a fixed pattern of human life to which human beings are forever confined. Rather, the Creator has made human beings free and intelligent, and it is precisely this intelligent freedom that *is* human nature and the foundation of natural moral law.

Human intelligence, however, is not disembodied; it depends on a brain and a body that have a specific structure. In caring for their total health, persons not only have the right but the obligation to understand their psychological and biological structure and to improve themselves, even in ways that may seem novel to past generations. Such improvement is good stewardship of the share in divine creativity with which God has endowed humankind.

Hence; our *eighth conclusion:* Genetic engineering of the human genome of phenotype is well within the realm of ethical research and therapy provided it is properly designed to protect human dignity and does not use as a source of stem cells embryonic material from human fetuses.

SUMMARY

As human power over our genetic constituents increases, the ability to change human design and function will also increase. Hence it is extremely important that we start to ask the important questions about human reconstruction now. Are there limits to the power we have over human engineering? Do we have the right to do something simply because we have the power to do something? Science can destroy the world and all its people, as well as improve life for every person. The choice is an ethical one. We believe that an ethical choice for the future of human development should follow the Christian principles applied in this chapter.

QUESTIONS

1. How would you explain this statement: "An artificial means of improving human function is an acceptable method of cooperating with God the Creator"?

2. If one person may freely give a kidney for transplant to another person, would it violate the principal of totality to give an eye to another person?

3. What are the various stages of sexual development, and what factors at each stage might inhibit a person's normal development?

CASES

1. As a research scientist working with DNA splicing, you are requested to participate in research that will improve human hearing by changing the genotype of the human person. What conditions would you stipulate concerning the research project before joining the team that will carry on the research?

2. Don and Dan are identical twins. After Don suffers kidney failure, Dan is requested by his brother's wife to donate one of his healthy kidneys to Don. Does Dan have any obligation to surrender one of his healthy kidneys to his brother? Under what condition would you defend Dan's decision not to surrender his kidney?

3. You and your spouse each have a nephew who has Down's syndrome. What criteria will you use to determine whether you will have children? Would you take part in a genetic screening program before conception occurs?

4. A research scientist from the United States seeks to cure a genetic defect in a native of Africa by means of recombinant DNA (gene splicing) that supplements a defective gene in the genotype of the patient. A federal agency declares his efforts unethical and cancels his research funds. When and under what conditions will such research be ethically acceptable?

11

Mental Illness: Medical and Psychiatric Therapies

OVERVIEW: Human beings suffer from psychological as well as physiological impairment. When the psychological function of the human personality is not working properly, the person needs therapeutic help to overcome or tolerate the illness or malady in question.

To present the ethical issues associated with mental therapy, this chapter first describes how psychological illness, often called mental illness, differs from physiological illness. Then we discuss the main methods of therapeutic assistance for psychological dysfunction, namely, the medical model and psychotherapeutic models. Finally, we consider addiction, a very common form of psychological illness in our society. Although the ethical principles used in this section stress the need for the therapist to develop the subject's inner freedom, the principles of growth through suffering and of human dignity are also operative.

11.1 MENTAL ILLNESS

In dealing with ethical problems in psychiatric medicine, a very special problem arises: What is the difference between mental illness and ordinary physical illness? In our model of the human personality, its *psychological* dimension is closely interrelated with its *physical* dimension but also clearly distinct from it, as well as from its ethical and spiritual dimensions. The failure in the history of medicine to make these distinctions has been a source of vast confusion, and it remains a source of current controversy. In the past, mental illness was often thought to be possession by the devil. Recently, some people have maintained that it is a social construct, because behavior in one society thought to be aberrant is often tolerated in another society.

Thus, a group of psychiatrists has made a strong, if exaggerated, case against the whole concept of mental illness and the medical model of psy-

159

chiatry. These psychiatrists argue that the greater number of psychiatric ill-nesses are really social maladjustments between the behavior of a noncon-formist individual and the demands of a social system. The cause of these maladjustments is to be located in the modern social system, which is unable to deal with individual differences. The line between normal behavior and abnormal behavior thus turns out to be only a question of who is deciding what *they* want *us* to do.

This warning should be heeded, but the outcries against the system should not be allowed to confuse the problem of medical care. Thus, it is nec-essary to hold firmly to the fact that there is such a thing as human behavior that is dysfunctional and that is caused by organic and physiological defects. There can be no doubt that lesions of the central nervous system and a wide variety of other physiological disorders can make it difficult or impossible for human beings to sense and perceive the world correctly—or to live in a state of emotional balance and sensitivity, to think clearly, and to make deci-sions free from uncontrollable impulses. Moreover, there is increasing evi-dence that there may be a genetic basis for mental illnesses, particularly for schizophrenia and manic-depressive psychosis.

What is optimal or normal for mental functioning is not easy to deter-mine objectively. There is a natural range of acuteness of the senses, of sen-sitivity of effective response, and of "general intelligence" that the intelli-gence quotient is supposed to measure. Subnormal intelligence, however, is generally determined by the fact that a person is incapable of being educated independently to make reasonable judgments about basic problems of life. For example, a person with Down's syndrome may be able to do simple jobs routinely but may need the help of others to select a job suitable for his or her capacities.

Such chronic mental deficiencies, however, are quite different from *psy-chosis*, in which a person with normal intelligence can no longer distinguish between reality and imagination. A similar although less severe problem is raised by *neuroses*, in which the person's judgement is impaired about certain matters by excessive fears, or by *addiction*, which occurs when impairment is due to an habitual, overwhelming desire for a particular physical pleasure. From an ethical perspective, what is most significant about these conditions, especially psychoses, is that freedom is impaired if not altogether restricted.

Insofar as chronic mental deficiency with a physiological basis is con-cerned, it is now difficult to improve the functioning of such persons. How-ever, it is not impossible that the neurological repair of these conditions may become possible. At present, the ethical issues involved in caring for such peo-ple are to ensure that their capacities are developed, that they find suitable employment and activities, and that their human dignity is protected, above all by protecting them from abuse and exploitation. Society has a role to play in this effort to treat impaired persons ethically, as is outlined in chapter 7.

There are, however, several forms of treatment for psychoses, neuroses, and addiction. If successful, these treatments free the person for moral autonomy and for the responsibility that is essential to human fulfillment. Persons have a right to treatment, and the community has an interest and a responsibility to provide it. The goal of treating mental illnesses, parallel to that of treating other physiological illnesses, is optimal functioning of human mental capacities of sensation, affectivity, abstract thought, and freedom of choice. The criteria for success for this latter form of therapy are:

- relief from undesirable symptoms (i.e., excessive anxiety or fear),
- increased productivity in the person's work,
- adjustment and satisfaction in interpersonal relations and sexual relations,
- increased ability to endure the stresses of life, and
- increased freedom to make realistic decisions about these and other matters necessary to attain the goal of human fulfillment.

This last point is important for ethics. Mental health is a prior condition requisite for dealing with ethical problems of moral right and wrong, because only to the degree that a person is free can there by the possibility of moral choice and moral responsibility. Because human personality is complex yet requires integration, it is not surprising that no human person is totally free, as we shall explain below. In sum, it is not the aim of the therapist to make patients virtuous but to help them to trust others so that they may act freely, and use such virtues as they may have or acquire them.

Thus, the *first conclusion*: Mental illness sometimes results from physical impairment, but it also results from the faulty development of human affective and cognitive capacities.

11.2 THERAPIES FOR MENTAL ILLNESS

Therapies to treat mental illness can be divided into two main approaches, depending upon whether the illness has mainly a physiological or psychological basis. Insofar as illnesses with a physiological basis are concerned (e.g., Down's syndrome), we have indicated that the therapy for such persons should enable them to develop the capacities that they possess and to help them strive for human dignity, as much as they are able.

More subject to improvement are people with mental illness that mainly has a psychological basis. Insofar as these people are concerned, there are two therapeutic approaches: One follows a medical model, and the other follows a psychotherapeutic model. We shall consider the medical model first, and then the psychotherapeutic model.

Therapies of the Medical Model

Therapies that follow the medical model presuppose that there is physiological defect that disposes for, or causes, the mental illness. In this model, there are three main approaches: (1) psychoactive drugs, (2) shock therapy, and (3) psychosurgery.

Treating mental illness by means of psychoactive drugs is by far the most common method in contemporary medical practice. Even if a health care professional will later use psychotherapeutic methods, he or she will begin therapy by means of psychoactive drugs. Their use has become so prevalent that one of the largest clinics for therapy and training in psychotherapy, the Menninger Foundation in Topeka, Kansas, recently listed the preponderant use of psychoactive drugs to treat mental illness as one of the reasons for its closing.

Psychoactive drugs, sometime called psychotropic drugs, alter emotions, perceptions, and imagination so that the patient is able to pursue a more normal pattern of behavior. Some forms of psychoactive agents have been used since the beginning of civilization. Alcoholic beverages were invented at the same time as cereal agriculture. Opium in one form or another has been used as a pain reliever for centuries. Aspirin, the first of the wonder drugs, has been used for more than 100 years to treat pain and anxiety.

However, in the past fifty years the study of psychopharmacology has expanded and led to the development of treatment for specific disorders. Moreover, the potential for the future development of pharmaceuticals to treat mental illness is even more impressive than what has happened in the past fifty years. As knowledge of the interaction between the brain and behavior increases, it is likely that we will develop knowledge of neurochemical and neurophysiological bases for memory, learning, moral aggression, appetite, and sexual lust. Hence, the treatment of major psychiatric disorders has become more pharmocologic and less psychotherapeutic.

Psychotropic drugs have proved highly effective in tranquilizing patients in manic states or with uncontrollable anxiety, reducing the condition of mental confusion and dissociation especially in schizophrenia, and lifting certain types of depression. These effects may be symptomatic rather than truly curative, but they raise hope that as these underlying organic causes are understood, more successful therapies and preventatives for mental illness can be developed. It is also clear, however, that drugs can never be the total answer to mental health because there are so many social factors involved in psychological development.

In sum, from an ethical point of view, the increasing reliance on pharmacotherapy seems justified by its results. However, we offer the following ethical admonitions for health care professionals insofar as the use of psychoactive drugs is concerned:

- Observe the principle of free and informed consent before prescribing psychoactive drugs.
- Do not succumb to the temptation to give pills, rather than to carefully diagnose and monitor the patient.
- Do not let prejudice in favor of the medical model of therapy lead to a neglect of psychotherapy when a need for it is indicated.
- Do not neglect assessing and monitoring the side effects of psychoactive drugs.
- Promote continued research to determine the value of psychoactive drugs and their safety.

Two main forms of therapy that follow the medical model, psychosurgery and electroconvulsive therapy (ECT), are not as frequently used at present because of the success of psychotherapeutic drugs. Nonetheless, we shall consider them briefly.

Psychosurgery or lobotomy is a surgical destruction of certain parts of the brain for the purpose of treating psychiatric conditions. Arguments on the ethics and merits of psychosurgery vary from severe condemnation to modified enthusiasm. One of the results of this surgical procedure is a blunting of human emotional response. Because of the dramatic effects of this form of behavior control on the emotional life of the patient, psychosurgery fell into disuse when psychoactive drugs became more effective ways to treat severe psychosis. Modern procedures, for example, ultrasound, electrical coagulation, or implanted radium seeds, are more localized and less destructive. Despite indications that these less severe interventions are helpful for severely depressed people, many scientists and physicians denounce all forms of psychosurgery. Those who argue in favor of it in specific cases cite the fact that some forms of epilepsy or severe depression in the elderly cannot be mitigated through the use of psychoactive drugs.

Lobotomy is an irreversible and drastic procedure, and lobotomized patients generally have inhibited, one-dimensional personalities. For this reason, we would discourage the use of this form of the medical model because it holds little hope of improving the mental health of the patient.

Another form of therapy using the medical model is ECT (or electrical stimulation of the brain). This form of treatment was initiated in the mid–twentieth century, and the theory was that violent stimulation of the brain would cause the readjustment of the neural patterns. Although shock therapy was sometimes effective, it could be dangerous, causing broken bones or heart attacks. When used again and again, it was said to leave the patient in the same condition as a lobotomy. After ECT became more widely used, it was criticized as being too brutal and invasive by psychiatrists who favored "talk therapy."

Today, ECT is administered more carefully, and it is accepted as preferred treatment for severe depression that will not yield to drugs, when the patient cannot tolerate drugs, or when the patient's condition is difficult to manage without rapid improvement. Among the elderly, it is often used to combat depression. Obtaining informed consent for the use of ECT is often a problem, because the patient may often be so depressed that he or she cannot respond adequately to the situation at hand, even though the patient may be aware and cognizant of the proposals presented by the health care professionals.

The reasons for efficacy of ECT are still unknown conclusively. What is certain, however, is that these procedures induce temporarily a severe loss of memory and a general state of psychic disorganization. Apparently, this makes it possible for some patients to break out of fixed patterns of fantasy and feeling and to respond to life situations in a more normal way. ECT is certainly a less invasive form of therapy than psychosurgery, but it should not be utilized unless informed consent, either of the patient or the guardian, is obtained. And it should never be applied without careful consideration of the potential outcome for the patient.

The *second conclusion*: Psychoactive drugs, which are less invasive and drastic then the other therapies of the medical model, psychosurgery and electroconvulsive therapy, may be considered an ethical way to treat mental illness. However, informed consent and greater emphasis upon research and safety are needed in their administration to patients with mental illnesses.

Therapies of the Psychotherapeutic Model

At present, although there is a plethora of psychotherapeutic methods, two very different conceptions of human psychological development are reflected in the two main schools of psychotherapy. These are *insight* therapy and *action* therapy. In practice, these therapies overlap, but they have different theoretical and clinical sources.

The insight therapies derive largely from Sigmund Freud and the psychoanalytical school, although they have now moved on to include a great variety of therapeutic methods other than psychoanalysis, and especially to take into consideration the social-group aspect of behavioral disorders. What characterizes these therapies is that they aim to help individuals *understand* ("gain insight into," "get in touch with") their own behavior and its affective sources and thus learn how to deal with life situations in an effective way. Thus, psychotherapy of this type deals with the lack of coordination between the rational level (and in the case of the therapy of Carl Jung, perhaps also with the spiritual level) and the psychological level of the personality. Normal persons have this coordination between rational and subrational processes, whereas neurotic or psychotic persons do not.

Action therapy is the outcome of the behaviorist school of psychology, which rejects or bypasses the whole notion of the subconscious because it does not consider the notion of consciousness to be of any great help in psychological theory. Human beings behave as they do because they live in a physical and social environment that has taught them to behave in a certain way through a kind of education that consists of an ordered series of rewards and punishments (positive and negative reinforcements) that favor some forms of behavior and eliminate others. Action therapy, therefore, is a process of reconditioning the person to a more self-consistent, socially acceptable type of behavior. Its methods do not depend on growth in insight in the subjects, need not explore how their malconditioning has arisen or even how the therapy works, but are aimed simply at removing undesirable behavior patterns and developing new ones.

These two points of view, which are often obscured by bitter polemics, are not necessarily contradictory. Action therapy reflects the fact that human behavior, which at first may be conscious and deliberate, quickly takes on a patterning and becomes automatic and subconscious. Thus, when a person is learning to drive a car or play the piano, each motion is conscious and deliberate. But once the habit is acquired, these actions can be performed without conscious attention. This applies also to motivation, because in general it is easier and more pleasant to perform in a habitual manner and more difficult and even painful to go against a habit or routine response.

Furthermore, in psychosocial development, the formation of such habits in the child precedes the time when the person is mature enough to have full self-consciousness and control. Action therapy, which is based on a highly developed theory of learning through conditioning, seeks to reeducate the patient by extinguishing undesirable patterns of behavior and establishing or strengthening desirable ones.

The insight therapists agree with the action therapists that the human being has many automatisms and that aberrant adult behavior is basically due to faulty conditioning in early childhood, when the organism is highly impressionable and the power of the ego to resist environmental influences is low. The emphasis of insight theories, however, is on the emergence of the ego or self as controlling behavior in an adaptive manner in the face of the natural and social environments. However, Freud and the psychoanalytic school too quickly assumed that a person who understands why he or she acts irrationally will spontaneously be free to act rationally.

Conversely, the goals of action therapy seem too limited because they are based on a narrow behavioristic conception of human life. Consequently, for the therapist simply to correct faulty habits in the client only treats symptoms. The real problem is to help patients develop a strong ego and to understand how they came to have faulty habits, so that they will be able under their own choice to form better ones. Hence, effective therapy requires at least some measure of exploration of the past and a growing insight into one's own personality structure.

It seems, therefore, that the two therapies can complement each other. Clients who have acquired insight into their own behavior and unconscious motivation may still need to be taught how to recondition themselves and to be aided by others in so doing. Thus, insofar as it is distinct from medical therapy, psychotherapy is not so much a process of healing a defective organic structure as of reeducation, not at the level of fully rational behavior, but rather at the level of automatic, conditioned, or subconscious behavior. Its purpose is to free the individual from undesirable patterns of behavior, especially those that are inconsistent with normal behavior, so that rational, free decisions become easier.

Goals of Psychotherapy

After surveying the bewildering array of insight therapies available, one therapist wrote that most therapies must settle for the following results to consider themselves successful:

1. The patient's weak ego is supported by the therapist's stronger ego.
2. The patient's lack of realism is corrected by the therapist's more realistic attitude.
3. The patient comes to see that many things he or she fears are not so terrible.
4. The patient learns to be more patient in solving problems, and less impulsive and panicky.
5. The patient acquires a greater or new faith, or "life-myth," from the example of the therapist, who represents a hope for health.
6. The patient gets a more objective perspective on his or her problems from discussing them with the therapist or with a therapy group.
7. The patient focuses his or her floating anxieties on the outcome of the therapy process, so as to feel less isolated and helpless.

At present, psychotherapeutic methods do not have a clear record of efficiency. Psychoanalytical methods are extremely time-consuming and expensive. The action therapists have argued that the insight therapists have very little objective proof that their methods succeed better than natural processes; furthermore, the success they have seems largely independent of the mode of therapy and mainly dependent upon the personal relation with a therapist who is a sensitive, realistic, and caring person.

The action therapists claim to have a better and more demonstrable record of success, but on examination this success mainly appears in rather restricted areas of phobias, and its permanence is often questioned. Furthermore, it often fails to achieve the ultimate aim of developing a strong autonomy in the patient. It must be concluded that this type of problem is very complex, and that knowledge about it and the ability to cure are still very limited. Nevertheless, there is no doubt that therapy is sometimes successful. Perhaps this is not so different from any other areas of medical care, let alone of ethical and spiritual guidance. It can never be stressed too much that all modes of therapy are only of service to facilitate the inherent power of the human beings as organisms and persons to heal themselves.

The *third conclusion:* Using the aforementioned goals, we can describe mental health as psychological freedom that is based on a realistic perception and understanding of the world, and that involves self-understanding, self-consistency, and self-control.

Human Freedom

Mental health is a prior condition requisite for dealing with ethical problems of moral right and wrong, because only to the degree that a person is free can there be the possibility of moral choice and moral responsibility.

In view of the multidimensional and integral character of human personality, it is important to emphasize that no human being is totally free. Human freedom is limited (1) by innate biological structure, determined genetically, with its innate needs and drive; (2) by unconscious conditioning of the sort described above; (3) by one knowledge of the world and self, set largely by the culture in which one lives; and (4) by the scope of experience and education. Psychotherapy deals principally, but not exclusively, with the limitations of human freedom that arise from the level of unconscious conditioning.

At the psychological level, the area of freedom is very limited in the psychotic person who is out of touch with reality. Most psychotic persons, however, have some area of human freedom at least sometime; that is why they can be reached by psychotherapy or chemotherapy. Neurotic persons are decidedly more free but have some areas of unfreedom that do not occur in normal persons. The normal person has limited areas of freedom, but its limits lie near the level of behavior that is compatible with normal freedom. The normal person is usually able to acknowledge his or her limits of freedom and, indeed, at times is able to see humor in these limitations.

Freedom demands not only trust between persons but within social groups. Recently, more methods of group therapy are becoming common, not only because of the expense of individual therapy but because mental illness is in part a disturbance of social relations and can be adequately treated only by learning social communication skills. In particular, family therapy—in which a family is treated as a dynamic system, whose malfunctions are reflected in the psychological problems of individual members— promises a radically effective approach to many mental problems that originate in the family.

Such methods raise special ethical issues, chiefly those of confidentiality and of adequate professional control. The frank communication required within the group can easily lead to an abuse of the privacy of individual members, and if the therapist does not remain fully in charge and sufficiently sensitive to the needs of each member, some especially fragile participants may be more hurt than healed by the experience.

Modern therapy has tended to move from the treatment of sexual neuroses, which were once common as a result of the Victorian refusal to recognize basic biological needs, to the treatment of anxiety, which is now common as a result of the excessive demands of a work-oriented society that fails to recognize human needs for leisure and intimacy. Hence, therapy deals more with neuroses of emptiness or lack of meaning as a result of society's failure to recognize the creative and spiritual sides of personhood. In all these cases, psychological therapy can only go so far to awaken the person's full capacity for freedom.

11.3   ETHICAL ISSUES IN PSYCHOTHERAPY

Punishment

On the basis of the distinctions just made, the first point about the ethics of psychotherapy is to reject any use of psychotherapy as punishment (although it must be admitted that the neurotic patient may at first perceive it as punishment, no matter what the therapist intends). Punishment and reward (in the proper sense of these words) belong only to ethical acts, that is, free, responsible acts. This, of course, requires penological reforms, by which the courts decide first on the facts of a criminal action and then separately on the moral responsibility of the person who has committed the act. In this second decision, expert testimony from psychiatrists should be admitted, but it should be directed toward determining whether the defendant's freedom was so limited by psychological factors as to remove his or her freedom with regard to this particular class of acts.

It must be remembered that the essential question in judging moral responsibility is not rationality in the sense of knowledge or in the sense of capacity to reason logically; nor is it voluntariness (i.e., whether one wills an action) but *moral freedom*, (i.e., the capacity to consider alternatives with their consequences and to choose one or the other without external or internal compulsion). This moral freedom can be destroyed mental confusion that makes it impossible to consider alternatives, by an emotional compulsion (overwhelming fear, pain, or passion) that compels the choice of one alternative, or perhaps by a pathological incapacity to foresee the consequences of one's actions or to appreciate them emotionally (sociopathy).

Therefore, psychiatrists called on in court for expert testimony, insofar as the present confusion of the law permits them, should be primarily concerned to make clear to the jury why, in their expert opinion, the accused's chronic or temporary psychological condition did or did not render him or her so unfree that he cannot be held responsible for the act of which he or she is accused, or if he or she is partially or remotely responsible for it, then in what degree or in what respect.

When a defendant is acquitted on the basis of lack of responsibility, then the court—in an entirely different process—should decide the question of involuntary commitment for treatment or of confinement to prevent the person from harming others or themselves. Such confinement, however, should not be dealt with as if it were punishment, because it would be unjust to punish someone for acts for which he or she was not morally responsible.

The question then arises whether psychiatrists should play any role in the process of punishment itself. It seems that their role should be limited to two functions: (1) Psychiatrists could diagnose prison inmates who develop mental illnesses and require occasional treatment exactly on the same basis as for medical ills; and (2) psychiatrists could act as consultants to penologists in setting up prison routines that make for good mental health and discipline, but they should not be engaged in staffing these services.

One authority states that the difficulty is that the psychiatric profession (1) does not like to take their own scientific criteria for mental illness to gather the necessary data to apply the criterion and (2) confines itself in court to stating its conclusions. What is necessary is that it gather the data on which a judgment can be made by the lay jury and that it present these data to the jury in such a way that the jury can make its own judgment of the validity of the expert conclusion. Only in this way can the adversarial process be applied so that juries can decide between conflicting expert opinions.

Informed Consent for Psychiatric Therapy

Granted that therapy has been carefully distinguished from punishment, which has no part in the therapeutic profession, what of the problem of the patient's informed consent? Clearly, here, as in other medical questions, the patient's free and informed consent is required if he or she is competent. The special problem, of course, is that mentally disturbed patients (1) may be unable to understand the purposes or risks of the treatment and (2) may not be truly free to make a decision even if they understand, because personal freedom is removed by irrational fear of the treatment or of the consequences of refusal, because of masochistic tendencies that lead a patient to submit to treatment out of a desire to suffer or be humiliated, or simply because of a narcissistic desire to be the center of attention.

Patients once self-committed to a hospital may then find themselves in a situation where in fact freedom to withdraw from highly traumatizing treatment is no longer practically possible. Yet every psychiatric institution must be dedicated to the proposition that it is therapeutic only to the degree that it really respects and seeks to enlarge the patient's capacity for freedom. If it lessens this capacity, it is countertherapeutic; it is making people ill rather than well.

Conversely, where it is rightly judged that free consent, at least in the area of treatment, is impossible, then a commitment must be made by the patient's guardian, and with scrupulous observance of due legal process. It is obvious that the guardian (usually a member of the family) may be biased, because of selfishness, ignorance, or more often through unconscious factors that may very well be part of the client's own breakdown.

If the treatment is carried out without the patient's consent, then a primary objective of the treatment must be to bring the patient as soon as possible to the level of mental integration where at least some self-determination becomes feasible. This means, of course, that the use of drugs or psychosurgery simply as a method of controlling patients or tranquilizing them cannot of themselves be legitimate therapeutic objectives. Undoubtedly, those who must care for patients who are out of control are strongly tempted to pacify them so that they "don't make trouble." This, of course, is permissible to prevent the patient from harming him- or herself or harming the therapist or others, but such self-defense is not *therapy*. It is only preliminary to therapy.

Value Systems and Psychotherapy

Perhaps the most serious issue for psychotherapy is whether the therapist is permitted to change the client's value system. The common answer is that a therapist should not change this system but should try to adjust the patient to the system. This answer, however, is somewhat disingenuous. As the existentialist psychoanalysts have pointed out, distortions in the patient's value system often underlie the disorder. Furthermore, the source of many problems is the patient's superego, which is in part the value system of the parents or society that has been incorporated into the unconsciousness of the child. Yet it is clear that if the psychological and ethical dimensions of human personality are distinct, as we have argued, then it cannot be the therapist's role to indoctrinate the patient in a value system.

In answer to this difficulty, we must say that there are certain values on which the very relation of patient to the therapist depends, and these values must be reinforced by therapy. Thus, the therapist must help the client to become more trustful, more honest, more hopeful, more courageous, more patient, and more realistic.

The effort of the therapist, then, is to extend the area of freedom for patients. As patients become freer, they must make free ethical decisions, and they will do so according to their own conscious, rational system of values. At this point, the therapist is nondirective, in the sense that it is not the therapist's task to give the patient ethical advice, but only to help the patient be free of illusion and neuroses in making decisions.

This limitation of the therapist's task may mean that the therapist sometimes thinks that the client's decisions are not ethically good, objectively speaking. In such a case, the therapist may point out that the client's decisions are questionable, or refer the client to an ethical counselor (a member of the clergy, a lawyer, or a friend), but the therapist should be careful not to take any responsibility for the person's decision. Thus, the therapist should refer the client to ethical or spiritual advisers if it becomes apparent that the client's value system is inconsistent or inadequate.

Persons undergoing therapy therefore should not change their system of values, divorce their partners, give up their religious vocation, or change their religion or their professional vocation merely under the influence of the psychotherapeutic process. Such changes should be made only when a real degree of psychological freedom has been reached and then under guidance that acts as a countervailing force to the possible ideology of the psychotherapeutic tradition. Thus, the tendency to transform one of the many forms of therapy (including the various mystical cults that are now so popular) into a religion is a violation of the lines between the psychological level of personality and the ethical and spiritual levels, and is doomed to end in disillusionment.

A deeper problem, however, is raised by contemporary critics of psychotherapy, especially of psychoanalysis. Is it possible that the whole system of insight therapy as it originated with Freud inculcates a built-in system of values or ideology? Thus, some have accused psychoanalysis in particular of being essentially a product of the middle class in opulent capitalist countries. Freud himself saw all of civilization as the imposition of social controls on humanity's infinite and even contradictory drives.

Consequently, according to Freud, every social system is a delicate balance between the repressive controls necessary for social life and work and the explosive drives of the id. If these critics are correct, the inherent ethic of psychoanalytical theory is to produce autonomous, hedonistic, goalless, conscienceless persons—the very sort that ethicists have always condemned as selfish, loveless, and empty. Obviously, such persons are individualistic in the extreme, because they are uncommitted to any social goal except the achievement of freedom to do what they please. These accusations are serious, but it seems that they are offset by leaders in the field of insight therapy and psychoanalysis in particular, such as Erik Erikson and Erich Fromm, who opt for a socially aware person, bent upon fulfilling genuine human needs as the goal of insight therapy.

Given the ethical issues that arise in psychotherapy, we reach the *fourth conclusion:* Therapists must be aware of the goal of psychiatry, namely, to make free moral decisions in accord with personal human needs. Freeing the patient from his or her neuroses or psychoses will require honesty and compassion on the part of the therapist.

11.4 ADDICTION

Generally speaking, addiction is habituation to some harmful practice. Although the term *addiction* usually refers to habituation to drugs, one can also be addicted to other detrimental substances or activities; for example, one can be addicted to alcohol or excessive food or to too much sleep, too much work, or too much pursuit of sexual pleasure. Although many people use all these things in ways that do not destroy human equilibrium, some persons, for a variety of reasons not fully understood, become addicted to them so that their whole life is more and more absorbed by a single activity that distorts the personality, consumes physical and psychic energy, and often results in an intense self-centeredness, personality deterioration, and an inability to communicate with others.

One component of chemical dependency, and the most obvious, is its hedonistic character, although persons who are in other respects very ascetic may fall victim to it, precisely because they lack healthy pleasures in their lives. The disposition for addiction to some pleasurable activity is an inability to gain pleasure from beneficial human activities. Too often, creative pleasures, such as reading, writing, and viewing works of art, are lacking in people's lives, and as a result, they are unable to seek pleasure above the sense level. For a well-balanced person, creative pleasure is as necessary as the pleasure that is associated with good food or a warm fire on a cold evening.

In the face of every difficulty of life, every tension or frustration, the chemically dependent person runs away from the loss of normal satisfaction and achievement by indulging in the physical pleasure, relaxation, and euphoria of the addicting experience. The search for pleasure alone does not constitute addiction, but rather the increasing guilt and helplessness that begin to accompany each overindulgence—with the result that the incipient addict begins to indulge not for the sake of pleasure itself but to blot out the guilt and remorse for the consequences of previous indulgences.

Furthermore, this vicious circle is reinforced by the use of psychological coping mechanisms of rationalization and denial that victims need to suppress guilt and pain, so that they become less and less able to perceive the real consequences of their behavior. Persons of very different personality types can become addicted, but a common feature is excessive dependency needs, which are not infrequently masked by outward aggressiveness and competitiveness. Moreover, recent research demonstrates that chemical dependency can affect people of all backgrounds. Often the gifted, talented, wealthy, and successful succumb to this severe personality problem.

Chemical dependency or addiction may be broadly classified as physiological or psychological. *Physiological addiction*, which causes a modification or need in the addict's physiological system, usually requires constantly increasing doses of the addicting substance to obtain the same physiological effect. *Psychological dependency* itself results from a learned conditioned behavior pattern that leads the victim to anticipate the pleasure and release of tension, even when the substance does not notably modify the physiological system. Both forms of addiction may exist in the same person and from the same activity.

Would chemical addiction be less of a problem in this country if it were considered a medical or social problem rather than a moral and legal one? Removing the moral stigma from addiction to alcohol has been helpful in assisting many people to overcome this addiction. Would a similar response to the use of drugs, plus legalization of narcotics for sustaining treatment of addicts, be beneficial over a long time? On the one hand, therapists speak of addiction as a "disease" to reduce its moral opprobrium and to achieve a more sympathetic attitude on the part of nonaddicts. On the other hand, it is always an important part of therapy to get addicts to accept moral responsibility for the harm they have done themselves and others through addiction.

This ambiguity can be cleared up if two points are kept in mind. First, chemical dependency is always a psychological disease, because it involves an abnormal behavior pattern accompanied by the neurotic coping mechanisms of rationalization and denial. It can also be a physiological disease, because it sometimes produces physiological dependency and usually produces widespread organic changes that greatly aggravate the condition.

Second, *voluntary* acts must be distinguished from *free* acts. Addictive behavior is voluntary in the sense that it proceeds from an inner compulsion, and the pleasure derived therefrom is pleasing to the addict. But addiction always involves a restriction of freedom, because the addict becomes less and less able to perceive alternatives of action or to choose among them. In times of addictive need, the practical conscience of the addict is concerned totally with the need for a drink or a fix. He or she acts voluntarily, compulsively, but without fully free choice.

Hence, the actual consumption of addictive substances by addicts is seldom in itself a morally culpable act, and the guilt felt afterward is unrealistic and neurotic. Even the acquisition of the addiction often proceeds so gradually and subtly that it is difficult to judge that the addict chose addiction knowingly and deliberately. Nevertheless, it would be a mistake to think that all of the guilt felt by addicts is illusory. If it were, it would be hard to explain why admission of responsibility has proved so important a part of therapy.

The truth seems to be that the real moral responsibility of the addicted person lies in the obligation to ask and receive help from others when this is offered, because therapy cannot be effective until the addict accepts help. Hence, it is a mistake to reduce this complex situation either to a purely moral question or to a purely sociological or medical one. To deny all moral responsibility or capacity to change is to degrade addicts as persons, yet to pass judgment on their degree of responsibility is to not see the many ways in which they are victims of forces beyond individual control.

Unfortunately, there is a tendency today to treat all problems of addiction as though they were medical problems that may be cured through hospitalization and drugs. Yet the most successful therapy program for addicts, namely, Alcoholics Anonymous (AA), and the several programs that follow the Twelve-Step AA philosophy require neither hospitalization nor drugs. Rather, AA requires one to acknowledge the existence of a higher power, to ask for forgiveness from the people one has hurt, and to rely upon a community of friends for enlightenment and support.

Students of addiction emphasize that the earlier in the addiction therapy takes place the better, but they also point out that family and employers commonly contribute to the problem by covering up, excusing, or attempting to endure addictive behavior, hoping that the addict will finally come to his or her senses. In fact, this spontaneous self-insight on the part of addicts is very rare, and family, friends, and employers have a serious ethical responsibility to face the facts realistically and intervene decisively and persistently until the addict accepts treatment. Intervention is best done by those who can be supportive rather than judgmental but who can also face the addict with detailed evidence of the seriousness of his or her condition.

Human beings grow as persons by facing the difficulties and struggles of life realistically, "bearing one another's burdens" (Gal 6:2) as free people, not as slaves to a pleasure ethic. In saying this, we are not proposing an exaggerated stoicism as the Christian ideal, but a realistic effort to overcome the actual causes of suffering, rather than an escape into unconsciousness. As was mentioned above, AA, which has led the way in the most successful methods of therapy for chemical dependency, has always emphasized that the addict cannot recover without reaching out for a higher power and being willing to repair the damage done to others and to be of service to others, especially to fellow victims of addiction.

Our *fifth conclusion:* Although addiction has many elements resembling a disease, recovery from addiction depends to a certain extent upon the addicted person and upon the community of persons that will assist the person in recovery. Today, addiction to drugs and alcohol is rampant in our society. This is another indication, it seems, of the extreme individualism that characterizes our thinking.

SUMMARY

Given these various methods of therapy for mental illness and addiction, we suggest seven ethical principles that should govern their use, all of which apply the general principle of human dignity in community, which requires that social control enhance the dignity of the members of the community, not reduce them to mere means of political manipulation.

First, no form of treatment may be used that will destroy human freedom. In *The Human Body*, Pius XII stated this well when he wrote:

> In exercising one's right to dispose of oneself or one's faculties and organs, the individual must observe the hierarchy of individual goods to the extent demanded by the laws of morality, so, for example, a person cannot perform upon him or herself or allow medical operations, either physical or somatic, which beyond doubt do remove serious defects or physical or psychic weaknesses, but which entail at the same time permanent destruction of or a considerable lasting lessening of freedom, that is to say, of the human personality in its particular and characteristic functions. (Pius XII 1979, 199)

Thus, any form of psychosurgery, personality manipulation, or use of psychoactive drugs that would remove or severely limit human freedom or destroy human personality could not be permitted and could need legal control.

Second, if the purpose of the therapy for mental illness is therapeutic, then the benefit to the patient must be proportionate to the damage or risk to be endured. A frontal lobotomy, for example, should be performed only as a last resort and with some indication that the patient will benefit. As a general rule, signs of organic brain pathology should be present before psychosurgery is approved.

Third, if the purpose of the treatment is therapeutic, the long-range effect of the treatment must be considered, as well as the short-range alleviation of some particular difficulty. Simply because a particular therapy alleviates or eliminates a symptom does not mean that it is ethically acceptable. Most of the drugs currently available for the relief of anxiety and tension carry some danger of dependency, habituation, and addiction. Such dependency diminishes human freedom and dignity and hence is to be avoided. Thus, the practice of using psychoactive drugs to treat psychological difficulties when the disorder lacks a physiological or organic basis must be questioned. Would it not be better to treat the causes of anxiety or depression through counseling or increased self-awareness than to depend on pills that merely treat the symptoms? Questions such as this are fundamental in developing a philosophy of health care, and they are too often neglected in the search for easier, but less beneficial, solutions.

Fourth, if behavior controls are used, the rules of free and informed consent apply, including the right to refuse treatment. Thus, psychoactive drugs and psychotherapy should not be inflicted or imposed upon people.

Moreover, children, prisoners, and people with limited awareness should not be subjected to experimental behavioral control, nor should proxy consent be given unless the treatment is truly therapeutic for them.

Fifth, the principle of professional communication as regards confidentiality must be applied with special care in psychotherapy, because the patient's trust in the therapist is of fundamental importance.

Sixth, experimental research on behavioral control should conform to the norms explained above in the section on human experimentation.

Seventh, the use of behavioral control procedures to improve such human capabilities as memory, intelligence, and sexual abilities would seem to be licit if free consent is given, if there is no other way to achieve the same goal, and if the action is in accord with the integrity of the human person. In itself, human betterment or human improvement is ethically acceptable and beneficial. Care must be exercised, however, to make sure that the basic integrity of the person is not violated and that addiction does not result in the course of seeking self-improvement.

We have the ethical goals to help people overcome mental illness or harmful behavior. However, both forms of therapy must be analyzed carefully, lest individuals' rights be violated or the freedom of the person be weakened or destroyed. Care must be exercised, then, when helping the mentally ill regain their health, so that the person's higher needs and functions are considered.

QUESTIONS

1. What are the relationships among mental illness, human freedom, and personal sin?
2. What is the meaning of the term a *normal person*, and what criteria determine whether or not a person is normal?
3. What is the proper attitude of a counselor or psychotherapist in relation to the value system of a neurotic or psychotic patient? Who sets the goals for therapy, and why?
4. What is the process of acquiring addictive behavior, and what moral responsibilities does the subject have at various stages of the process? Are the present methods of drug rehabilitation founded upon practices that are psychically and ethically sound?

CASES

1. A halfway house for recovering psychiatrics and patients is proposed for your neighborhood. Your neighbors, fearing for their safety and

property values, protest the location of the facility in your area. What arguments would you use to help them reconsider their decision?

2. Whenever we make an ethical evaluation of a human activity, it is essential that we have a firm notion of its purpose. For example, when evaluating the practice of medicine, it is important to realize that the purpose of medicine is not simply to prolong life as long as possible, but rather to prolong life in a manner that is beneficial for the patient. In the practice of psychiatry, therapists all have different ideas about the purpose of their therapy. Using the concepts contained in the earlier chapters of this book, how would you describe the goals of psychotherapy for the patient; for the therapist?

3. Jerry is forty years old and has been a priest for fifteen years. He is experiencing severe anxiety about the effectiveness of his priestly ministry and dissatisfaction with his present parochial assignment. He approaches his bishop with these problems. The bishop responds that Jerry is not praying enough; otherwise, he would be a happy priest. Jerry comes to you as a friend; how would you seek to help him?

4. Mary, a mother and housewife, enjoys several martinis before preparing dinner for her husband and four children. After she burns the main course three nights in a row, Harry, her husband, suggests that she might have a problem with alcohol. Mary violently rejects the idea, but later asks your opinion. Is Mary's reaction to be expected? How should Harry proceed in his dialogue with Mary?

12

Death and Dying

OVERVIEW: This chapter explores several ethical issues that are associated with dying and death. First, we probe the mystery of death and view it from the perspective of faith. Then we consider the biological signs that should be used to determine the fact of death. The need to care for the dying in a Christian manner leads to the following considerations:

1. **Should dying persons be told the truth about their condition?**
2. **Is euthanasia or assisted suicide part of Christian health care?**
3. **May life support be withheld or withdrawn from patients?**
4. **Who should make decisions concerning the use of life support?**
5. **What effort may be made to alleviate pain as death approaches?**
6. **What care should be given the body of a person who has died?**

12.1 THE MYSTERY OF DEATH

Although each person will experience death and the physical and psychic suffering associated with death, death is the great human mystery. Why does a merciful God allow suffering and death? "Death was not God's doing; he takes no pleasure in the extinction of the living. To be—for this he created all"(Wis 1:13–14). God had not wished to include suffering and death in human destiny. Whence, then, came suffering and death? Saint Paul says, "Through one man sin entered the world and with sin death, death thus coming to all men inasmuch as all sinned" (Rom 5:12).

This original sin was essentially a sin of pride, the will to be like God, not by using God's gifts to come closer to God in community, but by using these gifts to set up the human individual in self-centered domination of the world apart from God. It is this misuse of God's gifts from the beginning of the human race to this day that has prevented humankind from overcoming the natural causes and transformed natural death—which might have been a joyful completion of this life and a serene passage into a greater life—into a blind, terrifying mystery.

People have turned their backs on God, yet he has not turned from them but has offered them forgiveness and restoration. In his mercy, however, he cannot deny their human freedom but has called them to return to him, not simply by restoring them to their innocent beginnings, but through a long history of struggle and learning from experience, an experience in which suffering is inevitable. For the Christian and for all who travel the same road in less clear ways, God has revealed in Christ the direction of their journey and the power of grace by which it can be traveled. In baptism, according to Saint Paul (Rom 6:1–11), humankind has died and been reborn in a new creation that will be completed in the resurrection of the body in eternal life.

Men and women live now in such unity with Christ that all the events of their lives take on meaning from his life and death. Consequently, both the joy and the suffering of this life have a Christian meaning: Its joys are signs of the hope for everlasting life in his kingdom, which is already present here on earth in promise; and its sorrows are a sharing in his cross, through which a victorious resurrection is to be achieved.

Jesus came to conquer suffering and death. In what sense has he succeeded? People still get sick and continue to suffer, and death is inevitable. He conquered sickness, suffering, and death in the sense that he gave them a new meaning, a new power. By believing in Jesus as Savior, by joining suffering and death to his, humankind overcomes the evil aspect of suffering and death. Through his sacrifice, human beings are able to conquer the evil that is associated with suffering and death. Although the results of original and actual sin are still present in life, they no longer dominate it and they no longer serve as punishment for one who suffers with Christ. Rather, suffering and death are transformed into the very actions that help men and women fulfill their destiny.

At one time, death was defined as the separation of body and soul. Although this definition is true, it is no longer adequate. In their attempts to specify more clearly what it means to die, modern theologians have concentrated on death as a personal act of a human being—an act that terminates earthly existence but that also fulfills it. Hence, the person is not merely passive in the face of death, and death is different for the just and the sinner.

In the view of Karl Rahner, a view accepted and developed by many theologians, death is an active consummation, a maturing self-realization that embodies what each person has made of himself or herself during life. Death becomes a ratification of life, not an inevitable meaningless process. It is an event, an action in which the freedom of the person is intimately involved. Dying with Christ is an adventure, a consequence of, but not a penalty for, sin. This is a new approach to death, yet it is thoroughly in keeping with the Christian tradition. Indeed, this view of death seems to describe more clearly the experience of Christ, who offered his life, rather than have it taken from him, who completed his love and generosity in the final act of obedience to the Father.

Our *first conclusion:* Although death, from a human perspective, will always be a mystery, its ultimate meaning may be known through faith; death is the act by which we culminate our lives and prepare for transformation into eternal life.

12.2 DETERMINING THE MOMENT OF DEATH

When biologists speak of the death of any living organism, they refer to that inevitable and critical moment when an organism ceases to function as a specific, unified, homeostatic system and becomes disorganized into a mere collection of heterogeneous chemical substances. Sometimes, however, even after this moment, some tissues or cells of the former living organism may continue temporarily to carry on some minimum of life functions before they cease to live or are artificially sustained in the laboratory.

From a biological point of view, the death of a human organism is like any death and is determined in much the same way, by various signs that the unifying life force is no longer united to the matter with which it was at one time unified. Usually, the separation of spirit and body is verified by a body's lack of sensation and self-movement. But people believe that human death is something more than the absence of sensation and unified activity. Human death has a mystery about it, because at death we lose touch irrevocably with a person who previously was able to communicate and to share our human community of thought, of love, of freedom, and of creativity. Human death is not merely a decay of an organism; it is the departure of a member from the human community.

All over the world, people have interpreted this departure of someone known and loved as the separation of a spiritual soul from its body. Certainly, science is unable to close the door on such an explanation. Christians are convinced that the departed person will return in their fully, bodily personhood in a transformed existence, as Jesus did. In any case, people often have the painful responsibility of determining when the death of another has occurred, because the time of death influences many other human decisions, such as inheritance, the legal and moral rights of the dying person, spiritual care for the dying person, and the possibility of an organ transplant.

Dying is a process, but death is an event. We can be certain this event has not yet occurred as long as a person can communicate through speech or gesture. When such communication ceases, we can only judge by signs that the person is no longer distinctly and specifically human. Yet we do not dare to conclude quickly that death has occurred merely because specific human signs are no longer evident, as becomes very clear when we observe some-one wake from sleep or a coma.

Consequently, we are obliged morally to treat anybody who is appar-ently human, even in the fetal state, as a human person with human rights until we are sure that this body has become so disorganized that it no longer retains its human unity. To know this, we must be reasonably sure of three things: (1) that the body does not now exhibit specific human behavior, (2) that it will not be able to function humanly in the future, and (3) that it no longer has even a radical capacity for human functions because it has lost the basic structures required for human unity. This third condition is required because medical experience has shown that persons who have been in a prolonged, apparently irreversible coma nevertheless have sometimes recovered full human consciousness. Such resuscitation is possible as long as the radical structures of the human organism remain and the causes that inhibit their normal function can be removed. This is why some speculate that in the future the human body may be able to be frozen and revived cen-turies later.

Yet there is no reason to deny that after true human death some cells or even organs of the human body may for a time (perhaps indefinitely, if arti-ficially supported) continue to exhibit some life functions that are not those of the human organism as a unified entity but merely a residual life at a level of organization comparable to that of plants and lower animals. Hence, the essential point about determining human death is not to decide whether *any* life is present, but whether human life in the most radical sense of a unified human person is still present.

Signs of Death

Certainly, some signs of human death are always easy to identify. If rigor mortis or putrefaction has set in, then even nonprofessionals are able to rec-ognize that the human organism is irreversibly dysfunctional and dead. Other less conclusive signs of death are the absence of breathing and heart-beat, although these signs might be reversed by resuscitation. When resus-citation fails, death is judged to have occurred. Physicians are required to pronounce the patient dead on the basis of such evidence and to certify the time of death for legal purposes such as inheritance. Thus, the irreversible cessation of spontaneous heart and lung functions are known as the *clinical* signs of death.

In recent times however, two developments have led to the proposal of a new set of clinical signs for determining the fact of human death. First of all, mechanical devices have been perfected to aid heart and lung functions artificially or to enable a person to be resuscitated after these functions have ceased for a short time. People often recover full and spontaneous functions after being temporarily assisted by such devices, proving that the radical structures of the unified human organism had not been destroyed.

Such mechanisms have been able to maintain heart and lung activity, and to send profuse blood through the body (at least temporarily) even after the unity of the organism has ceased to exist. Yet although this mechanical assistance may keep some of the organs alive for awhile, and the living individual organs may simulate unity, unity is no longer present because the organs would cease to function if the mechanisms were removed.

Thus, artificially sustained heart and lung activity is not proof that human life still remains. Yet as long as these organs are sustained mechanically, it is impossible to verify the traditional signs of human death. Therefore, the question arose: Are there other clinical signs that can be used, not to constitute a new definition of death, but rather as alternative, complementary ways to establish the same essential fact, namely, the irreversible cessation of *spontaneous* heart and lung functions.

The second, and perhaps more important, reason for seeking new clinical signs of death has been the recent advancement of techniques of transplanting organs, especially the kidney and heart. Such transplants are more likely to be successful if the organs are harvested from a body through which blood is circulating, although this is not absolutely necessary. Hence, surgeons prefer to keep the body of a "dead" donor "alive" on a respirator. How, then, is it possible to be sure that the donor is in fact dead?

Is the Person Dead?

Three issues must be addressed before a person can be declared dead. First, the traditional cardiovascular clinical signs are basic and sufficient and should be retained; the new brain death criteria should be employed only when such signs cannot be used because the dying person depends on a respirator or other form of artificial maintenance. If brain death is permitted to become the exclusive definition (as is the increasing tendency in some states), the tendency will be to require elaborate tests in a hospital before declaring a person dead, even though the dying person will not be an organ donor. Current moral dilemmas about how to determine death are in large part the result of excessive reliance on technology; this reliance should be moderated rather than encouraged.

Second, the new brain death criteria must be ascertained by well-trained professionals. Human error and even carelessness must be anticipated and avoided. How can errors be prevented when human life is at stake? The *Harvard Criteria for Brain Death* (1968), one of the original statements in the United States concerning the criteria for brain death, envisions a process of observation for no less than twenty-four hours. Moreover, the persons using the electroencephalogram (EEG) must be trained to recognize such conditions as hypothermia and drug-induced coma, which may produce a flat EEG in a patient who can recover, because the flat EEG alone is not an infallible sign of death. Today, shorter intervals of observation are allowed (e.g., six hours), and the EEG may be replaced by an angiogram to test blood flow in the cerebellum.

Third, and most serious, is the issue of the nature of brain death itself. It is critical that the criteria used to certify brain death establish that the person is dead, not merely dying or in a deep coma. Although the medical profession has accepted the general idea of using the brain as the main criterion in some cases to establish human death, just which specific signs should be used to determine that human death has occurred have not been agreed upon by all. Thus, one group of physicians maintains that irreversible cessation of brain functions is not sufficient to signify human death because that does not indicate that the brain has been destroyed. Most neurosurgeons would respond that if the brain has ceased irreversibly to function, then it is destroyed because blood is not circulating effectively, even though the brain may not have lost all signs of cellular activity. It is not our purpose to settle any of the differences of opinion in regard to medical matters. However, our *second conclusion:* When total and irreversible function of brain activity is proved through accepted clinical signs, then the person in question is dead because the principle of life (soul) is no longer able to inform the matter (body). To date, many states have approved this method of discerning human death in so-called definition of death legislation, and the need for national legislation in this regard has been recommended. The legislation of the various states requires that the signs indicate that total, not merely partial, death of the brain has occurred.

Partial Brain Death

Would it be possible to change medical and legal requirements and declare a person dead if only some part of the brain—that is, the higher or neocortical centers on which it appears specifically human thought processes depend—ceased to function? Support for this position has arisen recently because of the desire to use anencephalic infants as organ donors before death occurs. Anencephalic infants are born with a severely depleted or undeveloped cerebral cortex because of a neural tube anomaly during pregnancy. They die shortly after birth. Some lawyers and philosophers (but few transplant surgeons) recommend taking organs from these infants before death, so that other infants may have their lives prolonged as a result of the transplant. Of course, the anencephalic infants would be killed as a result of losing vital organs. The basis for allowing anencephalic infants to be organ donors is founded upon consequentialist reasoning—they will die soon anyway, and great good will result from using them in this way)—or from the theory that cortical death constitutes human death.

Despite some support for the position that cortical death constitutes human death, this position presents several difficulties. First, if people with spontaneously functioning hearts and lungs, but no other vital signs, are declared dead, what about people who have weak signs of "human life"? If those in a deep and irreversible coma are declared dead insofar as human life is concerned, what about people who are mentally retarded or senile? Do they show sufficient signs of human life to be kept alive? Or should minimal care be given only to those who no longer have the functioning signs of human life that are associated with activity of the cortical center of the brain? Persons who argue for the elimination of the retarded, senile, infirm, and debilitated in certain circumstances believe partial brain death should be accepted as a proper clinical sign for human death. But society must go very slowly in accepting such a definition unless it is willing to bury people when they are still breathing and their hearts are pulsating spontaneously.

If the criteria of partial brain death were to be used as a sufficient evidence of death, ethical responsibility would require certitude about three matters of fact. First, the radical structures necessary and sufficient to constitute the unified organism of the human person would have to be found in the human brain separated from the rest of the body.

Second, most of the brain would have to be considered unnecessary for the specifically human functions of thinking and willing but existing only to maintain and move the body and supply the higher brain centers with nourishing materials. It is generally recognized today that the brain is a system of subsystems that are intimately interdependent. Although it is possible to localize such functions as speech and sight in particular parts of the brain, this is not proof that only one such part is involved in the function or even that it is its primary center, because inhibition of a merely secondary or auxiliary part of a system may impede its function.

Third, if it were certain that these higher centers are sufficient for the radical unity of the human organism, it would be very difficult to determine their exact condition without an autopsy. The mere absence of function would not establish their condition. Some day, it may be possible to determine when in special cases such centers are totally destroyed, but at present this is not the case.

Thus, our *third conclusion:* Although total brain death is a sufficient criterion for human death, partial brain death is not a sufficient criterion. Thus, we do not believe that death should be certified as long as patients are able to maintain spontaneous breathing and a heartbeat, because this constitutes strong evidence that the brain as the seat of the radical unity of the human body is still living, even if there is no evidence of its higher functions.

Although even then there may be reasonable doubts, the benefit of the doubt should be given to the person in question.

12.3 TELLING TRUTH TO THE DYING

"What to tell the patient?" has been considered one of the more difficult and delicate ethical questions for health care professionals. The principle of professional communication is relevant here. In the not-too-distant past, some physicians and other health care professionals thought that the less the patients knew about their condition, the better would be their chances of recovery. Moreover, some professionals would even withhold information about impending death, fearing that such knowledge might lead a person to despair. Because of an awakened moral sense on the part of professionals and a sharper realization that patients have legal and moral rights that must be respected, today there is a much greater tendency to be open and honest with patients concerning their condition. In general, patients have the right to the truth concerning their condition, the purpose of the treatment to be given, and the prognosis of the treatment. The *Ethical and Religious Directives for Catholic Health Facilities* (hereafter, the *Directives*; see appendix 1) declare:

> Persons in danger of death should be provided with whatever information is necessary to help them understand their condition and have the opportunity to discuss their condition with their family members and care providers. They should also be offered the appropriate medical information that would make it possible to address the morally legitimate choices available to them. (directive 55)

Clearly, information concerning serious sickness or impending death is to be furnished even if the individual does not ask for it. Legal precedent as well as moral concern prompts this realization. Hence, physicians and other health care professionals may not defend their lack of communication on the grounds that the patient did not wish to know and did not ask questions. Although health care professionals usually respect patients' rights insofar as providing the proper information is concerned, difficult situations often arise, and health care professionals hesitate to tell patients their true condition.

Even though the medical personnel might fear untoward results if patients are informed of their true condition, this does not mean that patients should not be given an accurate assessment of their condition. Indeed, in these situations, health care professionals should remember that the depression that often afflicts a patient after being diagnosed with a fatal disease may be due to the patient's lack of knowledge.

Hence, the medical team, along with a friend of the patient or a member of the family, should work together and prepare the patient so that he or she will be able to accept the truth. Interviews with people who are seriously ill and with dying patients have revealed that they do not wish to be kept continually in doubt about their condition; however, they do not want to find out about it abruptly or brutally.

The *fourth conclusion:* Increased knowledge of psychology and greater regard for the subjective process that accompanies sickness and dying has changed the ethical question in regard to truth telling. As Elisabeth Kübler-Ross (1969, 183) declares: "The question should not be 'should we tell?' but rather, 'How do we share this with the patient?'"

12.4 EUTHANASIA AND SUICIDE

The word "euthanasia" is derived from two Greek words that mean "good death" or "happy death." For centuries, the term referred to an action by which a person was put to death painlessly, usually to avoid further suffering from an incurable disease or to end an irreversible coma. *Webster's New International Dictionary* (3d ed.), for example, defines euthanasia as "a mode or act of inducing death painlessly as a relief from pain." Euthanasia in this sense is often called "mercy killing" or even "death with dignity." In this more traditional meaning of the term, it could be performed with or without the consent of the person to be put to death. In the Judeo-Christian moral tradition, euthanasia without the consent of the patient is murder, and with consent of the patient is both suicide and murder. Today, the proponents of euthanasia generally defend it in this latter form, in which the patient's consent is given or at least presumed. Thus our ethical analysis needs to begin with the question of whether suicide is ever permissible or whether it exceeds the limits of rightful control over one's own life.

It is important to be clear that the issue here is not whether persons who commit suicide are to be morally condemned. No doubt the great majority of persons who take their own lives do so because they are so emotionally disturbed that they act compulsively, or at least their perception of objective reality is so distorted by their anguish and depression that their freedom of choice is greatly restricted. Psychiatrists who specialize in suicide and the conditions of mind that lead to it regard suicide as an irrational act resulting from a state of depression or despair. Consequently, either the act of suicide is not to be evaluated ethically at all, or at least it may be assumed that persons who commit suicide act in good faith and are subjectively guiltless. Can this assumption really be made, or is there the possibility that the decision about whether to live or to take one's life may be a genuine ethical issue for some people who have the capacity to make a free and sane choice? Only in such cases does it make any sense to talk about the morality of suicide.

The monotheistic religions of Judaism, Christianity, and Islam have always opposed suicide because they regard life as God's gift, which his children are to use as faithful stewards. Moreover, these monotheistic religions, unlike others, hold that eternal life is not the survival of a disembodied soul, nor endless reincarnation, but resurrected life with God. Consequently, Christians cannot escape accounting to God for stewardship of the human life given them on earth, nor can they reject the body, which will always be part of them. This view was already anticipated by the great Greek philosopher Plato, who argued that suicide is a rejection of a person's duty to his or her body; to the community of which the person is a part; and to God, who gave the person life. In a very different way, another great philosopher, Immanuel Kant, argued that suicide is the greatest of crimes because it is a person's rejection of morality itself, because a person must be his or her own moral lawgiver. To kill oneself is to treat oneself as a thing (a means) rather than as a person.

It is probable that the personal reasons for suicide often underlie the social arguments. Basically, persons kill themselves because "there is no other way out." The question, therefore, is whether this can ever be reasonably said to be true. There is no doubt that one can feel this way easily enough, but can one conscientiously judge that it is really the case?

Essentially, humans are historical beings oriented to the future. As long as there is hope for a future, suicide is clearly unreasonable. When this hope is closed off, however, suicide may look like a rational thing to do. Yet in a Christian scheme of values, hope in God grounds the future. By God's providence, even the most painful situations not only can be endured but also may be extremely important events in the completion of earthly life. In a humanist system this may not be true, but Christians should wait on the God who gave them life, because he knows best how to prepare them for the mystery of eternal life with him.

Granted that suicide is intrinsically wrong, it also becomes clear that active euthanasia is also wrong, although many today, mainly because they see no value in suffering, would contest this issue. When sufferers freely choose to die and ask to be killed, they are not only committing the crime of suicide but are also compounding it by making another a partner in the crime. To yield to such a request is false compassion. To have true compassion for the person who has made such a decision is to realize that the person is hopeless, alienated from community, and doubtful of God's love. The mercy killer in such a case is really adding a final rejection to the many rejections that have already driven the person to that point of despair.

But if the sufferer is no longer really free to make a truly human decision and is pleading to be put out of the pain or depression that has taken away the sufferer's capacity to think straight, then the mercy killer is simply a murderer putting to death someone no longer able to protect himself or herself.

Moreover, if the person who carries out the killing is a physician, he or she destroys the trust that must be the basis of an effective patient–physician relationship in society.

If the motives of mercy killers are examined, their claim that they did it for the victim's sake cannot be easily accepted. The real motive may well be that the relative did not want to accept the responsibility of loving the dying person to the end. Often the killer says, "I loved my mother, I couldn't bear to see her suffer!" It is true in such a case that the killer could not bear to see her suffer, but the quality of that love is not so certain. No doubt, however, sometimes mercy killers are themselves not free enough from tortured feelings to make a sane decision.

The *fifth conclusion:* Euthanasia, whether voluntary (suicide) or involuntary (mercy killing) is contrary to the good of human persons as well as a denial of God's providential care for human beings. Hence, it is an unethical action, even though subjective guilt for the act of suicide or mercy killing may be mitigated by reason of emotional disturbance or despair.

12.5 ALLOWING A PERSON TO DIE

For the Christian, human life is a gift from the Creator, control of which implies stewardship, not absolute autonomy. It is like the talents given by the master to his servants, which he expects them to invest to gain him a proper return (Mt 25:14–30). Hence, this gift of human bodily life in this existence must be used for a good purpose. Such life, however, is not the ultimate value for the Christian, which is to be found only in serving God and living with him forever.

The time may come, therefore, when someone is reasonably convinced that life is coming to an end, and a prolongation of dying by additional complicated medical treatment is not the best investment the person can make of what time remains. Hence, if further therapy "does not offer a reasonable hope of benefit or imposes an excessive burden" (*Directives*, directive 56) insofar as attaining the spiritual purpose of life is concerned, it may be refused. It would be better, one might judge, to use the remaining time to compose oneself for death than to extend life in a profitless way that would only add to suffering and confusion of spirit for oneself and for relatives and friends.

To reject such additional medical efforts is not to reject life itself, or the God who gave it, but simply to reject well-meant efforts that will not help in completing the task of striving to fulfill the purpose of life. A decision to allow oneself to die in such circumstances is not the equivalent of suicide. On the contrary, it should be considered as the acceptance of the human condition, or as a wish to avoid the application of a medical procedure disproportionate to the results that can be expected, or as a desire not to impose excessive expense on the family or the community.

Notice then that the determination of what offers no hope of benefit or an excessive burden is not to be made solely by assessing the physiological function, the physical pain, or the monetary expenditure associated with the therapy. Prolonged physiological function, physical pain, and the money involved are to be evaluated insofar as they affect an individual's ability to serve God and neighbor (strive for the spiritual purpose of life). Unless one keeps the spiritual purpose of life in mind when evaluating life-prolonging measures, ultimately one uses physiological function or economic criteria (cost-benefit ratio) as the sole standard for making difficult ethical decisions.

In the same way, the relatives and the medical professionals who care for a dying person who is unable to make competent decisions may judge that any further efforts to preserve life will be ineffective or of no significant benefit and may even make it more difficult for the person to finish the course of life in peace, composure, and union with God. Hence they can make the decision to terminate the supports that prolong the dying process and allow the person to die more quickly.

Finding the right words to express the judgment that efforts to prolong life are no longer beneficial is difficult. We wish to avoid saying that a person has "a right to die," as many seem to be doing today or that human beings exist "to get to heaven," or that one may be allowed to die if "life is useless." All these terms can lead to faulty conclusions. For example, some means of prolonging life may be useless, but human life is never useless because of the dignity of the gift and the transcendence of the Giver. Moreover, if one admits there is "a right to die," then some would conclude that suicide is licit, which is not to be easily conceded.

In discussing the decision to allow oneself or another to die, it is wise to avoid all slogans and spell out completely what one implies by this ethical terminology, recognizing that the distinction is difficult to define. Each case should be decided on its own merits. No class of persons should be refused therapy. The decision to withhold or remove life support should not be made unless a fatal pathology is present; that is, an illness or disease from which the person will die if therapy is not utilized. Hence, life support should not be withheld from the retarded or severely debilitated simply because they are disabled.

After discerning the presence of a fatal pathology, one or two questions should be asked. The first is:

1. Does the therapy offer hope of benefit insofar as helping the person strive for the goods and goals of life (the spiritual purpose of life)?

If death is judged to be imminent and inevitable no matter what, life support is used, or if the person cannot be restored to cognitive-affective function, then the life support may be judged ineffective. Only if the response to the first question is affirmative, the second question—about the degree of burden that the life-supporting therapy will impose—should be asked:

2. Will the burden resulting from the therapy impede significantly the person's quest to fulfill the goods and goals of life (the spiritual purpose)?

Answering this second question will involve more subjective response on the part of the patient. Some persons, if forced to live as a quadriplegic and be respirator dependent for the rest of life, would choose to have the respirator removed, even though death would ensue. Others would declare that this form of therapy does not impose an intolerable burden and not wish the respirator removed. This method of removing life support is based upon the Christian view of the purpose of human life; a principle that should be the basis for all our free decisions.

A final principle concerning the removal of life support is that the intention of the people removing the life support should never be to kill the patient. In actual clinical cases, it is clear that when patients, physicians, and families determine to remove life support, they do not have the intent to kill the patient. If possible, they would prolong the life of the patient if there were some hope of benefit or no excessive burden. Rather, their intention is to stop doing something futile (therapy with no hope of benefit) or to remove a burden imposed by the therapy (burdensome therapy). Death is the result of an indirect intention.

Ordinary and Extraordinary Means to Prolong Life

In the tradition of Catholic moral theology, the terminology *ordinary and extraordinary means to prolong life* is used most frequently to describe medical therapy that must be utilized or that may be omitted. However, the use of these terms is often misleading, for three reasons. First, as is explained in the next section, ethicists and physicians often use these terms with different meanings. Second, the terms are often used as principles, rather than conclusions. No medical therapy may be judged to be ordinary or extraordinary until the two questions noted above (does the therapy offer hope of benefit, or is it an excessive burden?) have been answered. Answering these questions accurately requires a thorough diagnosis and prognosis of the illness and a knowledge of the patient's spiritual condition. Third, some people use the terms ordinary and extraordinary in the abstract. Thus, they speak about medical procedures or technology as being ordinary or extraordinary before referring the procedure or technology to a particular patient. A respirator or tube feeding may not be defined as ordinary or extraordinary until the medical condition of the patient is known and the possible use of the therapy is evaluated in relation to the patient's ability to strive for the spiritual purpose of life.

Because of the confusion often present when the terms ordinary and extraordinary are used, a relatively recent document of the Catholic Church, *Declaration on Euthanasia* (Congregation for the Doctrine of the Faith 1980a) advised that perhaps the terms "proportionate" or "disproportionate" would be good substitutes for ordinary and extraordinary. In our opinion, however, the new terms have the same problems unless they are used with reference to the medical diagnosis and prognosis of the illness and spiritual condition of the patient. Hence, we prefer to use the traditional terms, ordinary and extraordinary, but to insist they be used as conclusions, not as principles in the ethical analysis of the use of life support.

When therapy is ineffective or imposes a severe burden, ethicists have little problem approving the decision to remove life support, even if a person is allowed to die. Many physicians and nurses in the same situation, however, are unwilling to remove life-support systems if it entails allowing a person to die. The reasons for this attitude can be summarized in the following three observations: (1) It is difficult to know when death is imminent and further therapy would be futile. (2) Even though a patient may be desperately ill, some physicians will not give up hope of doing some good; indeed, they would identify "doing something to help" as their role. (3) Some physicians, wishing to avoid malpractice suits, are hesitant to remove life-sustaining means, even though they may no longer be useful.

Clearly, physicians and ethicists approach the dying patient with different emphases, the ethicist being more concerned with how the person lives as death approaches and the physician being more concerned with how to prolong life. We believe that there need not be any radical disagreement between physicians and ethicists, however, if three truths are understood clearly.

1. Physicians and moralists often use the terms ordinary means and extraordinary means with different connotations. Physicians use these terms insofar as the means to prolong life is standard and accepted or experimental and unproved. Ethicists, conversely, look to the way in which the therapy will affect the person's ability to function at the spiritual level of human potential. If the therapy is useless or a severe burden insofar as the spiritual function is concerned, then it is extraordinary. Thus, one might reject brain surgery to prolong life a few weeks if it might render one comatose for the remainder of one's life.

2. Although the physician has the expertise and the right to make decisions concerning the usefulness or medical effects of some particular medical procedure, the patient (or the family of the patient) has the right to determine whether a particular medical procedure is ordinary

or extraordinary from an ethical viewpoint. Thus, the decision to use or remove life support is a collaborative decision.

3. If the means in question are determined to be ordinary from an ethical viewpoint, then they must be employed; if extraordinary, they may or may not be employed. The decision should be made by the patient (or the family) in consultation with the physician, but ordinary care should continue.

In maintaining that one is free to decide not to prolong life because a grave burden would result, even though prolonging life is possible, we are affirming that, though human life is a great good, it is not the greatest good. The greatest good is friendship with God, charity. Thus, if prolonging life would seem to interfere—directly or indirectly—with friendship with God, life need not be prolonged. This is the practical meaning of the words "no hope of benefit" and "excessive burden." Therapy with no hope of benefit is that therapy that will impede a person's ability to strive for eternal life. Therapy that imposes an excessive burden is that therapy that may extend the person's life, but at the same time imposes such a burden that striving for the purpose of life is rendered too difficult. Pope Pius XII expressed this thought in a statement, "On the Prolongation of Life," that is quoted by non-Catholics as well as Catholics:

> Natural reason and Christian morals say that man (and whoever is entrusted with the task of taking care of another) has the right and duty in case of serious illness to take the necessary treatment for the preservation of life and health. This duty that one has toward himself, toward God, toward the human community, and in most cases toward certain determined persons, derives from a well-ordered charity, from submission to the Creator, from social justice and even from strict justice as well as from devotion toward one's family.
>
> But normally one is held to use only ordinary means—according to the circumstances of persons, places, times and cultures—that is to say, means that do not involve any grave burdens for oneself or another. A more strict obligation would be too burdensome for most men and would render the attainment of a higher, more important good too difficult. Life, health, all temporary activities are in fact subordinated to spiritual ends. On the other hand, one is not forbidden to take more than the strictly necessary steps to preserve life and health, as long as he does not fail in some more serious duty. (Pius XII 1957, 396)

Do these principles ever make it easy to determine when to remove respirators or tube feeding? No, they do not. The practical difficulties in applying the ordinary and extraordinary distinction will always remain. Determining whether it is time to allow oneself to die, or to allow another to die, will always be complex. This is especially true if the decision involves discontinuing a means already used or withdrawal of life-support systems from newborns with birth defects, for instance. But following the above-mentioned principles provides a basis for compassionate and ethical decisions in any circumstance.

The Patient Decides

Who decides that life should or should not be prolonged and that a certain means is ordinary or extraordinary? Some place the burden primarily on the physician; some believe it should be the courts' duty to protect incompetent patients' rights. Clearly, the physician is deeply involved in the decision and must consider the patient's condition and determine the medical prognosis, that is, whether the means in question will cure, help appreciably, or have no effect on the dying patient. But other circumstances must be considered in addition to the medical effectiveness of the means. What about expense, pain, and inconvenience? What about the spiritual condition of the patient? Only the patient or the family can decide these circumstances. Hence, the radical right to make a decision on what would be an ordinary means and what would be an extraordinary means from an ethical point of view belongs to the patient. Following the principles of human dignity, informed consent, and professional communication, with the guidance of the physician, and consultation with relatives, the patient decides what actions should be performed and what should be omitted. The physician and patient relationship is expressed aptly by Pope Pius XII in this manner:

> The rights and duties of the doctor are correlative to those of the patient. The doctor, in fact, has no separate or independent right where the patient is concerned. In general, he can take action only if the patient explicitly or implicitly, directly or indirectly, gives him permission. (Pius XII 1952, 201)

Proxy Consent

The most difficult problems arise when patients are incompetent to decide and others must decide for them. Special care must be taken to defend the right to life of such persons. Some physicians are tempted, for example, to judge too easily that newborns who suffer from a serious handicap are not to be treated despite the fact that parents, once they come to know and love such handicapped children, find their lives very precious. Conversely, parents who have just been informed that a newborn is handicapped may too quickly decide to allow such children to die. Patients who are severely depressed may also refuse treatment that they would have accepted in a better frame of mind. Treating severe burn victims is difficult because they often ask to be allowed to die, even though many later declare they are happy that therapy was utilized. Hence, the norms of informed consent are not rigid and legalistic and must be interpreted in accord with the patient's condition.

To ensure that proxies and physicians will act in the best interest of patients, a series of legal documents known as advanced directives have been formulated. These directives are the living will and the durable power of attorney for health affairs. Although the latter is more useful than the former, both documents may facilitate decision making, provided that:

1. The advanced directive does not preempt the physician's moral responsibility to offer a diagnosis and prognosis directed toward patient benefit.
2. The proxy realizes that her responsibility is to act in the best interest of the patient, not merely to convey a request made in the past when the circumstances of the present were not known.

Not all lawyers, physicians, and ethicists would agree with this latter admonition. But sound reason makes us realize that the decisions concerning the removal of life support made by proxies must be made in the light of actual circumstances now, not in the light of some past statements of the then-conscious patient that no longer fit the circumstances.

Striving for the Purpose of Life, Persistent Vegetative State, and Advanced Dementia

What of the patient medically judged to be in an irreversible coma, in a persistent vegetative state (PVS), or suffering from advanced Alzheimer's disease. Do these people still have the potential to strive for the purpose of life, which we have posited as a condition for the moral obligation to prolong life? Patients in this condition suffer from a dysfunctional cerebral cortex (higher brain), and their recovery is deemed, at best, highly improbable. In other words, patients in this condition are not able to perform human acts (acts of intellect and will), nor do they have the potential to perform these acts in the future, and it is by means of human acts that humans are able to pursue the purpose of life (cf. *Summa Theol.*, Aquinas 1947, I-II, q. 1, a. 1). As our prior considerations indicate, patients in this condition should not be put to death, but when they contract a fatal pathology, overcoming or resisting that pathology would usually involve extraordinary or disproportionate means. Thus, if a person with PVS or advanced Alzheimer's disease is unable to eat without artificial hydration and nutrition, it is reasonable to maintain that such therapy need not be utilized.

Some Catholic ethicists would not agree with this opinion, maintaining either that artificial hydration and nutrition for people who cannot assimilate food and liquid naturally is comfort care, not a medical therapy, or that prolonging life, even in a state of mere physiological function, is of "great benefit" to the patient. The Council on Ethics and Judicial Affairs of the American Medical Association declared, however, that artificial hydration and nutrition a medical therapy and may be withdrawn if a patient is in an irreversible coma, with care being taken to verify the accuracy of this diagnosis.

Care for patients "who require medically assisted nutrition and hydration" is summed up in the *Directives*:

> There should be a presumption in favor of providing nutrition and hydration to all patients, including patients who require medically assisted nutrition and hydration, as long as this is of sufficient benefit to outweigh the burden involved to the patient. (directive 58)

In our opinion, for patients who will not recover the ability to perform human acts, there is no benefit resulting from artificial nutrition and hydration, and thus the presumption in favor of using an artificial means to prolong their life yields to contrary fact.

Those caring for patients with severely debilitated mental function should make sure that the patient is given standard nursing care. Although the comatose person is not conscious of this care, it is required by human dignity and respect for the feelings of others.

Moreover, if the intention of the family in removing artificial hydration and nutrition were to cause the death of the patient, it would be unethical. In practice, however, this is seldom the intention of the family. Rather, they decide that the therapy does not offer hope of benefit and they wish to stop applying therapy that is futile, or they determine that the therapy imposes an excessive burden upon the patient or themselves. Thus, they are intending a good, namely withdrawing a burden, even though they apprehend that an evil, the death of a person, will follow from the good action. When therapy is withdrawn because it imposes a serious burden, it is an application of the principle of double effect.

People who oppose the withdrawal of medically supplied hydration and nutrition often do so because they fear that permitting the removal of such tubes and thereby allowing comatose people to die becomes a first step toward creating a pro-euthanasia mentality in the country. Certainly it is true that all abuses that lead to the acceptance of euthanasia are to be rejected. Nevertheless, if a person will not be able to strive for the purpose of life as a result of the therapy, then the therapy is extraordinary and may be withheld. Feeding of this sort is usually unable to prevent increasing debilitation, and the use of intubation is merely prolonging the dying process for patients unable to use that time for any beneficial activity. Even if the patient can be maintained in a comatose condition indefinitely, it is difficult to claim that a long period of comatose life is of human value for the patient.

The *sixth conclusion:* Life support may be removed even though the patient will die if the therapy is ineffective or imposes an excessive burden. Usually, the terms ordinary and extraordinary means, if used accurately, are helpful in discerning the ethical issues concerning the use of life support. The decision to remove life support should be made collaboratively by the medical team, patient, and family.

12.6 PAIN AND DYING

The principle of growth through suffering has been considered in chapter 2, but five observations are relevant with regard to pain at the time of death. First, pain is not an absolute human evil. Although suffering is truly an ontological evil to be alleviated whenever possible, it is not of itself a moral evil nor without supernatural and human benefits when rightly used. The theological teaching of the church in regard to the nature of evil and the permissive will of God are valuable in understanding the place of suffering and death in human life.

Some will scoff at this view of life, but the Christian tradition holds that great good can come out of suffering when this is joined to the suffering of Jesus. Although Christian teaching in this regard is often misrepresented, it does not imply a masochistic desire for pain, nor does it stand in the way of medical progress. As one group of Christians that has investigated the situation maintains, "A terminal illness can be transformed into a time for which everyone concerned is grateful" (Amulree 1975, 20).

Second, alleviating pain by medicine or even by surgery does not constitute active euthanasia, even if the suffering person's life might be shortened by the pain-alleviating medical or surgical procedure. In this case, the direct object of the act is to relieve pain; if life is shortened, it is an accidental, even though foreseen, result. This view is expressed succinctly in the *Directives:* "Medicines capable of alleviating or suppressing pain may be given to a dying person, even if this therapy may indirectly shorten the person's life so long as the intent is not to hasten death" (directive 61).

The opportunity to use suffering as a means of spiritual growth is not destroyed if painkilling drugs are used. Rather, the individual and those who care for him or her have the right to use such drugs to permit the best use of the patient's remaining energies, times of consciousness, and so forth, so that the patient can complete life with maximum composure.

Third, in recent years, medical and psychological breakthroughs have occurred in regard to severe pain. Medically speaking, pharmaceutical and surgical procedures make it possible to control and alleviate severe pain in the hospital and at home. Severe and excruciating pain, then, is hardly a realistic excuse for direct euthanasia or suicide. Moreover, an even more startling discovery in the control of pain has been made by people in the hospice movement.

Case studies demonstrate that pain is alleviated and controlled more easily when human concern and care are given to the hopelessly ill and dying. The ultimate human pain seems to be loneliness and the feeling of dying alone. If these feelings are overcome, it seems that pain is not such a prominent factor, even for those who are dying of debilitating diseases.

Fourth, if the patient is unable to make the pertinent decisions, then the family, in consultation with the physician, should have the right and obligation to determine whether aggressive pain control is ordinary or extra-ordinary and whether extraordinary means will be used. In making this decision, the family decides as would the patient and for the patient's bene-fit, not solely for the family's benefit.

Fifth, such documents as the *Advance Directives for Future Healthcare Deci-sions: A Christian Perspective* (de Blois, McGrath, and O'Rourke 1991) may be used by patients as a means of informing family and physician and as a help in preparing for death. A federal law, the 1991 Patient Self-Determination Act, encourages the use of advance directives.

The *seventh conclusion:* Pain resulting from illness may be used by a per-son to draw closer to Christ, but efforts to relieve pain are warranted when-ever the patient, or proxy, requests such help.

12.7 CARE FOR THE CORPSE AND CADAVER

When a human being dies, the body is no longer informed and unified by the life-giving principle or soul by which it is a constituted human person. The cadaver of a person, then, is not a *human* body in the proper sense of the word. Insofar as is possible, the remains of a person should not be referred to as though the human person existed *in* the human body or was, so to speak, limited by the human body.

Language of this nature is misleading, because it implies a duality in human existence; in a certain sense, the living human person *is* the living human body. When persons die, they exist in a new form, which in a sense is incomplete, because they no longer have a body. While existing in this life, the human person is a substantial unity of spirit (form) and body (matter), not an accidental juxtaposition of two distinct entities. Although the remains of a human body may resemble for a time the body of a living person, and although this resemblance may be prolonged through embalming, the remains are not a *human* body but a mass of organic matter, decomposing into constitutive, organic elements.

If the corpse of a human person is not a human body, then why are peo-ple so concerned about proper care for the remains of the deceased person? Why treat it with the respect and reverence it usually receives? Respect and reverence are due the remains of a human being because of the sacredness of human life that once informed the now inert mass still bearing the per-son's bodily image. To mourn the fact that the person will no longer be pre-sent in the same human manner as before, the people who remain perform certain reverential spiritual actions to express their love. Respect for the dead body, then, signifies respect for human life—respect for the Author of life, respect for the person who now exists in a different modality, and respect for the family and friends of the deceased person. Hence, the ceremonial actions that people follow when caring for the body of a deceased person have a meaning beyond their physical impact.

Although the ceremonies of wake, funeral, and burial have been criticized for their gross and inhuman excesses, fundamentally this process has a meaning and worth in accord with the Judeo-Christian tradition. Having friends share the burden through liturgical services is also a source of strength and support for bereaved people. Hence, the legitimate customs of people at the time of death are not signs of superstition or blind fear; rather, they bespeak a noble belief about life, its purpose, and the enduring strength of human love.

In accord with the respect due to the remains of a human person, no organs should be removed from a corpse, nor should the body be dismembered unless a sufficient reason justifies such an action. Usually the next of kin or the person to whom the corpse is committed for care has the legal right to determine if organs may be removed from the body and if an autopsy may be performed. The right of the next of kin in regard to caring for the human body is not absolute. It may be superseded by statements made by the person while still alive, for example, through the Uniform Anatomical Gift Act, or by the needs of society, for example, when an autopsy might help stave off a contagious disease.

The Anatomical Gift Act is "designed to facilitate the donation and use of human tissues and organs for transplantation and other medical purposes and provide a favorable legal environment for such activities." At present, all fifty states have enacted the gift act, thus enabling persons who are of sound mind and eighteen years of age or more to give all or part of their bodies to persons or institutions authorized to practice or perform research medicine, or to engage in tissue banking, with the gift to take effect upon death. This law also recognizes the right of the next of kin to donate the body or any part for the same purpose, but in most states the law declares that if there is a conflict between the donor and the next of kin, the wishes of the donor have precedence.

From a Christian point of view, the practice of donating organs and one's body for scientific research is ethical and even to be encouraged if a true need exists. Hence, we are in favor of laws that enable organs to be retrieved from the remains of dead people who have not signed statements donating the organs. Such laws, which presume consent for organ donations, are common in Europe and have been enacted in certain states for people killed in accidents.

Another ethical question, however, does not admit of such easy solution: Is it immoral to accept or solicit payment for the gift of certain organs? Although some have defended such practices, others maintain that abuses could spring up very quickly if cadaver organs were sold or contracted for money. We agree with this latter opinion. If society is to live in a humane manner, then generosity and charity, rather than monetary gain and greed, must serve as the basis for the donation of functioning organs. Recent federal legislation has outlawed the sale of human organs for transplant.

An autopsy is the examination of a cadaver performed in order to provide greater medical knowledge concerning the cause of death. Occasionally, an autopsy will have the benefit of providing knowledge about a rare or contagious disease. In such cases, the good of the community would overrule the rights of the next of kin, and if the next of kin were not willing, the court could order that an autopsy be performed. In cases of violent death or unattended death, an autopsy is required by law, no matter what wishes are expressed by the next of kin.

Usually, however, the purpose of an autopsy is not to trace the etiology of a rare disease but to discover unknown or violent causes of death. Frequently, autopsies are performed to help health professionals achieve a higher level of efficiency in the care of the living. The autopsy rate of a hospital is usually a good sign of concern for quality medical care and offers a gauge of professional integrity and interest in scientific advancement. Through autopsies, the diagnosis and treatment a person received can be evaluated and staff members encouraged to observe a high level of proficiency. For this reason, autopsies should be encouraged, and people should be encouraged to look upon them as an ordinary part of the medical care process. Needless to say, the human remains of a person should always be treated with the utmost respect during an autopsy.

In the Judeo-Christian tradition, respect for the dead has usually been shown by burying the corpse in the ground or in a mausoleum. The cremation of the remains, although not a common part of this tradition, has never been considered as totally disrespectful. For a long time, however, cremation was forbidden in the Catholic Church because anti-Christian groups in the eighteenth century advocated cremation as a means of denying externally the immortality of the human person and the resurrection. Thus—not because it was immoral in itself, but rather because of what it might signify— cremation was not an acceptable form of caring for the remains of a person in the Catholic Church. In modern times, however, the church has withdrawn opposition to cremation and allows it as part of the rite of Christian burial for any good reason.

The *eighth conclusion:* Autopsies are to be encouraged, and because cremation is no longer associated with a denial of religious truth, although burying the dead is encouraged as the usual procedure, the total remains or an amputated member may be cremated if there is a serious reason; for example, if the custom of the country favors cremation, if there is danger of disease, or if a suitable gravesite cannot be obtained at a reasonable cost.

SUMMARY

Because of our weakened nature, death will never be something that we welcome. But through grace, we can accept it as the way to union with God. As we view the health care scene in our country, one is struck by "the denial of death." To overcome the fear of death and help oneself as well as other people die well, one must learn to conquer the emotional strain that accompanies suffering and death and deal with the ethical issues that are often encountered.

It takes more than words to accomplish this transformation of attitude with regard to suffering and death. One must be willing to surrender to God through the person of Jesus Christ every day if one wishes to give new meaning and power to suffering and death. In short, one must enter into a lifelong love affair with God. The small deaths one dies every day prepare a person for the larger and more important deaths and, finally, for the ultimate moment of meaning and power.

The perfection of Christian suffering and death is to accept it with joy. This is not possible unless one works at it faithfully, relying on the unfailing grace of God. To communicate the meaning and power of death to patients effectively, health care professionals must have some experience of its reality themselves. Thus, health care is more than a job, more than knowledge and technique. Basically, in its fullness, it is a way of life that sees beyond the hurt, the sickness, the anguish; a way of life that enables one to look beyond the drudgery of daily reality, beyond the suffering in the hospital ward and the emergency room; a way of life that is centered in God's love for his children, the suffering of Christ for all human beings, and his victorious resurrection.

QUESTIONS

1. How would you respond to a person who maintains that all sickness would be eliminated if people would believe more strongly in Jesus Christ?
2. We know the reality of life and death by observing activities (signs) of the being in question, be it vegetable, animal, or human. What are the activities or signs that indicate that human life is present? What medical criteria enable us to measure these activities?
3. Distinguish clearly between mercy killing of a patient and allowing a patient to die.
4. Distinguish the different connotations of the terminology *ordinary and extraordinary means to prolong life* from a medical and ethical perspective.

5. Respond to this statement: "Christians should refrain from alleviating pain at the time of death because God has willed that people suffer."

CASES

1. In the oncology ward at Saint Joseph's Hospital, health care professionals experience "burn out" more frequently than in other service areas within the hospital. As a pastoral care person, you are requested to explain this phenomenon and to present a program to alleviate the problem.

2. Carl, a young father with three children, is dying, but his life would be prolonged indefinitely with a heart transplant. Tom, who has been injured critically in a motorcycle accident, is admitted to the emergency room. Normal procedure calls for using a respirator on Tom, but the emergency room physician realizes that Tom will die no matter what care is given. Thus, wishing to provide a heart for Carl, he withholds the respirator from Tom, thinking that this would hasten his death. Is the physician acting ethically? What norms would ensure ethical procedures in such cases?

3. Millie is severely depressed, and her family feels she may become suicidal if she is told that she is dying. Her attending physician does not believe that Millie is clinically depressed and asks you, a fourth-year medical student and a friend of Millie, to inform her of her condition. What ethical norms will you follow in your dialogue with Millie?

4. Ken—a character in the movie *Whose Life Is It Anyway?*—is a young artist who is quadriplegic as a result of being severely injured in an automobile accident. He wishes to have a catheter draining his kidneys removed to hasten his death from uremic poisoning. Evaluate his desire from an ethical viewpoint.

13

Spiritual Ministry and Health Care

OVERVIEW: When we discuss the human person and the capacities and needs of the human person, it becomes clear that human health involves not only the biological, physiological, and social functions of the human person, but also a person's creative or spiritual life. That is, his or her deepest concerns and commitments, his or her worldview and value systems. Total health requires the balanced and effective functioning of all human potentialities. Thus, no one is truly healthy if his or her spiritual life is atrophied, stunted, or pathologically conflicted.

In this chapter, we consider how health care professionals can contribute to the spiritual well-being and growth of their patients in the process of medical therapy and care. We seek to show that from a spiritual point of view the work of physicians and nurses is truly a healing ministry in which they act as ministers of God, who is the Author of all life and health. More attention, however, is devoted to the efforts of pastoral care professionals. The task of pastoral care professionals is made more difficult because of shorter stays in hospitals. But more attention is being devoted by pastoral care professionals to the spiritual ministry of people in long-term care facilities, in home health care, and in hospices.

In books on medical ethics, spiritual care is usually considered as something pertinent only in the care of the dying. We stress that it is a dimension of all health care and that all sick people need and deserve it. The principles applied in this chapter are mainly those associated with hope, that is, the principles of stewardship and of growth through suffering. But the principles of human dignity and of a well-formed conscience also apply.

13.1 THE PURPOSE OF PASTORAL CARE

Most Catholic and many community health care facilities have a pastoral care department whose staff have a fourfold role: to heal, to sustain, to guide, and to reconcile. Hence, the pastoral care team seeks to afford help at the spiritual and social levels, just as other health care professionals offer help at the physiological and psychological levels.

Trained pastoral care staff are a great asset for a health care facility, but their presence also presents a difficulty not often realized by health care personnel and administrators. Because ministers, sisters, priests, and laity trained in pastoral care all are present in a hospital, physicians, nurses, and technicians often feel that the patient's spiritual needs are not their concern. Thus, they act as if the patient could be divided effectively into parts and cared for at only one level of personality.

As we have indicated, however, every human act affects each level of human function, even though that act may be primarily concerned with only one level of function. Our human faculties and powers are not related as floors in a building but rather as dimensions of a building. The height, length, and depth of a building cannot be separated. Too many health care professionals care for only one dimension of a patient's need. True, many health care professionals may not have the training to respond to spiritual needs, but there is a basic level of spiritual care that any person can offer. A patient being wheeled into the surgery suite will benefit considerably if a technician, nurse, or physician asks, "Would you like to offer a prayer with me?" Health care professionals who are not members of the pastoral care team have a wonderful opportunity to be concerned about their patients' spiritual needs.

The *first conclusion:* The first task of those involved in pastoral care is to heighten the awareness of other health care professionals so that they are sensitive to patients' social and spiritual needs and that they minister to this level of need whenever possible.

13.2 SPIRITUAL COUNSELING

Pastoral care professionals contribute to patients' overall health in two ways: through spiritual counseling and through sacramental ministry. When offering care, pastoral personnel, in a manner similar to other health care professionals, must realize that there is more to a patient's personality than the dimension to which they minister. Hence pastoral care personnel must be well trained in their own specialty and be able to answer accurately the question, "What do you do to help the patient?" But they must also have some appreciation of medical procedures and practice. Conversely, pastoral care personnel must be careful not to offer opinions about medical care or give anything resembling medical advice, because they are simply unprepared to do so.

When acting as spiritual counselors, the pastoral care person, like a psychotherapist, is a listener and a reflector through whom the realities of the patient's situation become clearer to the patient and more manageable. Furthermore, like the psychotherapist, the minister listens not just to what the patient seems to be saying verbally but to what the patient, perhaps unconsciously, is trying to say nonverbally and symbolically. The psychotherapist, however, is listening for the message that rises from the patient's subconscious emotional drives, whereas the minister as a spiritual therapist is listening for a message that comes from a still deeper level, from what the Scriptures call the "heart," that is, from the spiritual interior of the person's being, where the person is committed to some sort of ultimate values and to some fundamental insight into reality.

In most patients, as in most everyone, this commitment and vision is dim and confused indeed, and yet it is the source of all personal life, where people really live and where they really die. "Out of the depths I call to you O Lord; O Lord hear my voice" (Ps 130:1–2). It is this voice *de profundis* to which the minister must listen. Moreover, a spiritual guide is not looking, as is the psychotherapist, for the psychic energies and motivations that flow from human instinctual needs, but rather for the work of the Holy Spirit in the patient, the signs of faith, hope, and charity, and the spiritual forces of sin and alienation that oppose these. This is the spiritual level of human functioning.

The patient may raise these questions directly by saying, "Why has this happened to me? Have I sinned? Am I going to be punished? What will happen to me if I die?" or "I don't seem to be able to pray now that I am sick," and so forth. Today, in a secularized society, such questions are seldom asked directly. Even if they are, the counselor may very well suspect that they do not really come from the spiritual level of personality but are merely the pious language that some people use when speaking of purely physical or psychological problems. Or the patient may think that this is the way you are supposed to converse with a pastoral care person who is supposed only to talk that kind of religious language. Therefore, the pastoral care person must listen to religious questions inherent in secular language or to secular problems inherent in pseudoreligious language. In both cases, counselors must go deeper to find the really spiritual level in the patient.

This requires patience, and certainly it is usually a mistake to begin asking spiritual questions of a patient with whom the needed level of trust has not yet been established. Conversely, experienced spiritual counselors learn how to cut through other levels of small talk and psychological talk to the issues with which they must deal. Simple directness is ordinarily not resented by patients. Directness is not bluntness or insensitivity. It is, rather, a form of respect for a patient, a refusal to play games.

The counselor as well as the patient must trust in God's providence. God is using the patient's experience of illness as an occasion of possible spiritual growth. The spirit of God is already at work in the sufferer in ways that are not labeled religious. The minister must recognize this growth process and cultivate it, helping patients to understand this in their own terms.

A specific responsibility for pastoral care personnel is not only to deal with the patient's spiritual problems, but also to help him or her become vividly aware of the real presence of God and of the church as the People of God in the patient's life in this very event of sickness where the patient may feel abandoned and isolated. Counselors are themselves a visible sign or sacrament of this presence, incarnating God, as it were, in a tangible, human, imperfect, but real form.

Nor is it enough that counselors provide this witness of God's presence only to members of their own church. Too many ministers assume that they have a responsibility only to their own parishioners or to those of their own denomination, and that others will resent their presence. Usually, however, this is not the case. Most laity are less ecclesiastically defined than they used to be. For them any minister or rabbi is still a "man of God," and as such ought to have some interest in them as "children of God." Even the humanist is seldom content with the silence of humanism in the face of the ultimate questions and is resentful if the religious minister writes him or her off as a nonbeliever.

The *second conclusion:* The spiritual counselor's primary task is really a very simple one. It is to say, as much or more by presence, attitude, and non-verbal symbols as by the exhortatory word, that God is present to sick persons in their fear or suffering—that God as loving, caring Father, as cosuffering Lord Jesus, as Healing Spirit, is present and acting, but present in mystery. The sick person, like Job, feels guilty and yet is not clear how he or she is guilty. There is a sense of judgment. The counselor should not deny this. Indeed, a counselor symbolizes this judgment. But the counselor also overcomes judgment by being a sign of mercy and reconciliation.

13.3 CELEBRATING THE HEALING PROCESS

Sickness may be the time of genuine conversion in which persons truly find God for the first time in their lives or after a long time of forgetfulness and separation. The counselor must affirm the reality of this invitation of divine mercy, but that is not the whole of the minister's responsibility. Conversion is the beginning of a new life, but that life has to be lived authentically or it will be lost again. Consequently, one of the chief aims of spiritual counseling is to assist people to begin to grow daily in the Christian life and to plan practically to continue that growth once they have returned to the routine situations of everyday life.

It is important also that the counselor, in helping sick persons realize God's presence, also make clear to them that he or she is a sign of the concern of God's people, of the Christian community or church, for a suffering brother or sister. Sickness is in Old Testament terms a kind of "uncleanness," and the patient may experience the "leprosy" of loneliness, alienation, and "excommunication" of the outcast from life and the human community. The minister removes this excommunication and reunites the lonely one with the community that is praying for him or her. Recall how Jesus, healing a leper, sent him to a priest to be readmitted to the Jewish community (Mk 1:44).

The specific spiritual task of pastoral care, however, is not exhausted simply by the counseling situation. It must not be confined to talking about the presence of God, but it must deepen into experiencing that presence in prayer, worship, celebration, and communion.

Today, when most chaplains are well trained in clinical pastoral education, they sometimes feel a tension between the model of the chaplain as a pastoral counselor whose main task is to engage in a therapeutic and psychological process with the patient and the older model of the pastor as the one who reads the Scriptures, prays with and exhorts the patient, and administers the sacraments. These two models seem opposed to each other. In particular, one seems aimed at removing feelings of guilt and giving feelings of interpersonal warmth and confidence and getting clients "in touch with their feelings," whereas the other tends to generate guilt and to impose a formalized religious response that covers up a patient's real experience.

Actually the two models, when they are well understood, are complementary and can reinforce each other. The Word of God first came to humans, not in the text of the Bible that records his coming, but in the incarnation of Jesus Christ, the man who came to the sick and suffering, shared their suffering, and healed them by his touch. Ministers, because they are sent by Jesus, are the living witnesses, "another Christ," a sign of Christ's care for the patient.

Therefore, everything that the minister does to witness to this tender concern, this ability to empathize, listen, and not judge, is a sacrament of Jesus's presence. Even humor and light banter, if its purpose is precisely to establish real communication, is like the wit that Jesus constantly displayed in his preaching and parables. Above all, the down-to-earthness—the freedom from stuffiness, self-righteousness, and elitism that can be the curse of the clerical state—are in imitation of Jesus, who did not hesitate to eat with sinners in simple fellowship.

Thus, when chaplains read the Scriptures with patients, they should already have placed the Scriptures in the kind of human relational context in which the Word of God can be truly understood. Prayer also must grow out of this living context; that is, it should be natural for two people who have come to share a common concern to give it prayerful expression. The chaplain should not be praying in front of an embarrassed patient who feels as if something is "being laid on" him or her in which the patient has no part. An opening for prayer will come, however, only if the patient senses that the minister's concern for her goes deep, deeper than mere professional interest. Moreover, the Scriptures that are read should be chosen just because they help to make real the presence of Jesus, especially in his power to forgive, heal, and lead on into the fullness of life.

The Anointing of the Sick and Reconciliation

The Catholic priest is more likely than the Protestant minister or the rabbi to be concerned about administering the sacraments in the health care setting. But these, too, must be understood not as some ritual intruding into a real situation but as a ritualization of a process of healing that is already going on. The primordial sacrament is the touching that Jesus used when he healed the leper. It indicates the intimate presence, the care, the community, the power of life between Jesus and the sick and outcast. When a chaplain gives reassurance that the patient is not alone, that is the primordial sacramental rite on which all the other sacraments are based—human bodily contact as a sign of spiritual presence.

In administering the sacraments, using the new rites that the Catholic Church has recently improved precisely for this purpose, priests must try to enhance this character of human contact already present in the counseling situation. What priests have done as good pastoral counselors, they now deepen and intensify by a sign that combines the verbal word of the Scriptures with the nonverbal sacramental act.

The new rite for the Anointing of the Sick brings this out clearly. It is not merely for the dying, as formerly, but for any person who is seriously ill ("seriously" should be judged here not merely in physical terms, but also in psychological terms). Thus, when anyone is physically sick enough that the priest suspects that the thought of possible death with its deep anxiety has entered his or her mind and produced fear and the threat of despair, then the spiritual and perhaps physical healing of the sacrament is needed and should be given. Whenever there is question of major surgery or of any disease that patients know sometimes leads to death and thus raises this fear in their own minds, priests can anoint. They should not anoint when the illness is one in which recovery is ensured and that consequently does not appear to contain any serious threat.

What is the meaning of this rite? First, it is not merely something done by a priest to a patient. Even when priests are alone, they are there to represent not only God, but also the Christian community. In fact, God is the center of the Christian community, so the priest is there to represent the Trinitarian community, into whose Second Person all Christians are incorporated by their baptism. The anxiety of sick persons is that by their illness they are outcasts, aliens to this community. Patients experience this by their isolation from usual daily life and by the threat of death, which might take them away forever.

What such anxious patients need is the reassurance that their people and their God are still with them. The priest supplies the sign of this by touching a patient. This touch means "presence," "acceptance," and as such is common to all the sacraments. But it is a special kind of touch in this case, a healing touch because it is the "anointing with oil," a common kind of healing remedy that has the sense of soothing pain and infusing life and movement. Its significance as a spiritual healing is given by the words that are spoken.

But this actual form of the sacrament is also preceded by brief scriptural passages, which can be expanded, in keeping with the general principle of the new rites that each sacrament should begin with a proclamation of God's Word of faith, because it is faith that opens the person to God's work and is the beginning of God's gifts.

It is essential to realize that the sacraments are not performed merely in the ritual moment. Rather, they are the celebration of a culminating moment (not necessarily the last) of the saving work of God that has gone on for some time through what are apparently merely secular events. Therefore, it is fitting not only that physicians and nurses be present at the anointing, but also that they participate in it by reading the Scriptures, or saying some of the prayers and by imposing hands on the patient or signing with the cross. Priests in their instruction and commentary and by additions to some of the prayers, if necessary, should thank God for the healing gifts and work of the medical staff. It would also be very appropriate at this time for patients to express their thanks to the doctors and nurses.

The proper rite for the dying patient is not the Anointing of the Sick but the reception of Viaticum, or final communion. This is the expression of the sick person's communion and unity with the church on earth, which prays for his or her swift passage to the eternal banquet. Hence this communion should be shared with others present, if possible.

Laypeople as Ministers

What should ministers do who are not priests? These days, religious sisters and brothers and lay people share in the sacramental ministry. It is perfectly possible for nonordained persons, sisters, and laypersons to hold a service of healing consisting of Scripture readings, prayers, and the laying on of hands for the sick. It can even make use of blessed oil as a sacramental.

It would seem, however, that in such services it should be made clear to all that what is taking place is not a sacrament in the strict sense. By this is not meant that it is inefficacious (all true prayer is efficacious), but that it is preparatory to the full public visit of the priest to the sick as a representative of the Christian community. Just as the arrival of physician completes the care given to patients by nurses—although in fact the physician does nothing additional except to approve and confirm what has already been done—so the priest approves and confirms the healing prayer of a local group and of auxiliary ministry. However, the priest adds to what has already been done by sacramental anointing and, as appropriate, sacramental absolution, which may precede it. This is not a mere formality but an expression of the unity and public witness of the church.

The Sacrament of Reconciliation for the sick can also take place in the form of a penance service in the hospital chapel or even in the ward, with the invitation to all who wish to make individual confession and receive absolution. Such a service is an opportunity for the priest to deal with the question of sin and guilt and the meaning of suffering and to alleviate neurotic guilt. When confession is made on a ward, it should be remembered that if it is difficult to achieve sufficient privacy the penitent can be instructed simply to make a general acknowledgment of sins and to speak of them in detail in a future confession. Diocesan regulations sometime limit the practice of general confession, but it should be recognized as a possibility in accord with Canon Law (canons 961–62) and other church norms.

It also should be remembered that deacons, sisters, brothers, and other visitors, although they cannot give absolution, can truly help a sick person to conversion and reconciliation with God and neighbor in an efficacious way. We are not proposing revival of the "confession to a layman," which was common enough in the Middle Ages when a priest was not available, but are emphasizing that today in pastoral counseling such confession often takes place spontaneously.

When confession does happen, the ministers who are not priests should help such patients make an act of contrition and then encourage them to go to the sacrament when it becomes possible, but should also assure them here and now that the mercy of God is truly present in prayer, and that with this trust in God's mercy they should be at peace. The reason for confession later is to ratify and complete by the public acknowledgment of the priest as a representative of the church a conversion that has already taken place, and also to provide sacramental absolution as needed. There is no reason for nonordained ministers to feel that because they are not ordained they cannot help patients achieve this reconciliation here and now.

The *third conclusion:* The pastoral care person helps patients experience the presence of God through prayer, worship, celebration and communion. Laypeople as well as the ordained may have a role in this ministry.

13.4 BAPTISM AND THE EUCHARIST

Baptism

Today, some Catholics are raising doubts about infant baptism. This, however, seems to have Pelagian overtones, because it implies that the grace of God can be received only on one's initiative. Baptism, however, is a sign of the pure gift from God, the gift of faith and justification that comes to people without any merit on their part if they do not reject it. Before an infant is born, it is already subject to the grace of God through the prayers of the church. Infant baptism is the public ratification that the infant, alienated from God through no fault of its own but by the sins of society (original sin), is now being drawn by the Holy Spirit through Jesus Christ and his redeemed community of the church into union with the Father.

This act of incorporating the infant into the life of the human community begins biologically and sociologically from the moments of conception and birth. Why, then, should not the infant also be incorporated into the redeemed community of the church? Consequently, it is certain that baptism can be validly conferred on the child from the moment of conception and probable that it can be conferred on any unconscious adult (although not certain, because the person may have positively rejected the grace of God that he offers to all). From this, some theologians in the past concluded that it is essential that all children in danger of death, even in utero, should be baptized, and encouraged the baptism of all doubtfully baptized adults who had not actually refused baptism.

Today, theologians still maintain the principle that persons can only be saved by Christ through the church, but they see the prayer of the church as efficacious even when it cannot be ritually expressed in the sacraments (cf. 1 Cor 7:14). Thus, it is very probable that the infant dying before baptism has already been justified through the prayer of the church (especially of the child's family) and will enter into the intimate mystery of God. The *Instruction on Infant Baptism* states: "As for infants who have died without baptism, the Church can do nothing but commend them to the mercy of God," as in fact it does in the funeral rite designed for them (Congregation for the Doctrine of the Faith 1980b).

Nevertheless, it still is important to administer baptism to manifest the concern of the church and thus to keep alive the consciousness of the dignity of the human person from the first moments of existence. Consequently, nurses and physicians should baptize infants who are in danger of death and even miscarried fetuses who exhibit human form and some sign of life. They should pour water on the child (on the head, if possible), touch the skin, and say, "I baptize you in the name of the Father, Son, and Holy Spirit." In this way, they have expressed Christian reverence and fellowship with this little person who will forever be part of the Trinitarian community.

For the dying unconscious person, it is permissible also to perform such a baptism with the condition, "If you are not baptized, I baptize you." Clearly this is not a grave obligation unless the person has asked to be baptized before lapsing into unconsciousness, and should not be done in a merely mechanical manner (trying to baptize everyone in the hospital, etc.), but as part of the nurses' care for particular persons in their charge whom they believe have given some indication that they might wish such an administration. Again, the reason is to show the church's concern for a person who has providentially come under the care of the Catholic community.

The Eucharist

The Eucharist is the supreme sacrament and sign of the Christian community, indicating that such patients remain a part of that community, even when absent from the public worship assembly, and that they are destined for eternal life with the community. It is a life-giving, health-giving sacrament, because eating the bread and drinking the wine are the basic symbols of the power to live. After Jesus raised the daughter of Jairus, "He told them to give her something to eat" (Lk 8:55). Again, Saint Paul believed (1 Cor 11:27–31) the unworthy reception of the Eucharist leads to sickness and death because this hypocrisy cuts a person off from the God of the living.

Today, the Eucharist is often distributed by auxiliary ministers, not by a priest. This is not inappropriate, because in the earliest days communion was taken from the public assembly to the homes of the sick. In a hospital, it would be appropriate when possible to have the patients who so wish listen to the mass in the chapel on closed circuit radio or television, then to be brought communion immediately afterward. In this way, the union between mass and communion would be emphasized. It is essential in any case that communion for the sick, no matter where they might be, should not be reduced to a routine in which someone pops in and out of a room to place a wafer in a sleepy patient's mouth. We would suggest at least a card containing Scripture readings and prayers that a patient can use while preparing for communion.

The *fourth conclusion:* What we have been saying about Baptism and the Eucharist may sound liturgical rather than ethical, but it sums up the ethical message of this book, namely, that medical ethics has to do not merely with certain rules about forbidden procedures, but rather with a healing process, throughout which the dignity of every human person in all its dimensions is respected by the community and by which the sick person is restored to full life in community. Unethical behavior tends to exclude persons from the deepest sharing of communal life centered in the Trinity. Ethical behavior fosters this communion. This ethical vision with its perception of the true scale of values is summed up and expressed in the sacraments, especially in the Eucharist. The sacraments represent for us how Jesus went about treating sick people.

SUMMARY

To be fully healthy, we must fulfill human needs in an integrated and balanced manner. Caring for the spiritual needs of sick and dying people is the work of the pastoral care team. Other health care professionals should contribute to this effort, but the primary responsibility for spiritual care lies with the pastoral care team. Ministering adequately in the service of pastoral care requires more than a degree in theology or training in clinical pastoral education. Pastoral care, like all forms of health care, requires a knowledge and love of the person to whom care is being given. Only if the patient is recognized and valued as a unique, worthwhile individual is health care truly human and humanizing. Thus the person who is a pastoral care worker is an integral member of the health care team, and counseling and sacramental celebration are integral elements of health care.

QUESTIONS

1. Why would a priest or minister need special preparation, in addition to the preparation required for ordination, to offer pastoral care to people who are ill?
2. Why are most people reluctant to speak about spiritual realities, even though those realities are important in our lives?
3. What can the pastoral minister do to help the patient "experience the presence" of God when receiving the sacraments?
4. Explain the healing potential of the Eucharist.

CASES

1. Research indicates that many physicians look upon pastoral care as an intrusion in the healing process. Other physicians look upon pastoral care as another form of psychotherapy or social work. In your capacity as chief executive officer of a Catholic hospital, how would you respond to those opinions?
2. Jane, a lay minister of the pastoral care department, does not wish to be assigned to care for AIDS patients. Although she realizes that there is no danger of contagion, she feels that her inability to accept homosexual activity, which is sometimes related to this disease, makes her a poor counselor for such patients. Analyze her attitudes from a pastoral care perspective.
3. Albert, a young Protestant minister serving in a home for retired people, finds that the people make him uneasy because of the respect they offer him. Albert wishes they would look upon him as a friend rather than as a clergyperson. What thoughts can you offer to help Albert feel more at home in his ministry?
4. Although Fred is on a respirator, he is declared brain dead. His parents want you, as a priest, to give him the last rites of the church. In addition to the Sacrament of Anointing, they wish you to administer Viaticum to him, arguing that he can still digest the host. What is your response?

Epilogue

"Wherever Jesus put in an appearance, in villages, in towns, or at crossroads, they laid the sick in the marketplace and begged him to let them touch just the tassel of his cloak. All who touched him got well" (Mk 6:36). Jesus is the Great Physician of body and soul, and he came to show us that his Father wants health for all his children. That means God wants us, with all the science and technology we can develop through research, to share in Jesus's ministry of healing of body and of mind, and with the same attitudes of compassion and of respect for the dignity of every child of God that he had. Thus, we share in Jesus's ministry mainly by internalizing the values Jesus presented in the Gospels, which makes following the teaching of the church more of a benefit than a burden.

This vocation to health is given to every one of us, and we all have personal responsibility for the health of our own minds and bodies. But we are also called to help one another to achieve health and to care for one another in times when health fails. As Christians, we realize the communal aspect of every human endeavor. As citizens, we have a great responsibility to do what we can to bring about peace and justice not only in our own country but throughout the world. We must seek to preserve the ecology of our planet and to cleanse it of the pollution it has suffered from unwise technology, so that our environment may become healthy. And we must strive to establish economic and political conditions where famine, poverty, contagious disease, and destructive violence will be overcome, so that healthy life for all may be possible. We must strengthen families through responsible parenthood achieved in ways that respect the gift of sexuality and the gift of children as God has given these gifts, because only out of healthy families will a healthy future develop.

As Christians, we also know that this better, healthier world cannot be achieved simply by human power. Our sins as a human community and as individuals go very deep, and we cannot heal ourselves, because we are like surgeons operating with diseased hands. Even in trying to do good, we do much harm. Yet there is good news and certain hope. If we faithfully follow our vocation to share in the healing work of Jesus, the Great Physician, we can accomplish all these works of healing with ultimate success.

Nevertheless, if we are to achieve success through him, we must also share his cross, and that means that in the work of health care we must be ready to meet scorn and opposition from the sin-sick society in which we live. In our society, far beyond the limits of the Christian community, the Holy Spirit of God is at work, and there are many waiting for our witness to give them courage to speak up for the values that the Spirit has led them to appreciate in their own hearts but that they feel very much alone in defending.

We must have the courage to rally all these men and women of goodwill who stand for a deep respect for human dignity and human rights, so that we may stand together against the self-destructive spirit of a world that today seems bent on destroying the environment, wasting its resources, breaking up the family, denying the value of children, destroying life in the womb, exalting lust and violence, wasting the powers of science on instruments of destruction, producing luxuries rather than necessities, prolonging dying, and neglecting the poor and powerless—a sick world that must reach out to touch Jesus if it is ever to be healed.

Appendix 1

Ethical and Religious Directives for Catholic Health Care Services

National Conference of Catholic Bishops
Fourth Edition

PREAMBLE

Health care in the United States is marked by extraordinary change. Not only is there continuing change in clinical practice due to technological advances, but the health care system in the United States is being challenged by both institutional and social factors as well. At the same time, there are a number of developments within the Catholic Church affecting the ecclesial mission of health care. Among these are significant changes in religious orders and congregations, the increased involvement of lay men and women, a heightened awareness of the Church's social role in the world, and developments in moral theology since the Second Vatican Council. A contemporary understanding of the Catholic health care ministry must take into account the new challenges presented by transitions both in the Church and in American society.

Throughout the centuries, with the aid of other sciences, a body of moral principles has emerged that expresses the Church's teaching on medical and moral matters and has proven to be pertinent and applicable to the ever-changing circumstances of health care and its delivery. In response to today's challenges, these same moral principles of Catholic teaching provide the rationale and direction for this revision of the *Ethical and Religious Directives for Catholic Health Care Services*.

These Directives presuppose our statement *Health and Health Care* published in 1981.[1] There we presented the theological principles that guide the Church's vision of health care, called for all Catholics to share in the healing mission of the Church, expressed our full commitment to the health care ministry, and offered encouragement to all those who are involved in it. Now, with American health care facing even more dramatic changes, we reaffirm the Church's commitment to health care ministry and the distinctive Catholic identity of the Church's institutional health care services.[2] The purpose of these *Ethical and Religious Directives* then is twofold: first, to reaffirm the ethical standards of behavior in health care that flow from the Church's teaching about the dignity of the human person; second, to provide authoritative guidance on certain moral issues that face Catholic health care today.

The *Ethical and Religious Directives* are concerned primarily with institutionally based Catholic health care services. They address the sponsors, trustees, administrators, chaplains, physicians, health care personnel, and patients or residents of these institutions and services. Since they express the Church's moral teaching, these Directives also will be helpful to Catholic professionals engaged in health care services in other settings. The moral teachings that we profess here flow principally from the natural law, understood in the light of the revelation Christ has entrusted to his Church. From this source the Church has derived its understanding of the nature of the human person, of human acts, and of the goals that shape human activity.

The Directives have been refined through an extensive process of consultation with bishops, theologians, sponsors, administrators, physicians, and other health care providers. While providing standards and guidance, the Directives do not cover in detail all of the complex issues that confront Catholic health care today. Moreover, the Directives will be reviewed periodically by the United States Conference of Catholic Bishops (formerly the National Conference of Catholic Bishops), in the light of authoritative church teaching, in order to address new insights from theological and medical research or new requirements of public policy.

The Directives begin with a general introduction that presents a theological basis for the Catholic health care ministry. Each of the six parts that follow is divided into two sections. The first section is in expository form; it serves as an introduction and provides the context in which concrete issues can be discussed from the perspective of the Catholic faith. The second section is in prescriptive form; the directives promote and protect the truths of the Catholic faith as those truths are brought to bear on concrete issues in health care.

GENERAL INTRODUCTION

The Church has always sought to embody our Savior's concern for the sick. The gospel accounts of Jesus' ministry draw special attention to his acts of healing: he cleansed a man with leprosy (Mt 8:1–4; Mk 1:40–42); he gave sight to two people who were blind (Mt 20:29–34; Mk 10:46–52); he enabled one who was mute to speak (Lk 11:14); he cured a woman who was hemorrhaging (Mt 9:20–22; Mk 5:25–34); and he brought a young girl back to life (Mt 9:18, 23–25; Mk 5:35–42). Indeed, the Gospels are replete with examples of how the Lord cured every kind of ailment and disease (Mt 9:35). In the account of Matthew, Jesus' mission fulfilled the prophecy of Isaiah: "He took away our infirmities and bore our diseases" (Mt 8:17; cf. Is 53:4).

Jesus' healing mission went further than caring only for physical affliction. He touched people at the deepest level of their existence; he sought their physical, mental, and spiritual healing (Jn 6:35, 11:25–27). He "came so that they might have life and have it more abundantly" (Jn 10:10).

The mystery of Christ casts light on every facet of Catholic health care: to see Christian love as the animating principle of health care; to see healing and compassion as a continuation of Christ's mission; to see suffering as a participation in the redemptive power of Christ's passion, death, and resurrection; and to see death, transformed by the resurrection, as an opportunity for a final act of communion with Christ.

For the Christian, our encounter with suffering and death can take on a positive and distinctive meaning through the redemptive power of Jesus' suffering and death. As St. Paul says, we are "always carrying about in the body the dying of Jesus, so that the life of Jesus may also be manifested in our body" (2 Cor 4:10). This truth does not lessen the pain and fear, but gives confidence and grace for bearing suffering rather than being overwhelmed by it. Catholic health care ministry bears witness to the truth that, for those who are in Christ, suffering and death are the birth pangs of the new creation. "God himself will always be with them [as their God]. He will wipe every tear from their eyes, and there shall be no more death or mourning, wailing or pain, [for] the old order has passed away" (Rev 21:3–4).

In faithful imitation of Jesus Christ, the Church has served the sick, suffering, and dying in various ways throughout history. The zealous service of individuals and communities has provided shelter for the traveler; infirmaries for the sick; and homes for children, adults, and the elderly.[3] In the United States, the many religious communities as well as dioceses that sponsor and staff this country's Catholic health care institutions and services have established an effective Catholic presence in health care. Modeling their efforts on the gospel parable of the Good Samaritan, these communities of women and men have exemplified authentic neighborliness to those in need (Lk 10:25–37). The Church seeks to ensure that the service offered in the past will be continued into the future.

While many religious communities continue their commitment to the health care ministry, lay Catholics increasingly have stepped forward to collaborate in this ministry. Inspired by the example of Christ and mandated by the Second Vatican Council, lay faithful are invited to a broader and more intense field of ministries than in the past.[4] By virtue of their Baptism, lay faithful are called to participate actively in the Church's life and mission.[5] Their participation and leadership in the health care ministry, through new forms of sponsorship and governance of institutional Catholic health care,

are essential for the Church to continue her ministry of healing and compassion. They are joined in the Church's health care mission by many men and women who are not Catholic.

Catholic health care expresses the healing ministry of Christ in a specific way within the local church. Here the diocesan bishop exercises responsibilities that are rooted in his office as pastor, teacher, and priest. As the center of unity in the diocese and coordinator of ministries in the local church, the diocesan bishop fosters the mission of Catholic health care in a way that promotes collaboration among health care leaders, providers, medical professionals, theologians, and other specialists. As pastor, the diocesan bishop is in a unique position to encourage the faithful to greater responsibility in the healing ministry of the Church. As teacher, the diocesan bishop ensures the moral and religious identity of the health care ministry in whatever setting it is carried out in the diocese. As priest, the diocesan bishop oversees the sacramental care of the sick. These responsibilities will require that Catholic health care providers and the diocesan bishop engage in ongoing communication on ethical and pastoral matters that require his attention.

In a time of new medical discoveries, rapid technological developments, and social change, what is new can either be an opportunity for genuine advancement in human culture, or it can lead to policies and actions that are contrary to the true dignity and vocation of the human person. In consultation with medical professionals, church leaders review these developments, judge them according to the principles of right reason and the ultimate standard of revealed truth, and offer authoritative teaching and guidance about the moral and pastoral responsibilities entailed by the Christian faith.[6] While the Church cannot furnish a ready answer to every moral dilemma, there are many questions about which she provides normative guidance and direction. In the absence of a determination by the magisterium, but never contrary to church teaching, the guidance of approved authors can offer appropriate guidance for ethical decision making.

Created in God's image and likeness, the human family shares in the dominion that Christ manifested in his healing ministry. This sharing involves a stewardship over all material creation (Gn 1:26) that should neither abuse nor squander nature's resources. Through science the human race comes to understand God's wonderful work; and through technology it must conserve, protect, and perfect nature in harmony with God's purposes. Health care professionals pursue a special vocation to share in carrying forth God's life-giving and healing work.

The dialogue between medical science and Christian faith has for its primary purpose the common good of all human persons. It presupposes that science and faith do not contradict each other. Both are grounded in respect for truth and freedom. As new knowledge and new technologies expand, each person must form a correct conscience based on the moral norms for proper health care.

PART ONE: THE SOCIAL RESPONSIBILITY OF CATHOLIC HEALTH CARE SERVICES

Introduction

Their embrace of Christ's healing mission has led institutionally based Catholic health care services in the United States to become an integral part of the nation's health care system. Today, this complex health care system confronts a range of economic, technological, social, and moral challenges. The response of Catholic health care institutions and services to these challenges is guided by normative principles that inform the Church's healing ministry.

First, Catholic health care ministry is rooted in a commitment to promote and defend human dignity; this is the foundation of its concern to respect the sacredness of every human life from the moment of conception until death. The first right of the human person, the right to life, entails a right to the means for the proper development of life, such as adequate health care.[7]

Second, the biblical mandate to care for the poor requires us to express this in concrete action at all levels of Catholic health care. This mandate prompts us to work to ensure that our country's health care delivery system provides adequate health care for the poor. In Catholic institutions, particular attention should be given to the health care needs of the poor, the uninsured, and the underinsured.[8]

Third, Catholic health care ministry seeks to contribute to the common good. The common good is realized when economic, political, and social conditions ensure protection for the fundamental rights of all individuals and enable all to fulfill their common purpose and reach their common goals.[9]

Fourth, Catholic health care ministry exercises responsible stewardship of available health care resources. A just health care system will be concerned both with promoting equity of care—to assure that the right of each person to basic health care is respected—and with promoting the good health of all in the community. The responsible stewardship of health care resources can be accomplished best in dialogue with people from all levels of society, in accordance with the principle of subsidiarity and with respect for the moral principles that guide institutions and persons.

Fifth, within a pluralistic society, Catholic health care services will encounter requests for medical procedures contrary to the moral teachings of the Church. Catholic health care does not offend the rights of individual conscience by refusing to provide or permit medical procedures that are judged morally wrong by the teaching authority of the Church.

Directives

1. A Catholic institutional health care service is a community that provides health care to those in need of it. This service must be animated by the Gospel of Jesus Christ and guided by the moral tradition of the Church.
2. Catholic health care should be marked by a spirit of mutual respect among care-givers that disposes them to deal with those it serves and their families with the compassion of Christ, sensitive to their vulnerability at a time of special need.
3. In accord with its mission, Catholic health care should distinguish itself by service to and advocacy for those people whose social condition puts them at the margins of our society and makes them particularly vulnerable to discrimination: the poor; the uninsured and the underinsured; children and the unborn; single parents; the elderly; those with incurable diseases and chemical dependencies; racial minorities; immigrants and refugees. In particular, the person with mental or physical disabilities, regardless of the cause or severity, must be treated as a unique person of incomparable worth, with the same right to life and to adequate health care as all other persons.
4. A Catholic health care institution, especially a teaching hospital, will promote medical research consistent with its mission of providing health care and with concern for the responsible stewardship of health care resources. Such medical research must adhere to Catholic moral principles.
5. Catholic health care services must adopt these Directives as policy, require adherence to them within the institution as a condition for medical privileges and employment, and provide appropriate instruction regarding the Directives for administration, medical and nursing staff, and other personnel.
6. A Catholic health care organization should be a responsible steward of the health care resources available to it. Collaboration with other health care providers, in ways that do not compromise Catholic social and moral teaching, can be an effective means of such stewardship.[10]
7. A Catholic health care institution must treat its employees respectfully and justly. This responsibility includes: equal employment opportunities for anyone qualified for the task, irrespective of a person's race, sex, age, national origin, or disability; a workplace that promotes employee participation; a work environment that ensures

employee safety and well-being; just compensation and benefits; and recognition of the rights of employees to organize and bargain collectively without prejudice to the common good.

8. Catholic health care institutions have a unique relationship to both the Church and the wider community they serve. Because of the ecclesial nature of this relationship, the relevant requirements of canon law will be observed with regard to the foundation of a new Catholic health care institution; the substantial revision of the mission of an institution; and the sale, sponsorship transfer, or closure of an existing institution.

9. Employees of a Catholic health care institution must respect and uphold the religious mission of the institution and adhere to these Directives. They should maintain professional standards and promote the institution's commitment to human dignity and the common good.

PART TWO: THE PASTORAL AND SPIRITUAL RESPONSIBILITY OF CATHOLIC HEALTH CARE

Introduction

The dignity of human life flows from creation in the image of God (Gn 1:26), from redemption by Jesus Christ (Eph 1:10; 1 Tm 2:4–6), and from our common destiny to share a life with God beyond all corruption (1 Cor 15:42–57). Catholic health care has the responsibility to treat those in need in a way that respects the human dignity and eternal destiny of all. The words of Christ have provided inspiration for Catholic health care: "I was ill and you cared for me" (Mt 25:36). The care provided assists those in need to experience their own dignity and value, especially when these are obscured by the burdens of illness or the anxiety of imminent death.

Since a Catholic health care institution is a community of healing and compassion, the care offered is not limited to the treatment of a disease or bodily ailment but embraces the physical, psychological, social, and spiritual dimensions of the human person. The medical expertise offered through Catholic health care is combined with other forms of care to promote health and relieve human suffering. For this reason, Catholic health care extends to the spiritual nature of the person. "Without health of the spirit, high technology focused strictly on the body offers limited hope for healing the whole person."[11] Directed to spiritual needs that are often appreciated more deeply during times of illness, pastoral care is an integral part of Catholic health care. Pastoral care encompasses the full range of spiritual services, including a listening presence; help in dealing with powerlessness, pain, and alienation;

and assistance in recognizing and responding to God's will with greater joy and peace. It should be acknowledged, of course, that technological advances in medicine have reduced the length of hospital stays dramatically. It follows, therefore, that the pastoral care of patients, especially administration of the sacraments, will be provided more often than not at the parish level, both before and after one's hospitalization. For this reason, it is essential that there be very cordial and cooperative relationships between the personnel of pastoral care departments and the local clergy and ministers of care.

Priests, deacons, religious, and laity exercise diverse but complementary roles in this pastoral care. Since many areas of pastoral care call upon the creative response of these pastoral care-givers to the particular needs of patients or residents, the following directives address only a limited number of specific pastoral activities.

Directives

10. A Catholic health care organization should provide pastoral care to minister to the religious and spiritual needs of all those it serves. Pastoral care personnel—clergy, religious, and lay alike—should have appropriate professional preparation, including an understanding of these Directives.

11. Pastoral care personnel should work in close collaboration with local parishes and community clergy. Appropriate pastoral services and/or referrals should be available to all in keeping with their religious beliefs or affiliation.

12. For Catholic patients or residents, provision for the sacraments is an especially important part of Catholic health care ministry. Every effort should be made to have priests assigned to hospitals and health care institutions to celebrate the Eucharist and provide the sacraments to patients and staff.

13. Particular care should be taken to provide and to publicize opportunities for patients or residents to receive the sacrament of Penance.

14. Properly prepared lay Catholics can be appointed to serve as extraordinary ministers of Holy Communion, in accordance with canon law and the policies of the local diocese. They should assist pastoral care personnel—clergy, religious, and laity—by providing supportive visits, advising patients regarding the availability of priests for the sacrament of Penance, and distributing Holy Communion to the faithful who request it.

15. Responsive to a patient's desires and condition, all involved in pastoral care should facilitate the availability of priests to provide the sacrament of Anointing of the Sick, recognizing that through this sacrament Christ provides grace and support to those who are seri-

ously ill or weakened by advanced age. Normally, the sacrament is celebrated when the sick person is fully conscious. It may be conferred upon the sick who have lost consciousness or the use of reason, if there is reason to believe that they would have asked for the sacrament while in control of their faculties.

16. All Catholics who are capable of receiving Communion should receive Viaticum when they are in danger of death, while still in full possession of their faculties.[12]

17. Except in cases of emergency (i.e., danger of death), any request for Baptism made by adults or for infants should be referred to the chaplain of the institution. Newly born infants in danger of death, including those miscarried, should be baptized if this is possible.[13] In case of emergency, if a priest or a deacon is not available, anyone can validly baptize.[14] In the case of emergency Baptism, the chaplain or the director of pastoral care is to be notified.

18. When a Catholic who has been baptized but not yet confirmed is in danger of death, any priest may confirm the person.[15]

19. A record of the conferral of Baptism or Confirmation should be sent to the parish in which the institution is located and posted in its Baptism/Confirmation registers.

20. Catholic discipline generally reserves the reception of the sacraments to Catholics. In accord with canon 844, §3, Catholic ministers may administer the sacraments of Eucharist, Penance, and Anointing of the Sick to members of the oriental churches that do not have full communion with the Catholic Church, or of other churches that in the judgment of the Holy See are in the same condition as the oriental churches, if such persons ask for the sacraments on their own and are properly disposed.

   With regard to other Christians not in full communion with the Catholic Church, when the danger of death or other grave necessity is present, the four conditions of canon 844, §4, also must be present, namely, they cannot approach a minister of their own community; they ask for the sacraments on their own; they manifest Catholic faith in these sacraments; and they are properly disposed. The diocesan bishop has the responsibility to oversee this pastoral practice.

21. The appointment of priests and deacons to the pastoral care staff of a Catholic institution must have the explicit approval or confirmation of the local bishop in collaboration with the administration of the institution. The appointment of the director of the pastoral care staff should be made in consultation with the diocesan bishop.

22. For the sake of appropriate ecumenical and interfaith relations, a diocesan policy should be developed with regard to the appointment of non-Catholic members to the pastoral care staff of a Catholic

health care institution. The director of pastoral care at a Catholic institution should be a Catholic; any exception to this norm should be approved by the diocesan bishop.

PART THREE: THE PROFESSIONAL–PATIENT RELATIONSHIP

Introduction

A person in need of health care and the professional health care provider who accepts that person as a patient enter into a relationship that requires, among other things, mutual respect, trust, honesty, and appropriate confidentiality. The resulting free exchange of information must avoid manipulation, intimidation, or condescension. Such a relationship enables the patient to disclose personal information needed for effective care and permits the health care provider to use his or her professional competence most effectively to maintain or restore the patient's health. Neither the health care professional nor the patient acts independently of the other; both participate in the healing process.

Today, a patient often receives health care from a team of providers, especially in the setting of the modern acute-care hospital. But the resulting multiplication of relationships does not alter the personal character of the interaction between health care providers and the patient. The relationship of the person seeking health care and the professionals providing that care is an important part of the foundation on which diagnosis and care are provided. Diagnosis and care, therefore, entail a series of decisions with ethical as well as medical dimensions. The health care professional has the knowledge and experience to pursue the goals of healing, the maintenance of health, and the compassionate care of the dying, taking into account the patient's convictions and spiritual needs, and the moral responsibilities of all concerned. The person in need of health care depends on the skill of the health care provider to assist in preserving life and promoting health of body, mind, and spirit. The patient, in turn, has a responsibility to use these physical and mental resources in the service of moral and spiritual goals to the best of his or her ability.

When the health care professional and the patient use institutional Catholic health care, they also accept its public commitment to the Church's understanding of and witness to the dignity of the human person. The Church's moral teaching on health care nurtures a truly interpersonal professional–patient relationship. This professional–patient relationship is never separated, then, from the Catholic identity of the health care institution. The faith that inspires Catholic health care guides medical decisions in ways that fully respect the dignity of the person and the relationship with the health care professional.

Directives

23. The inherent dignity of the human person must be respected and protected regardless of the nature of the person's health problem or social status. The respect for human dignity extends to all persons who are served by Catholic health care.

24. In compliance with federal law, a Catholic health care institution will make available to patients information about their rights, under the laws of their state, to make an advance directive for their medical treatment. The institution, however, will not honor an advance directive that is contrary to Catholic teaching. If the advance directive conflicts with Catholic teaching, an explanation should be provided as to why the directive cannot be honored.

25. Each person may identify in advance a representative to make health care decisions as his or her surrogate in the event that the person loses the capacity to make health care decisions. Decisions by the designated surrogate should be faithful to Catholic moral principles and to the person's intentions and values, or if the person's intentions are unknown, to the person's best interests. In the event that an advance directive is not executed, those who are in a position to know best the patient's wishes—usually family members and loved ones—should participate in the treatment decisions for the person who has lost the capacity to make health care decisions.

26. The free and informed consent of the person or the person's surrogate is required for medical treatments and procedures, except in an emergency situation when consent cannot be obtained and there is no indication that the patient would refuse consent to the treatment.

27. Free and informed consent requires that the person or the person's surrogate receive all reasonable information about the essential nature of the proposed treatment and its benefits; its risks, side-effects, consequences, and cost; and any reasonable and morally legitimate alternatives, including no treatment at all.

28. Each person or the person's surrogate should have access to medical and moral information and counseling so as to be able to form his or her conscience. The free and informed health care decision of the person or the person's surrogate is to be followed so long as it does not contradict Catholic principles.

29. All persons served by Catholic health care have the right and duty to protect and preserve their bodily and functional integrity.[16] The functional integrity of the person may be sacrificed to maintain the health or life of the person when no other morally permissible means is available.[17]

30. The transplantation of organs from living donors is morally permissible when such a donation will not sacrifice or seriously impair any

essential bodily function and the anticipated benefit to the recipient is proportionate to the harm done to the donor. Furthermore, the freedom of the prospective donor must be respected, and economic advantages should not accrue to the donor.

31. No one should be the subject of medical or genetic experimentation, even if it is therapeutic, unless the person or surrogate first has given free and informed consent. In instances of nontherapeutic experimentation, the surrogate can give this consent only if the experiment entails no significant risk to the person's well-being. Moreover, the greater the person's incompetency and vulnerability, the greater the reasons must be to perform any medical experimentation, especially nontherapeutic.

32. While every person is obliged to use ordinary means to preserve his or her health, no person should be obliged to submit to a health care procedure that the person has judged, with a free and informed conscience, not to provide a reasonable hope of benefit without imposing excessive risks and burdens on the patient or excessive expense to family or community.[18]

33. The well-being of the whole person must be taken into account in deciding about any therapeutic intervention or use of technology. Therapeutic procedures that are likely to cause harm or undesirable side-effects can be justified only by a proportionate benefit to the patient.

34. Health care providers are to respect each person's privacy and confidentiality regarding information related to the person's diagnosis, treatment, and care.

35. Health care professionals should be educated to recognize the symptoms of abuse and violence and are obliged to report cases of abuse to the proper authorities in accordance with local statutes.

36. Compassionate and understanding care should be given to a person who is the victim of sexual assault. Health care providers should cooperate with law enforcement officials and offer the person psychological and spiritual support as well as accurate medical information. A female who has been raped should be able to defend herself against a potential conception from the sexual assault. If, after appropriate testing, there is no evidence that conception has occurred already, she may be treated with medications that would prevent ovulation, sperm capacitation, or fertilization. It is not permissible, however, to initiate or to recommend treatments that have as their purpose or direct effect the removal, destruction, or interference with the implantation of a fertilized ovum.[19]

37. An ethics committee or some alternate form of ethical consultation should be available to assist by advising on particular ethical situations, by offering educational opportunities, and by reviewing and

recommending policies. To these ends, there should be appropriate standards for medical ethical consultation within a particular diocese that will respect the diocesan bishop's pastoral responsibility as well as assist members of ethics committees to be familiar with Catholic medical ethics and, in particular, these Directives.

PART FOUR: ISSUES IN CARE FOR THE BEGINNING OF LIFE

Introduction

The Church's commitment to human dignity inspires an abiding concern for the sanctity of human life from its very beginning, and with the dignity of marriage and of the marriage act by which human life is transmitted. The Church cannot approve medical practices that undermine the biological, psychological, and moral bonds on which the strength of marriage and the family depends.

Catholic health care ministry witnesses to the sanctity of life "from the moment of conception until death."[20] The Church's defense of life encompasses the unborn and the care of women and their children during and after pregnancy. The Church's commitment to life is seen in its willingness to collaborate with others to alleviate the causes of the high infant mortality rate and to provide adequate health care to mothers and their children before and after birth.

The Church has the deepest respect for the family, for the marriage covenant, and for the love that binds a married couple together. This includes respect for the marriage act by which husband and wife express their love and cooperate with God in the creation of a new human being. The Second Vatican Council affirms:

> This love is an eminently human one. . . . It involves the good of the whole person. . . . The actions within marriage by which the couple are united intimately and chastely are noble and worthy ones. Expressed in a manner which is truly human, these actions signify and promote that mutual self-giving by which spouses enrich each other with a joyful and a thankful will.[21]
>
> Marriage and conjugal love are by their nature ordained toward the begetting and educating of children. Children are really the supreme gift of marriage and contribute very substantially to the welfare of their parents. . . . Parents should regard as their proper mission the task of transmitting human life and educating those to whom it has been transmitted. . . . They are thereby cooperators with the love of God the Creator, and are, so to speak, the interpreters of that love.[22]

For legitimate reasons of responsible parenthood, married couples may limit the number of their children by natural means. The Church cannot approve contraceptive interventions that "either in anticipation of the marital act, or in its accomplishment or in the development of its natural consequences, have the purpose, whether as an end or a means, to render procreation impossible."[23] Such interventions violate "the inseparable connection, willed by God . . . between the two meanings of the conjugal act: the unitive and procreative meaning."[24]

With the advance of the biological and medical sciences, society has at its disposal new technologies for responding to the problem of infertility. While we rejoice in the potential for good inherent in many of these technologies, we cannot assume that what is technically possible is always morally right. Reproductive technologies that substitute for the marriage act are not consistent with human dignity. Just as the marriage act is joined naturally to procreation, so procreation is joined naturally to the marriage act. As Pope John XXIII observed:

> The transmission of human life is entrusted by nature to a personal and conscious act and as such is subject to all the holy laws of God: the immutable and inviolable laws which must be recognized and observed. For this reason, one cannot use means and follow methods which could be licit in the transmission of the life of plants and animals.[25]

Because the moral law is rooted in the whole of human nature, human persons, through intelligent reflection on their own spiritual destiny, can discover and cooperate in the plan of the Creator.[26]

Directives

38. When the marital act of sexual intercourse is not able to attain its procreative purpose, assistance that does not separate the unitive and procreative ends of the act, and does not substitute for the marital act itself, may be used to help married couples conceive.[27]

39. Those techniques of assisted conception that respect the unitive and procreative meanings of sexual intercourse and do not involve the destruction of human embryos, or their deliberate generation in such numbers that it is clearly envisaged that all cannot implant and some are simply being used to maximize the chances of others implanting, may be used as therapies for infertility.

40. Heterologous fertilization (that is, any technique used to achieve conception by the use of gametes coming from at least one donor other than the spouses) is prohibited because it is contrary to the covenant of marriage, the unity of the spouses, and the dignity proper to parents and the child.[28]

41. Homologous artificial fertilization (that is, any technique used to achieve conception using the gametes of the two spouses joined in

marriage) is prohibited when it separates procreation from the marital act in its unitive significance (e.g., any technique used to achieve extra-corporeal conception).[29]

42. Because of the dignity of the child and of marriage, and because of the uniqueness of the mother–child relationship, participation in contracts or arrangements for surrogate motherhood is not permitted. Moreover, the commercialization of such surrogacy denigrates the dignity of women, especially the poor.[30]

43. A Catholic health care institution that provides treatment for infertility should offer not only technical assistance to infertile couples but also should help couples pursue other solutions (e.g., counseling, adoption).

44. A Catholic health care institution should provide prenatal, obstetric, and postnatal services for mothers and their children in a manner consonant with its mission.

45. Abortion (that is, the directly intended termination of pregnancy before viability or the directly intended destruction of a viable fetus) is never permitted. Every procedure whose sole immediate effect is the termination of pregnancy before viability is an abortion, which, in its moral context, includes the interval between conception and implantation of the embryo. Catholic health care institutions are not to provide abortion services, even based upon the principle of material cooperation. In this context, Catholic health care institutions need to be concerned about the danger of scandal in any association with abortion providers.

46. Catholic health care providers should be ready to offer compassionate physical, psychological, moral, and spiritual care to those persons who have suffered from the trauma of abortion.

47. Operations, treatments, and medications that have as their direct purpose the cure of a proportionately serious pathological condition of a pregnant woman are permitted when they cannot be safely postponed until the unborn child is viable, even if they will result in the death of the unborn child.

48. In case of extrauterine pregnancy, no intervention is morally licit which constitutes a direct abortion.[31]

49. For a proportionate reason, labor may be induced after the fetus is viable.

50. Prenatal diagnosis is permitted when the procedure does not threaten the life or physical integrity of the unborn child or the mother and does not subject them to disproportionate risks; when the diagnosis can provide information to guide preventative care for the mother or pre- or postnatal care for the child; and when the

parents, or at least the mother, give free and informed consent. Prenatal diagnosis is not permitted when undertaken with the intention of aborting an unborn child with a serious defect.[32]

51. Nontherapeutic experiments on a living embryo or fetus are not permitted, even with the consent of the parents. Therapeutic experiments are permitted for a proportionate reason with the free and informed consent of the parents or, if the father cannot be contacted, at least of the mother. Medical research that will not harm the life or physical integrity of an unborn child is permitted with parental consent.[33]

52. Catholic health institutions may not promote or condone contraceptive practices but should provide, for married couples and the medical staff who counsel them, instruction both about the Church's teaching on responsible parenthood and in methods of natural family planning.

53. Direct sterilization of either men or women, whether permanent or temporary, is not permitted in a Catholic health care institution. Procedures that induce sterility are permitted when their direct effect is the cure or alleviation of a present and serious pathology and a simpler treatment is not available.[34]

54. Genetic counseling may be provided in order to promote responsible parenthood and to prepare for the proper treatment and care of children with genetic defects, in accordance with Catholic moral teaching and the intrinsic rights and obligations of married couples regarding the transmission of life.

PART FIVE: ISSUES IN CARE FOR THE DYING

Introduction

Christ's redemption and saving grace embrace the whole person, especially in his or her illness, suffering, and death.[35] The Catholic health care ministry faces the reality of death with the confidence of faith. In the face of death—for many, a time when hope seems lost—the Church witnesses to her belief that God has created each person for eternal life.[36]

Above all, as a witness to its faith, a Catholic health care institution will be a community of respect, love, and support to patients or residents and their families as they face the reality of death. What is hardest to face is the process of dying itself, especially the dependency, the helplessness, and the pain that so often accompany terminal illness. One of the primary purposes of medicine in caring for the dying is the relief of pain and the suffering caused by it. Effective management of pain in all its forms is critical in the appropriate care of the dying.

The truth that life is a precious gift from God has profound implications for the question of stewardship over human life. We are not the owners of our lives and, hence, do not have absolute power over life. We have a duty to preserve our life and to use it for the glory of God, but the duty to preserve life is not absolute, for we may reject life-prolonging procedures that are insufficiently beneficial or excessively burdensome. Suicide and euthanasia are never morally acceptable options.

The task of medicine is to care even when it cannot cure. Physicians and their patients must evaluate the use of the technology at their disposal. Reflection on the innate dignity of human life in all its dimensions and on the purpose of medical care is indispensable for formulating a true moral judgment about the use of technology to maintain life. The use of life-sustaining technology is judged in light of the Christian meaning of life, suffering, and death. Only in this way are two extremes avoided: on the one hand, an insistence on useless or burdensome technology even when a patient may legitimately wish to forgo it and, on the other hand, the withdrawal of technology with the intention of causing death.[37]

Some state Catholic conferences, individual bishops, and the USCCB Committee on Pro-Life Activities (formerly an NCCB committee) have addressed the moral issues concerning medically assisted hydration and nutrition. The bishops are guided by the Church's teaching forbidding euthanasia, which is "an action or an omission which of itself or by intention causes death, in order that all suffering may in this way be eliminated."[38] These statements agree that hydration and nutrition are not morally obligatory either when they bring no comfort to a person who is imminently dying or when they cannot be assimilated by a person's body. The USCCB Committee on Pro-Life Activities' report, in addition, points out the necessary distinctions between questions already resolved by the magisterium and those requiring further reflection, as, for example, the morality of withdrawing medically assisted hydration and nutrition from a person who is in the condition that is recognized by physicians as the "persistent vegetative state" (PVS).[39]

Directives

55. Catholic health care institutions offering care to persons in danger of death from illness, accident, advanced age, or similar condition should provide them with appropriate opportunities to prepare for death. Persons in danger of death should be provided with whatever information is necessary to help them understand their condition and have the opportunity to discuss their condition with their family members and care providers. They should also be offered the appropriate medical information that would make it possible to

address the morally legitimate choices available to them. They should be provided the spiritual support as well as the opportunity to receive the sacraments in order to prepare well for death.

56. A person has a moral obligation to use ordinary or proportionate means of preserving his or her life. Proportionate means are those that in the judgment of the patient offer a reasonable hope of benefit and do not entail an excessive burden or impose excessive expense on the family or the community.[40]

57. A person may forgo extraordinary or disproportionate means of preserving life. Disproportionate means are those that in the patient's judgment do not offer a reasonable hope of benefit or entail an excessive burden, or impose excessive expense on the family or the community.[41]

58. There should be a presumption in favor of providing nutrition and hydration to all patients, including patients who require medically assisted nutrition and hydration, as long as this is of sufficient benefit to outweigh the burdens involved to the patient.

59. The free and informed judgment made by a competent adult patient concerning the use or withdrawal of life-sustaining procedures should always be respected and normally complied with, unless it is contrary to Catholic moral teaching.

60. Euthanasia is an action or omission that of itself or by intention causes death in order to alleviate suffering. Catholic health care institutions may never condone or participate in euthanasia or assisted suicide in any way. Dying patients who request euthanasia should receive loving care, psychological and spiritual support, and appropriate remedies for pain and other symptoms so that they can live with dignity until the time of natural death.[42]

61. Patients should be kept as free of pain as possible so that they may die comfortably and with dignity, and in the place where they wish to die. Since a person has the right to prepare for his or her death while fully conscious, he or she should not be deprived of consciousness without a compelling reason. Medicines capable of alleviating or suppressing pain may be given to a dying person, even if this therapy may indirectly shorten the person's life so long as the intent is not to hasten death. Patients experiencing suffering that cannot be alleviated should be helped to appreciate the Christian understanding of redemptive suffering.

62. The determination of death should be made by the physician or competent medical authority in accordance with responsible and commonly accepted scientific criteria.

63. Catholic health care institutions should encourage and provide the means whereby those who wish to do so may arrange for the dona-

tion of their organs and bodily tissue, for ethically legitimate purposes, so that they may be used for donation and research after death.

64. Such organs should not be removed until it has been medically determined that the patient has died. In order to prevent any conflict of interest, the physician who determines death should not be a member of the transplant team.

65. The use of tissue or organs from an infant may be permitted after death has been determined and with the informed consent of the parents or guardians.

66. Catholic health care institutions should not make use of human tissue obtained by direct abortions even for research and therapeutic purposes.[43]

PART SIX: FORMING NEW PARTNERSHIPS WITH HEALTH CARE ORGANIZATIONS AND PROVIDERS

Introduction

Until recently, most health care providers enjoyed a degree of independence from one another. In ever-increasing ways, Catholic health care providers have become involved with other health care organizations and providers. For instance, many Catholic health care systems and institutions share in the joint purchase of technology and services with other local facilities or physicians' groups. Another phenomenon is the growing number of Catholic health care systems and institutions joining or co-sponsoring integrated delivery networks or managed care organizations in order to contract with insurers and other health care payers. In some instances, Catholic health care systems sponsor a health care plan or health maintenance organization. In many dioceses, new partnerships will result in a decrease in the number of health care providers, at times leaving the Catholic institution as the sole provider of health care services. At whatever level, new partnerships forge a variety of interwoven relationships: between the various institutional partners, between health care providers and the community, between physicians and health care services, and between health care services and payers.

On the one hand, new partnerships can be viewed as opportunities for Catholic health care institutions and services to witness to their religious and ethical commitments and so influence the healing profession. For example, new partnerships can help to implement the Church's social teaching. New partnerships can be opportunities to realign the local delivery system in order to provide a continuum of health care to the community; they can witness to a responsible stewardship of limited health care resources; and they can be opportunities to provide to poor and vulnerable persons a more equitable access to basic care.

On the other hand, new partnerships can pose serious challenges to the viability of the identity of Catholic health care institutions and services, and their ability to implement these Directives in a consistent way, especially when partnerships are formed with those who do not share Catholic moral principles. The risk of scandal cannot be underestimated when partnerships are not built upon common values and moral principles. Partnership opportunities for some Catholic health care providers may even threaten the continued existence of other Catholic institutions and services, particularly when partnerships are driven by financial considerations alone. Because of the potential dangers involved in the new partnerships that are emerging, an increased collaboration among Catholic-sponsored health care institutions is essential and should be sought before other forms of partnerships.

The significant challenges that new partnerships may pose, however, do not necessarily preclude their possibility on moral grounds. The potential dangers require that new partnerships undergo systematic and objective moral analysis, which takes into account the various factors that often pressure institutions and services into new partnerships that can diminish the autonomy and ministry of the Catholic partner. The following directives are offered to assist institutionally based Catholic health care services in this process of analysis. To this end, the United States Conference of Catholic Bishops (formerly the National Conference of Catholic Bishops) has established the Ad Hoc Committee on Health Care Issues and the Church as a resource for bishops and health care leaders.

This new edition of the *Ethical and Religious Directives* omits the appendix concerning cooperation, which was contained in the 1995 edition. Experience has shown that the brief articulation of the principles of cooperation that was presented there did not sufficiently forestall certain possible misinterpretations and in practice gave rise to problems in concrete applications of the principles. Reliable theological experts should be consulted in interpreting and applying the principles governing cooperation, with the proviso that, as a rule, Catholic partners should avoid entering into partnerships that would involve them in cooperation with the wrongdoing of other providers.

Directives

67. Decisions that may lead to serious consequences for the identity or reputation of Catholic health care services, or entail the high risk of scandal, should be made in consultation with the diocesan bishop or his health care liaison.

68. Any partnership that will affect the mission or religious and ethical identity of Catholic health care institutional services must respect church teaching and discipline. Diocesan bishops and other church authorities should be involved as such partnerships are developed,

and the diocesan bishop should give the appropriate authorization before they are completed. The diocesan bishop's approval is required for partnerships sponsored by institutions subject to his governing authority; for partnerships sponsored by religious institutes of pontifical right, his *nihil obstat* should be obtained.

69. If a Catholic health care organization is considering entering into an arrangement with another organization that may be involved in activities judged morally wrong by the Church, participation in such activities must be limited to what is in accord with the moral principles governing cooperation.

70. Catholic health care organizations are not permitted to engage in immediate material cooperation in actions that are intrinsically immoral, such as abortion, euthanasia, assisted suicide, and direct sterilization.[44]

71. The possibility of scandal must be considered when applying the principles governing cooperation.[45] Cooperation, which in all other respects is morally licit, may need to be refused because of the scandal that might be caused. Scandal can sometimes be avoided by an appropriate explanation of what is in fact being done at the health care facility under Catholic auspices. The diocesan bishop has final responsibility for assessing and addressing issues of scandal, considering not only the circumstances in his local diocese but also the regional and national implications of his decision.[46]

72. The Catholic partner in an arrangement has the responsibility periodically to assess whether the binding agreement is being observed and implemented in a way that is consistent with Catholic teaching.

CONCLUSION

Sickness speaks to us of our limitations and human frailty. It can take the form of infirmity resulting from the simple passing of years or injury from the exuberance of youthful energy. It can be temporary or chronic, debilitating, and even terminal. Yet the follower of Jesus faces illness and the consequences of the human condition aware that our Lord always shows compassion toward the infirm.

Jesus not only taught his disciples to be compassionate, but he also told them who should be the special object of their compassion. The parable of the feast with its humble guests was preceded by the instruction: "When you hold a banquet, invite the poor, the crippled, the lame, the blind" (Lk 14:13). These were people whom Jesus healed and loved.

Catholic health care is a response to the challenge of Jesus to go and do likewise. Catholic health care services rejoice in the challenge to be Christ's healing compassion in the world and see their ministry not only as an effort to restore and preserve health but also as a spiritual service and a sign of that final healing that will one day bring about the new creation that is the ultimate fruit of Jesus' ministry and God's love for us.

NOTES

1. National Conference of Catholic Bishops, *Health and Health Care: A Pastoral Letter of the American Catholic Bishops* (Washington, D.C.: United States Catholic Conference, 1981).

2. Health care services under Catholic auspices are carried out in a variety of institutional settings (e.g., hospitals, clinics, out-patient facilities, urgent care centers, hospices, nursing homes, and parishes). Depending on the context, these Directives will employ the terms "institution" and/or "services" in order to encompass the variety of settings in which Catholic health care is provided.

3. *Health and Health Care*, p. 5.

4. Second Vatican Ecumenical Council, *Decree on the Apostolate of the Laity (Apostolicam Actuositatem)* (1965), no. 1.

5. Pope John Paul II, Post-Synodal Apostolic Exhortation, *On the Vocation and the Mission of the Lay Faithful in the Church and in the World (Christifideles Laici)* (Washington, D.C.: United States Catholic Conference, 1988), no. 29.

6. As examples, see Congregation for the Doctrine of the Faith, *Declaration on Procured Abortion* (1974); Congregation for the Doctrine of the Faith, *Declaration on Euthanasia* (1980); Congregation for the Doctrine of the Faith, *Instruction on Respect for Human Life in its Origin and on the Dignity of Procreation: Replies to Certain Questions of the Day (Donum Vitae)* (Washington, D.C.: United States Catholic Conference, 1987).

7. Pope John XXIII, Encyclical Letter, *Peace on Earth (Pacem in Terris)* (Washington, D.C.: United States Catholic Conference, 1963), no. 11; *Health and Health Care*, pp. 5, 17–18; *Catechism of the Catholic Church*, 2nd ed. (Washington, D.C.: United States Catholic Conference, 2000), no. 2211.

8. Pope John Paul II, *On Social Concern, Encyclical Letter on the Occasion of the Twentieth Anniversary of "Populorum Progressio" (Sollicitudo Rei Socialis)* (Washington, D.C.: United States Catholic Conference, 1988), no. 43.

9. National Conference of Catholic Bishops, *Economic Justice for All: Pastoral Letter on Catholic Social Teaching and the U.S. Economy* (Washington, D.C.: United States Catholic Conference, 1986), no. 80.

10. The duty of responsible stewardship demands responsible collaboration. But in collaborative efforts, Catholic institutionally based health care services must be attentive to occasions when the policies and practices of other institutions are not compatible with the Church's authoritative moral teaching. At such times, Catholic health care institutions should determine

whether or to what degree collaboration would be morally permissible. To make that judgment, the governing boards of Catholic institutions should adhere to the moral principles on cooperation. See Part Six.

11. *Health and Health Care*, p. 12.

12. Cf. *Code of Canon Law*, cc. 921–923.

13. Cf. ibid., c. 867, §2, and c. 871.

14. To confer Baptism in an emergency, one must have the proper intention (to do what the Church intends by Baptism) and pour water on the head of the person to be baptized, meanwhile pronouncing the words: "I baptize you in the name of the Father, and of the Son, and of the Holy Spirit."

15. Cf. c. 883, §3.

16. For example, while the donation of a kidney represents loss of biological integrity, such a donation does not compromise functional integrity since human beings are capable of functioning with only one kidney.

17. Cf. directive 53.

18. *Declaration on Euthanasia*, Part IV; cf. also directives 56–57.

19. It is recommended that a sexually assaulted woman be advised of the ethical restrictions that prevent Catholic hospitals from using abortifacient procedures; cf. Pennsylvania Catholic Conference, "Guidelines for Catholic Hospitals Treating Victims of Sexual Assault," *Origins* 22 (1993): 810.

20. Pope John Paul II, "Address of October 29, 1983, to the 35th General Assembly of the World Medical Association," *Acta Apostolicae Sedis* 76 (1984): 390.

21. Second Vatican Ecumenical Council, "Pastoral Constitution on the Church in the Modern World" (*Gaudium et Spes*) (1965), no. 49.

22. Ibid., no. 50.

23. Pope Paul VI, Encyclical Letter, *On the Regulation of Birth (Humanae Vitae)* (Washington, D.C.: United States Catholic Conference, 1968), no. 14.

24. Ibid., no. 12.

25. Pope John XXIII, Encyclical Letter, *Mater et Magistra* (1961), no. 193, quoted in Congregation for the Doctrine of the Faith, *Donum Vitae*, no. 4.

26. Pope John Paul II, Encyclical Letter, *The Splendor of Truth (Veritatis Splendor)* (Washington, D.C.: United States Catholic Conference, 1993), no. 50.

27. "Homologous artificial insemination within marriage cannot be admitted except for those cases in which the technical means is not a substitute for the conjugal act but serves to facilitate and to help so that the act attains its natural purpose" (*Donum Vitae*, Part II, B, no. 6; cf. also Part I, nos. 1, 6).

28. Ibid., Part II, A, no. 2.

29. "Artificial insemination as a substitute for the conjugal act is prohibited by reason of the voluntarily achieved dissociation of the two meanings of the conjugal act. Masturbation, through which the sperm is normally obtained, is another sign of this dissociation: even when it is done for the

purpose of procreation, the act remains deprived of its unitive meaning: It lacks the sexual relationship called for by the moral order, namely, the relationship which realizes 'the full sense of mutual self-giving and human procreation in the context of true love'" (*Donum Vitae*, Part II, B, no. 6).

30. Ibid., Part II, A, no. 3.

31. Cf. directive 45.

32. *Donum Vitae*, Part I, no. 2.

33. Cf. ibid., no. 4.

34. Cf. Congregation for the Doctrine of the Faith, "Responses on Uterine Isolation and Related Matters," July 31, 1993, *Origins* 24 (1994): 211–212.

35. Pope John Paul II, Apostolic Letter, *On the Christian Meaning of Human Suffering (Salvifici Doloris)* (Washington, D.C.: United States Catholic Conference, 1984), nos. 25–27.

36. National Conference of Catholic Bishops, *Order of Christian Funerals* (Collegeville, Minn.: The Liturgical Press, 1989), no. 1.

37. *Declaration on Euthanasia.*

38. Ibid., Part II, p. 4.

39. Committee for Pro-Life Activities, National Conference of Catholic Bishops, *Nutrition and Hydration: Moral and Pastoral Reflections* (Washington, D.C.: United States Catholic Conference, 1992). On the importance of consulting authoritative teaching in the formation of conscience and in taking moral decisions, see *Veritatis Splendor*, nos. 63–64.

40. *Declaration on Euthanasia*, Part IV.

41. Ibid.

42. Cf. ibid.

43. *Donum Vitae*, Part I, no. 4.

44. While there are many acts of varying moral gravity that can be identified as intrinsically evil, in the context of contemporary health care the most pressing concerns are currently abortion, euthanasia, assisted suicide, and direct sterilization. See Pope John Paul II's *Ad Limina* Address to the bishops of Texas, Oklahoma, and Arkansas (Region X), in *Origins* 28 (1998): 283. See also "Reply of the Sacred Congregation for the Doctrine of the Faith on Sterilization in Catholic Hospitals" (*Quaecumque Sterilizatio*), March 13, 1975, *Origins* 10 (1976): 33–35: "Any cooperation institutionally approved or tolerated in actions which are in themselves, that is, by their nature and condition, directed to a contraceptive end . . . is absolutely forbidden. For the official approbation of direct sterilization and, a *fortiori*, its management and execution in accord with hospital regulations, is a matter which, in the objective order, is by its very nature (or intrinsically) evil." This directive supersedes the "Commentary on the Reply of the Sacred Congregation for the Doctrine of the Faith on Sterilization in Catholic Hospitals" published by the National Conference of Catholic Bishops on September 15, 1977 in *Origins* 11 (1977): 399–400.

45. See *Catechism of the Catholic Church*: "Scandal is an attitude or behavior which leads another to do evil" (no. 2284); "Anyone who uses the power at his disposal in such a way that it leads others to do wrong becomes guilty of scandal and responsible for the evil that he has directly or indirectly encouraged" (no. 2287).

46. See "The Pastoral Role of the Diocesan Bishop in Catholic Health Care Ministry," *Origins* 26 (1997): 703.

Appendix 2

The Universal Declaration of Human Rights of the United Nations

United Nations

Article 1. All human beings are born free and equal in dignity and rights. They are endowed with reason and conscience and should act toward one another in a spirit of brotherhood.

Article 2. Everyone is entitled to all the rights and freedoms set forth in this Declaration, without distinction of any kind, such as race, colour, sex, language, religion, political or other opinion, national or social origin, property, birth or other status. Furthermore, no distinction shall be made on the basis of the political, jurisdictional or international status of the country or territory to which a person belongs, whether it be independent, trust, non-self-governing or under any other limitation of sovereignty.

Article 3. Everyone has the right to life, liberty and security of a person.

Article 4. No one shall be held in slavery or servitude; slavery and the slave trade shall be prohibited in all their forms.

Article 5. No one shall be subjected to torture or to cruel, inhuman or degrading treatment or punishment.

Article 6. Everyone has the right to a recognition everywhere as a person before the law.

Article 7. All are equal before the law and are entitled without any discrimination to equal protection of the law. All are entitled to equal protection against any discrimination in violation of this Declaration and against any incitement to such discrimination.

Article 8. Everyone has the right to an effective remedy by the competent national tribunal for acts violating the fundamental right granted him by the constitution or by law.

Article 9. No one shall be subjected to arbitrary arrest, detention or exile.

Article 10. Everyone is entitled in full equality to a fair and public hearing by an independent and impartial tribunal, in the determination of his rights and obligations and of any criminal charge against him.

Article 11. (1) Everyone charged with a penal offence has the right to be presumed innocent until proved guilty according to law in a public trial at which he has had all the guarantees necessary for his defense. (2) No one shall be held guilty of any penal offence on account of any act or omission which did not constitute a penal offence, under national or international law, at the time when it was committed. Nor shall a heavier penalty be imposed that the one that was applicable at the time the penal offence was committed.

Article 12. No one shall be subjected to arbitrary interference with his privacy, family, home or correspondence, nor to attacks upon his honour and reputation. Everyone has the right to the protection of the law against such interference or attacks.

Article 13. (1) Everyone has the right to freedom of movement and residence within the borders of each state. (2) Everyone has the right to leave any country, including his own, and to return to his country.

Article 14. (1) Everyone has the right to seek and to enjoy in other countries asylum from persecution. (2) This right may not be invoked in the case of prosecutions genuinely arising from non-political crimes or from acts contrary to the purposes and principles of the United Nations.

Article 15. (1) Everyone has the right to a nationality. (2) No one shall be arbitrarily deprived of his nationality nor denied the right to change his nationality.

Article 16. (1) Men and women of full age, without a limitation due to race, nationality or religion, have the right to marry and to found a family. They are entitled to equal rights as to marriage, during marriage and at its dissolution. (2) Marriage shall be entered into only with the free and full consent of the intending spouses. (3) The family is the natural and fundamental group unit of society and is entitled to protection by society and the state.

Article 17. (1) Everyone has the right to own property alone as well as in association with other. (2) No one shall be arbitrarily deprived of his property.

Article 18. Everyone has the right to freedom of thought, conscience and religion; this right includes freedom to change his religion or belief, and freedom, either alone or in community with others and in public or private, to manifest his religion or belief in teaching, practice, worship and observance.

Article 19. Everyone has the right to freedom of opinion and expression; this right includes freedom to hold opinions without interference and to seek, receive and impart information and ideas through any media, regardless of frontiers.

Article 20. (1) Everyone has the right to freedom of peaceful assembly and association. (2) No one may be compelled to belong to an association.

Article 21. (1) Everyone has the right to take part in the government of his country, directly or through freely chosen representatives. (2) Everyone has the right of equal access to public service in his country. (3) The will of the people shall be the basis of the authority of government; this will shall be expressed in periodic and genuine elections which shall be by universal and equal suffrage and shall be held by secret vote or by equivalent free voting procedures.

Article 22. Everyone, as member of a society, has the right to social security and is entitled to realization, through national effort and international cooperation and in accordance with the organization and resources of each State, of the economic, social and cultural rights indispensable for his dignity and the free development of his personality.

Article 23. (1) Everyone has the right to work, to free choice of employment, to just and favourable conditions of work and to protection against unemployment. (2) Everyone, without any discrimination, has the right to equal pay for equal work. (3) Everyone who works has the right to just and favourable remuneration ensuring for himself and his family an existence worthy of human dignity, and supplemented, if necessary, by other means of social protection. (4) Everyone has the right to form and to join trade unions for the protection of his interests.

Article 24. Everyone has the right to rest and leisure, including reasonable limitation of working hours and periodic holidays with pay.

Article 25. (1) Everyone has the right to a standard of living adequate for the health and well-being of himself and of his family, including food, clothing, housing and medical care and necessary social services, and the right to security in the event of unemployment, sickness, disability, widowhood, old age or other lack of livelihood in circumstances beyond his control. (2) Motherhood and childhood are entitled to special care and assistance. All children, whether born in or out of wedlock, shall enjoy the same protection.

Article 26. (1) Everyone has the right to education. Education shall be free, at least in the elementary and fundamental stages. Elementary education shall be compulsory. Technical and professional education shall be made generally available and higher education shall be equally accessible to all on the basis of merit. (2) Education shall be directed to the full development of the human personality and to the strengthening of respect for human rights and fundamental freedoms. It shall promote understanding, tolerance and friendship among all nations, racial or religious groups, and shall further the activities of the United Nations for the maintenance of peace. (3) Parents have a prior right to choose the kind of education that shall be given to their children.

Article 27. (1) Everyone has the right freely to participate in the cultural life of the community, to enjoy the arts and to share in scientific advancement and its benefits. (2) Everyone has the right to the protection of the moral and material interests resulting from any scientific, literary or artistic production of which he is the author.

Article 28. Everyone is entitled to a social and international order in which the rights and freedoms set forth in this Declaration can be fully realized.

Article 29. (1) Everyone has duties to the community in which alone the free and full development of his personality is possible. (2) In the exercise of his rights and freedoms, everyone shall be subject only to such limitations as are determined by law solely for purpose of securing due recognition and respect for the rights and freedoms of others and of meeting the just requirements of morality, public order and the general welfare in a democratic society. (3) These rights and freedoms may in no case be exercised contrary to the purposes and principles of the United Nations.

Article 30. Nothing in the Declaration may be interpreted as implying for any State, group or person any right to engage in any activity or to perform any act aimed at the destruction of any of the rights and freedoms set forth herein.

Sources

Amulree, Lord. 1975. *On Dying Well*. London: Church Information Service.

Aquinas, Thomas. 1947. *Summa Theologica*. 3 vols. New York: Benzinger.

Ashley, Benedict, and Kevin O'Rourke. 1997. *Health Care Ethics*, 4th ed. Washington, D.C.: Georgetown University Press.

Australian Research Committee. 1985. *Human Embryo Experimentation in Australia*. Canberra: Senate Committee on Human Experimentation, Australian Government Printing Office.

Beauchamp, Tom L., and James Childress. 1994. *Principles of Biomedical Ethics*, 3d ed. New York: Oxford University Press.

Catechism of the Catholic Church. 1997. 2d ed. Vatican City: Libreria Editrice Vaticana.

Collins, Francis. 1995. *The Human Genenome Project*. Washington D.C.: National Center for Human Genome Research, National Institutes of Health.

Congregation for the Doctrine of the Faith. 1974. *Declaration on Procured Abortion. Osservatore Romano*, Dec. 5.

———. 1980a. *Declaration on Euthanasia*, May 5. In *Vatican Council II: More Postconciliar Documents*, ed. by Austin Flannery, O.P. Northport, N.Y.: Costello Publishing.

———. 1980b. *Instruction on Infant Baptism*, Oct. 20. In *Vatican Council II: More Postconciliar Documents*, ed. by Austin Flannery, O.P. Northport, N.Y.: Costello Publishing.

———. 1987. *On Respect for Human Life*. Origins 16 (March 19): 40.

———. 1989. *The Moral Norms of Humanae Vitae*. Origins 16 (March 2): 38.

———. 1998. *To Defend the Faith* (*Ad Tuendam Fidem*). Origins 28 (July 16): 113.

Council for Secular Humanism. 1980. *A Secular Humanist Declaration*. Available at the council's website (http://www.secularhumanism.org).

CPHS (National Commission for the Protection of Human Subjects of Biomedical and Behavioral Research). 1978. *The Belmont Report: Ethical Perspectives and Guidelines for the Protection of Human Subjects of Research*. Washington, D.C.: U.S. Government Printing Office.

de Blois, Jean, Mary McGrath, and Kevin O'Rourke. 1991. *Advance Directives for Future Healthcare Decisions: A Christian Perspective*. Saint Louis: Virginia Publishing Co.

Flannery, Austin, O.P., ed. 1975a. *Decree on the Apostolate of Lay People*. In *Documents of Vatican Council II*. Wilmington, Del.: Scholarly Resources.

———. 1975b. *The Pastoral Constitution of the Church in the Modern World*. In *Documents of Vatican Council II*. Wilmington, Del.: Scholarly Resources.

Hardin, Garrett. 1974. "Living in a Lifeboat." *Biosciences* 24: 561–68.

———. 1993. *Living within Limits, Ecology, Economics, and Population Taboos*. New York: Oxford University Press.

Harvard Criteria for Brain Death. 1968. "A Definition of Irreversible Coma." *Journal of the American Medical Association* 205: 85.

Hinds, Stewart. 1975. "Triage in Medicine." *Triage in Medicine and Society* 3: 6–22.

"Humanist Manifesto." 1933. *The New Humanist*, June 1936. Reprinted in *The Humanist*, Jan.–Feb. 1973: 4–13.

"Humanist Manifesto." II. 1973. *The Humanist*. Sept.

John Paul II, Pope. 1981. "Instruction on the Human Family" ("Familiaris Consortio"). *Origins* 11 (Dec. 29): 28.

———. 1983. "The Ethics of Genetic Manipulation." *Origins* 12 (Nov. 17): 385–89.

———. 1984. *Reflections on the Encyclical "Humanae Vitae" of Pope Paul VI*. Boston: Saint Paul Editions.

———. 1992. "Address to the Congress on Transplant of Organs." *Dolentium Hominum* 3 (June 20): 12–13.

———. 1993. *The Splendor of Truth (Veritatis Splendor)*. *Origins* 23 (Oct. 14): 18.

———. 1995. *The Gospel of Life (Evangelium Vitae)*. *Origins* 24 (April 6): 42.

———. 1998. *To Defend the Faith (Ad Tuendam Fidem)*. *Origins* 28 (July 16): 8.

Katz, Jay, Alex Capron, and Elenor Swift-Glass. 1972. *Experimentation of Human Beings*. New York: Russell Sage Foundation.

Kübler-Ross, Elisabeth. 1969. *On Death and Dying*. New York: Macmillan.

Maritain, Jacques. 1929. *Three Reformers: Luther, Descartes, Rousseau*. London: Sheed and Ward.

Maslow, Abraham. 1964. *Religion, Values, and Peak Experiences*, Columbus: Ohio State University Press.

National Conference of Catholic Bishops. 1996. "Moral Principles Concerning Infants with Anencephaly." *Origins* 26, no. 17 (Oct. 10).

———. 2001. *Ethical and Religious Directives for Catholic Health Care Services*. Washington, D.C.: United States Catholic Conference. [Reproduced as appendix 1 of this volume.]

National Institute of Medicine. 2000. *To Err Is Human: Building a Safer Health System*. Washington, D.C.: National Academy Press.

———. 2001. *Crossing the Quality Chasm: A New Health System for the 21st Century*. Washington, D.C.: National Academy Press.

Osservatore Romano. 1989. "The Moral Norms of *Humanae Vitae*." March 2.

Paul VI, Pope. 1968. *On Human Life (Humanae Vitae)*. Encyclical Letter on the Regulation of Births. Washington, D.C. United States Catholic Conference.

Piccione, Joseph, and Gerald McShane. 1997. "Rape and the Peoria Protocol." *Ethics and Medics* 22 (Sept.): 9.

Pius XII, Pope. 1952. "The Intangibility of the Human Person." *The Human Body*, Sept. 13. Reprinted in 1960 by Saint Paul Press, Boston.

———. 1957. "On the Prolongation of Life." *The Pope Speaks*, Nov. 24, 1958, 4(4): 395–98.

———. 1979. *The Human Body*. Allocution to Congress of Histopathology, 1952. Boston: Saint Paul Editions.

Plato. 1955. *Republic*. London: Penguin Books.

Rawls, John. 1971. *A Theory of Justice*. Cambridge, Mass.: Harvard University Press.

United Nations. 1948. *Universal Declaration of Human Rights of the United Nations*. New York: United Nations. [Reproduced as appendix 2 of this volume.]

Wade, Nicholas. 2001. *Life Script*. New York: Simon and Schuster.

Warnock Commission. 1985. *Report of the Inquiry into Human Fertilization and Embryology Medical Research*. London: The Medical Council.

World Health Organization. 1946. "Nuremberg Code." In *Encyclopedia of Bioethics*, vol. 4. New York: Free Press.

———. 1958. *Constitution: The First Ten Years of the World Health Organization*. Geneva: World Health Organization.

———. 1967. "Geneva Declaration on Human Research." In *Encyclopedia of Bioethics*, vol. 4. New York: Free Press.

———. 1987. "A Prospective Multicenter Trial for the Ovulation Method of Natural Family Planning." *Fertility and Sterility* 47:765.

Index

A

abortion, 129–31
  autonomy and, 66
  case studies on, 70, 86, 140
  church teachings on, 64
  direct, 129–30, 131, 140, 231,
    235
  the *Directives* on, 231, 235,
    240n44
  disputed issues in, 131–32
  genetic counseling and, 152–53
  indirect, 130, 131, 140
  John Paul II on, 130, 138
  laws and, 6
  Second Vatican Council on, 130
  for stem cell research, 156
absolution, 209
abstinence, 133, 134
abstract thought, 161
abuse, 228
acquired immune deficiency syndrome (AIDS), 83, 113, 119
action therapy, 164–65, 166–67
actions
  circumstances of, 9–10
  evil effect and, 20–21
  intention of, 10–11
  intrinsically evil, 19, 22
  morality of, 48, 50, 62
  moral object of, 9, 10
  natural law and, 8
  prudence and, 18
  purpose of life and, 195, 196
  responsibility for, 66
  utilitarianism on, 5
  values and, 32
  voluntary vs. free, 173
Acts of the Apostles, 92
Ad Hoc Committee on Health
  Care Issues and the Church,
  236
Ad Tuendam Fidem, 8
addiction, 172–74
  alcohol, 173, 174, 177
  case study on, 177
  chemical/drug, 172, 173
  definition of, 160
  to eating, 59
  physiological vs. psychologi-
    cal, 173
  to pleasurable activities, 27,
    172
  stress and, 58–59
adoption, 123
advance directives, 66, 194–95,
  198, 227
advocacy, 222

affection, 62
affectivity, 161
AIDS (acquired immune deficiency syndrome), 83, 113,
  119
Albert the Great, 125
Alcoholics Anonymous (AA), 174
alcoholism, 173, 174, 177
allocation. *See* resource allocation
altruism, 4
Alzheimer's disease, 195–96
ambiguous genitalia, 147
American Medical Association,
  195
American Revolution, 2
amniocentesis, 151, 153
anatomical integrity, 144–45
anemia, Franconi, 150
anencephalic infants, 131–32,
  184–85
angelism, 50
animals
  development of, 125–26
  experimentation on, 41, 109
  for organ transplantation, 146
  rights of, 41, 109
anointing, 208–9, 213, 224–25
antinomianism, 49
anxiety, 166, 168, 177, 208
Aristotle, 3, 8, 34
Art perfects nature, 141
artificial insemination, 128,
  239n27, 239n29
artificial nutrition, 191, 195–96,
  233, 234
artificial reproduction, 128–29,
  230, 239n27
asceticism, 49
Asclepias, 75
assisted suicide, Supreme Court
  on, 12
asylum, 244
Augustine, Saint, 53
Australian Research Committee,
  106–7
authentic magisterium, 63–64
autonomy, 5, 66, 84, 90, 97
autopsy, 200

B

baptism, 180, 210–12, 219, 225,
  239n14
the Beatitudes, 7, 92
Beauchamp, Tom L., 5
beginnings of life, 121, 124–25,
  229–32
behavioral control, 175, 176

Belmont Report, 66–67, 99
beneficence, 5
benefit, 108, 109, 193
Bentham, Jeremy, 5
Billings Method, 134
bioethics. *See* ethical systems;
  ethics
biological health, 47–49, 55–56
biological needs, 38–39, 45, 51,
  168
birth control pills, 132
bishops, diocesan, 220, 236–37
blood transfusions, 42
bodies
  care of after death, 198–200
  donating for research, 199
  health of, 55–56
  modification of, 141–58
  sale of, 145
body–soul dualism, 47, 48–49, 57,
  145
  in death, 180, 181, 184, 198
brain, 142, 157
brain death, 183–86, 213
burial ceremonies, 199, 200
burnout, 202
Bush, George, 99

C

can vs. *ought*, 61
Canadian national health care,
  104
capitalism
  church teachings on, 37
  vs. functionalism, 93
  individualism and, 35
  market-oriented, centralized
    systems in, 94–95
  pluralist model and, 88, 89
  for-profit health care and, 80
castration, 146
categorical imperative, 4–5
Catholic Church. *See also* church
  teachings
  on body–soul dualism, 48–49
  ethical systems of, ix–x, 1,
    7–12
  healing mission of, 217–18
  on natural law reasoning, 7,
    8–12
  on religious legalism, 7
  social role of, 217
  teaching authority of, 7–8,
    62–64, 69, 220
  values of, 15
Catholic Health Care Association,
  101

Catholic health care institutions, 100–102, 103–4
  directives for. See Ethical and Religious Directives for Catholic Health Care Facilities
  genetic screening in, 153
  mission of, 218–19, 220
  social responsibility of, 221–23
  spiritual responsibility of, 223–26
caution, 18
celibacy, 28, 69, 123–24
cell lines, 107, 156
central nervous system development, 125–26
centralized model, 89–90, 94–95
chaplains, 207
character, 3
charity, 16, 30, 116, 144
chemical dependency, 172–73
children
  personhood and, 33
  research on, 111–12
  sex selection of, 148–49
  United Nations's Declaration on, 245
Childress, James, 5
choice
  faith and, 16
  of lifestyle, 58
  mental health and, 161
  morality and, 62
  of physicians, 67–69
  in research, 115
chorionic villi sampling, 151, 152
Christian social thought model, 90–91
Christianity. See also church teachings
  on body–soul dualism, 48
  on collectivism, 35
  on conscience, 62–64
  on disease, 57–58
  on health, 57–58
  on individualism, 35
  on informed consent, 66
  Nietzsche on, 69
  on personhood, 34
  principles of, 15, 17–30
  religious legalism and, 6
  values of, 15–17
Christians, as health care professionals, 76–77
Chronic Disease Hospital case, 106
church teachings
  on abortion, 64
  authority for, 7–8, 62–64, 69, 220
  on body–soul dualism, 48
  on capitalism, 37
  Christian social, 90–91
  on community, 36
  on conscience, 62–64
  on contraception, 64, 132–34
  on death, 57–58
  the Directives on, 63, 217
  dissent from, 64

Jesus Christ on, 62
  pastoral, 63
  on reproduction, 137–39
  on sexuality, 28, 137–39
circumstances, 3, 9–10
clinical death, 182–83
clinical trials, randomized, 112–13
Clinton, Bill, 99
cloning, 156
cocaine, 69
coercion, 21, 67, 111
collaboration, 222, 236–37, 238–39n10
collectivism, 35, 36
colonialism, 117–18
coma, 182, 184, 185, 195–96
commercialization of medicine, 75
Commission for the Protection of Human Subjects, 112
commitment to life, 56–58
common good
  debt to, 92
  definition of, 91
  the Directives on, 221
  needs and, 95–96
  norms for, 3
  organ transplantation and, 145
  poverty and, 92
  principle of, 23, 24
  research for, 110
  resource allocation and, 116–17
  social justice and, 37, 116–17
  utilitarianism on, 5
common sense, 2
communication
  with health care professionals, 81–83
  of knowledge, 72
  in peer relations, 83
  in physician-patient relationships, 80, 81–83
  principle of professional, 18, 22–23
  society and, 44–45
  trust in, 22
communion, 209, 212, 225
communism, 35, 90, 93
community. See also society
  global, 41, 115, 117–18
  good. See common good
  illness and, 207, 208
  love and, 35–36
  participation in, 24
  the person and, 34–36
  role of, 36
  sharing in, 40
  sins of, 215
  United Nations's Declaration on, 246
  values, 36–38, 40
  welfare of, 35
compassion, 237
competition, 88
compulsions, 47
conception, 124–25, 126–27, 128
  assisted, 128–29, 230, 239n27
  rape and, 136–37, 228

concern, 79
conditioning, 165
confession, 210
Confessions (Saint Augustine), 53
confidentiality
  AIDS and, 83
  communication and, 22–23
  the Directives on, 228
  in group therapy, 168
  in physician-patient relationships, 82, 83
  United Nations's Declaration on, 244
Confirmation, 225
Congregation for the Doctrine of the Faith
  Declaration on Euthanasis, 192
  The Moral Norms of Humanae Vitae, 138
  On Respect for Human Life, 126, 128–29, 151
conscience
  church teachings on, 62–64
  decision making and, 18–19, 61–62, 65–66, 69
  development of, 60–64
  inner freedom and, 27
  Kant on, 4
  principle of, 18–19
  sin and, 61
consequentialism, 5
consumers, 84, 90
contraception
  church teachings on, 64, 132–34
  the Directives on, 229–30, 232
  rape and, 137
contracts, 79
convalescence, 56
cooperation, 18, 21–22, 236–37
coping mechanisms, 172
corpse, 198–200
cortical death, 184–85
cosmic order, 122
costs, health care, 88
counseling. See also psychotherapy
  genetic, 152–54, 232
  psychological, 74
  spiritual, 101, 204–6
countertransference, 78
courage, 56, 67, 68
National Commission for the Protection of Human Subjects of Biomedical and Behavioral Research (CPHS), 98–99
creativity
  brain and, 142
  external and internal, 44
  health and, 50, 59–60
  human reconstruction and, 142, 143
  need for, 39, 45, 51
  principle of, 26–27, 143
  value of, 32
cremation, 200
criminal acts, 168–69, 244
Critique of Pure Reason (Kant), 4
Crossing the Quality Chasm, 84–85

culture, 32, 39, 100, 149

D
death, 179–86. *See also* dying
  allowing, 189–94
  body–soul separation in, 180,
    181, 184, 198
  brain death, 183–86, 213
  care after, 198–200
  case studies on, 202
  church teachings on, 57–58
  clinical, 182–83
  cortical, 184–85
  definition of, 180
  denial of, 201
  determination of, 181–86, 234
  the *Directives* on, 234
  vs. dying, 181
  Jesus Christ and, 180
  mystery of, 179–81
  right to, 190
  signs of, 182–83
  sin and, 179
  Saint Paul on, 57, 58, 179, 180,
    219
  suffering and, 29, 179–80
decentralization, progressive, 93,
  95
decision making
  actions and, 11
  case studies on, 12–13
  certitude in, 65
  circumstances in, 3
  conscience and, 18–19, 61–62,
    65–66, 69
  continuous, 95
  the *Directives* on, 227
  emotivism in, 3
  for end-of-life care, 86, 194–95
  ethical systems for, 1–13
  in health care teams, 96
  information in, 62, 65
  intuition in, 2, 5
  knowledge in, 61–62
  moral object of, 9, 10, 11
  needs and, 33, 40, 41
  pain control and, 197–98
  by patients, 97, 194–95
  physicians role in, 74, 96, 97
  power of, 95
  reason in, 1–2, 5
  responsibility for, 61–62, 65–66
  social, 24, 93–94
  values in, 62
Declaration of Independence, 2
Declaration on Euthanasia, 192
"Declaration on Procured Abortion," 126
*Decree on the Apostolate of Lay Peo-
  ple*, 101
To Defend the Faith, 8
delayed humanization, 125–28
dementia, 195–96
democracy, 35
denial, 68, 172, 177, 201
deontology, 4
dependence, 24, 76, 172–73
depersonalization, 72, 73

depression, 186, 202
Descartes, 50
destiny, 122
developing countries, 117–18
Dewey, John, 36–37
diagnosis
  incorrect, 79
  prenatal, 150–51, 231–32
dialysis, 65
Didache, 130
dignity
  biological drives and, 47–48
  the *Directives* on, 221, 226, 227,
    233
  patient's bill of rights on, 68
  personhood and, 31–32
  in physician-patient relation-
    ships, 82
  principle of, 23–24, 25
  psychotherapy and, 175
  religions on, 36
  research and, 38, 112
  respect for, 38
  United Nations's *Declaration*
    on, 41, 243
diocesan bishops, 220, 236–37
direct abortion, 129–30, 131, 140,
  231, 235
the *Directives*. *See Ethical and Religious Directives for Catholic
  Health Care Facilities*
disabled persons, 43
disadvantaged groups, 88, 95
discipline, 84, 85
discrimination, 23–24, 222–23, 244
disease. *See also* mental illness
  Christianity on, 57–58
  community and, 207, 208
  definition of, 43–44, 45–47, 52
  the *Directives* on, 237
  medical model of, 78–80, 82
  ontological concept of, 46–47
  physical vs. mental, 159–60
  physiological concept of, 46–47
  predisposition to, 155
  sin and, 50
  spirituality and, 206–7
Dolentium Hominum (John Paul
  II), 145
dominion, human, 59–60, 141–43,
  220
donors, organ. *See* organ donors
double-blind protocols, 112–13
double effect, principle of, 20–21,
  109–10, 196
Down's syndrome, 160
drives, biological, 47–48
drug addiction, 172, 173
drug development, 110
drugs, psychoactive, 162–63, 164,
  175
dualism, body–soul. *See* body–
  soul dualism
durable power of attorney, 195
duress, 21, 22
duty ethics, 4–5, 16
dying, 179, 186–88. *See also* death
  case studies on, 202

vs. death, 181
  the *Directives* on, 186, 232–35
  knowledge of, 186–87
  pain and, 197–98
  prolongation of, 189–94
  truth about, 186–87

E
EAB. *See* Ethics Advisory Board
Eastern religions, 36
eating, 51, 59
economics, 5, 35, 100
ecosystem, 26–27, 215
ectopic pregnancy, 131, 132, 231
education, 94, 97–98, 245–46
EEG (electroencephalogram),
  183–84
ego, 166
elderly, 87, 103
electroconvulsive therapy, 163–64
electroencephalogram (EEG),
  183–84
elitism, 72, 74, 90, 94
embryos. *See also* fetus
  development of, 125–28
  the *Directives* on, 232
  genetic screening of, 150–52
  manipulation of, 148–54
  research on, 106–7, 232
  sex selection of, 148–49
  sexual differentiation of, 147
  splitting of, 149–50
emotions, 2
emotivism, 3
employees, 222–23
employment, 245
end-of-life care, 86, 194–95,
  197–98. *See also* dying; life
  support treatment
end, ultimate, 9, 10, 11
An Enemy of the People (Ibsen), 69
the Enlightenment, 1–2
environment, 26–27, 44, 156, 215
equality, 34, 243–44
Erikson, Erik, 171
To Err Is Human, 84–85
errors, medical, 84–85
*Ethical and Religious Directives for
  Catholic Health Care Facilities*,
  ix, 101, 217–41
  on abortion, 231, 235, 240n44
  on artificial nutrition, 196, 233,
    234
  on artificial reproduction, 128,
    129, 230
  on baptism, 219, 225, 239n14
  on the beginnings of life,
    229–32
  on church teachings, 63
  on the common good, 221
  on confidentiality, 228
  on contraception, 229–30, 232
  on cooperation, 22
  on death, 234
  on decision making, 227
  on dignity, 221, 226, 227, 233
  on dying, 186, 232–35
  on embryos, 232

on euthanasia, 233, 234, 240n44
on family, 229–30
on the fetus, 232
on functional integrity, 227
on genetic counseling, 232
on health, 228
on health care teams, 226
on illness, 237
on infertility, 231
on informed consent, 227
introduction to, 218–21
on lay ministers, 219–20, 224
on life support treatment, 234
on life support withdrawal, 234
on living donors, 227–28
on marriage, 229–30
on organ donors, 234–35
on organ transplantation, 227–28, 234–35
on pain, 197, 232
on partnerships, 235–37
on pastoral care, 219–20, 223–26
on physician-patient relationships, 226–29
on poverty, 221, 222
on privacy, 228
on professional-patient relations, 226–29
on proxies, 227
purpose of, 218
on rape, 137, 228
on research, 222, 228, 232
on resource allocation, 221, 222
on science, 220
on social responsibility, 221–23
on spirituality, 223–26
on sterilization, 136, 232, 240n44
on stewardship, 221, 238–39n10
on suffering, 219, 234
on technology, 220, 233
on therapy, 228
on treatment refusal, 228
ethical systems, 1–13
    case studies on, 12–13
    Catholic Church, 1, 7–12
    emotivism, 3
    the Enlightenment and, 1–2
    formalism, 3, 4–5
    of Hume, 2–3
    Kantian, 4–5
    legalism, 6
    positivism, 6
    public policy and, 98–100
    utilitarianism, 3, 5
ethics
    duty, 4–5, 16
    education in, 97–98
    fulfillment of needs and, 33, 40
Ethics Advisory Board, 98–99
ethics committees, 12–13, 228–29
Eucharist, 209, 212, 225
eugenics, 153
euthanasia, 187–89
    autonomy and, 66

circumstances and, 10
definition of, 187
the Directives on, 233, 234, 240n44
justification of, 11
as murder, 187, 188–89
suffering and, 189
evil
    common good and, 91
    cooperation with, 21–22
    effect, 20–21
    emotions and, 2
    intrinsic, 10, 19, 22, 240n44
    intuition and, 2
    lesser, 20
    values and, 3
exercise, 59
existentialism, 3
experience, 2
experimentation. See research
expertise, 79
extraordinary magisterium, 63

F
fairness, 5
faith, 16, 17–23, 30, 181, 220–21
family
    the Directives on, 229–30
    John Paul II on, 122
    parental relationships and, 78, 215, 246
    sexuality and, 28, 122, 139, 215
    strengthening, 215
family planning, natural, 134–35, 229–30
family therapy, 167
federal research funds, 107, 108
feeding tubes, 191, 195–96, 233, 234
feelings, 2
fees, health care, 80–81, 88
fertility, 134, 135
fertilization, artificial, 99, 106, 128–29, 230–31
fetishism, 148
fetus
    baptism of, 211
    development of, 125–26
    the Directives on, 232
    research on, 106–7, 232
    treatment of, 23, 153
finis operantis, 10, 11, 19
finis operis, 9, 10, 19
food resources, 117–18
for-profit health care, 80–81, 103–4
forgiveness, 23
formalism, 3, 4–5
fortitude, 16, 19, 26, 27
Franconi anemia, 150
free and informed consent. See informed consent
free-market system, 88–89, 94–95. See also capitalism
freedom
    biological drives and, 47
    God and, 7, 16
    informed consent and, 67, 111

inner, 26, 27
mental health and, 161, 167–68, 171, 172, 175
morality and, 50
needs and, 32
protection of, 35
psychotherapy and, 168–69, 170, 171, 172, 175
responsibility and, 168–69
United Nations's Declaration on, 243, 244–45
Freud, Sigmund, 164, 171
friendship, 9
Fromm, Erich, 171
functional integrity, 45, 50, 51–52, 144–45, 227
functionalism, 93–96
functioning
    hierarchy of, 51–52
    optimal, 44, 45, 160, 161
functions vs. structure, 125
funding, 107, 108, 117
funerals, 199
futile treatment, 191
the future, 188

G
Galileo, 64
gamete interfallopian transfer (GIFT), 129
gender dysphoria syndrome, 146, 148
gender identity, 147, 148
general practitioners, 96
Genesis, 28, 123
genetic counseling, 152–54, 232
genetic engineering, 141, 143, 154–57, 158
genetic individualization, 127
genetic screening, 150–52
Geneva statement on research, 109
genitalia, ambiguous, 147
genotype, 156
GIFT (gamete interfallopian transfer), 129
gifts, 26–27
global community, 41, 115, 117–18
goals
    acquired vs. innate, 8
    conscience and, 18–19
    faith and, 17–18
    ultimate, 9, 10, 11
God
    dependence on, 76
    freedom and, 7, 16
    of healing, 75
    on human dominion, 60
    image and likeness of, 7, 23–24, 34, 220
    in religious legalism, 6–7
good, 2, 3, 20–21
goods, material vs. spiritual, 35, 37
The Gospel of Life (John Paul II), 130, 137–38, 144, 151
the Gospel, on social organization, 91–93

governments
    ethical guidelines by, 98–100
    health care regulation by, 89,
        104
    role of, 35, 36
    United Nations's *Declaration*
        on, 245
Greek God of healing, 75
group practice, 88
group therapy, 167–68
growth
    personhood and, 33
    through suffering, 26, 29, 197
guardians. *See* proxies
guidelines, ethical, 98–100
guilt, 206

H
habits, 165
handicapped persons, 43
happiness, 9, 29
Hardin, Garrett, 117
harm, 82–83, 84–85
harmony, 46
Harvard Criteria for Brain Death,
    183–84
healing
    definition of, 56
    God of, 75
    by Jesus Christ, 102, 215,
        218–19, 237
    mission, 217–18
    pastoral care and, 206–8, 213
    professions, 74
    touch and, 207–8
    trust and, 75
health, 43–53
    biological, 47–49, 55–56
    case studies on, 53
    Christianity on, 57–58
    commitment to, 56–58
    creativity and, 50, 59–60
    definition of, 40, 43–45, 52
    the *Directives* on, 228
    levels of, 49–50
    Old Testament on, 57
    physiological, 44, 53
    psychological, 57
    responsibility for, 55–70, 74, 91
    right to, 37–38, 91
    seeking, 31–42
    spirituality and, 50, 53, 59
    stewardship of, 59–60, 69
    subjectivity of, 55–56
    United Nations's *Declaration*
        on, 245
Health and Health Care, 217
health care
    centralized model of, 89–90,
        94–95
    Christian social thought model
        of, 90–91
    commercialization of, 75
    costs, 88
    for the elderly, 87, 103
    fees, 80–81, 88
    for-profit, 80–81, 103–4
    funding, 107, 108, 117

humanization of, 76
market-oriented, centralized,
    94–95
models of, 87–91
national, 94–95, 104
need for, 92
participatory model of, 90
patient-centered, 96
planning, 95
pluralist model of, 88–89, 94
responsibility for, 87–104
substandard, 68
trends in, x
United Nations's *Declaration*
    on, 245
universal, 87, 103
    health care ethics. *See* ethical
        systems; ethics
health care institutions. *See also*
    Catholic health care
    institutions
    corporations of, 102
    for-profit, 80–81, 103–4
    non-Catholic, 222, 235–37,
        238–39n10
    public, 104
health care professionals. *See also*
    physicians; professional-
    client relationships
    autonomy of, 84, 90
    burnout of, 202
    Christian, 76–77
    communication with, 81–83
    discipline of, 84, 85
    dying patients and, 186–87
    fees of, 80–81
    ideals of, 74–76
    identity of, 72
    informed consent and, 66–67
    knowledge of, 79–80
    on participatory models, 90
    peer relations of, 83–85, 97, 98
    personalizing, 77
    responsibilities of, 71–86
    role of, 71–74
    spiritual care and, 204
health care reform, 87
health care teams, 96–98
    decision making in, 96
    the *Directives* on, 226
    pastoral care and, 212–13
    peer relations in, 83–85, 97, 98
    trust in, 85
health insurance, 80
health maintenance organiza-
    tions, 68, 89
health promotion, 94, 95
heart/lung function, 182–83
heart transplants, 104, 143–44, 202
helping professions, 73
higher education, 94
Hinds, Steward, 115
Hippocratic tradition, 46, 58
Hitler, Adolf, 6
holism, 77
homeostasis, 44, 46
homosexuality, 147, 213
hope, 16, 25–29, 188

hospice, 197
hospitals. *See* health care
    institutions
The Human Body (Pius XII), 175
human dominion, 59–60, 141–43,
    220
Human Genome Project, 154
human laws, 6
human nature, 1, 60, 156–57
human person. *See* person;
    personhood
humanism, 2, 36, 37, 93
"Humanist Manifesto," 36–37
humanization, 73, 76, 125–28
Hume, David, 2–3, 4
humility, 67, 68
Hutcheson, Francis, 2
hydration, artificial, 195–96, 233
hypochondriacs, 68

I
Ibsen, Henrik, 69
identical twins, 127, 150, 158
identity, 72, 147, 148
illness. *See* disease
imagination, 59
in vitro fertilization, 99, 106,
    128–29, 230–31
Incarnation, 48
incest, 86
incompetent person, 66
indirect abortion, 130, 131, 140
individualism, 5, 35, 36, 127,
    174
induced labor, 231
industrial society, 71–72, 117–18
infanticide, 130
infants
    anencephalic, 131–32, 184–85
    baptism of, 210–11
    as organ donors, 235
infertility, 123, 134, 231
information, 22–23, 62, 65, 83
informed consent, 18, 19, 66–67
    the *Directives* on, 227
    in double-blind protocols, 113
    freedom and, 111
    guidelines for, 99
    knowledge and, 67
    life support treatment and,
        194–95
    in mental illness, 163, 164
    patient's bill of rights on, 68
    proxies and, 111–12
    for psychotherapy, 169–70,
        175–76
    for research, 108, 110–11, 113
injustice, 91
inner freedom. *See also* freedom
    principle of, 26, 27
insemination, artificial, 128,
    239n27, 239n29
insight therapy, 165, 166, 171
institutional review boards (IRB),
    107–8
Instruction on Infant Baptism, 211
"Instruction on the Human Fam-
    ily" (John Paul II), 121, 122

integrity
　anatomical, 144–45
　functional, 45, 50, 51–52,
　　144–45, 227
　principle of, 23, 25, 110, 144–45
　psychotherapy and, 176
intellect, 7, 16, 52, 142, 157
intelligence, subnormal, 160
intention, 10–11, 18–19, 20–21, 191
intrauterine devices, 132
intuition, 2, 5
involuntary commitment, 169
IRB. *See* institutional review
　　boards
is vs. *ought*, 2, 3
isolation, 207, 208

J
Jehovah's Witnesses, 42
Jesus Christ
　on celibacy, 124
　death and, 180
　healing by, 102, 215, 218–19, 237
　on human dominion, 60
　on life, 57
　on marriage, 123
　on poverty, 37
　on the sacredness of life, 130
　on sexuality, 28
　on social justice, 37, 91–92
　on teaching, 62
　three-fold ministry of, 102
　virtues of, 16
John Paul II
　on abortion, 130, 138
　on contraception, 133–34
　Dolentium Hominum, 145
　on embryo research, 107
　on family, 122
　on Galileo, 64
　The Gospel of Life, 130, 137–38,
　　144, 151
　"Instruction on the Human
　　Family," 121, 122
　on marriage, 123
　on organ transplantation, 144,
　　145
　on prenatal diagnosis, 151
　on Proportionalism, 11
　*Reflections on the Encyclical "On
　　Human Life" of Pope Paul VI*,
　　133–34
　on sexuality, 28, 121
　The Splendor of Truth, 9, 10–11
　on teleogism, 11–12
John XXIII, 230
Judaism, 57
judgment, 65, 75–76
Jung, Carl, 164
juries, 169
justice
　charity and, 30
　global, 118
　in resource allocation, 116–17,
　　118
　social, 37–38, 91–92, 116–17
　triage and, 115–17
　virtue of, 16, 23

K
Kant, Immanuel, 4, 188
knowledge
　communication of, 72
　in decision making, 61–62
　of dying, 186–87
　of health care professionals,
　　79–80
　Hume on, 2–3
　informed consent and, 67
　of professionals, 72, 73
　from research, 108, 109
　through experience, 2
Kübler-Ross, Elisabeth, 187

L
labor, induced, 231
labor unions, 94
language, 34, 44
Larrey, Jean, 115, 116
laws, 4, 6
　natural, 1, 7, 8–12, 143, 157
　United Nations's *Declaration*
　　on, 243–44
lay ministers, 209–10, 213, 219–20,
　　224
layperson. *See* consumers
learning, 165
legal norms, 6–7, 100
legalism, 6–7
life
　beginning of, 121, 124–25,
　　229–32
　commitment to, 56–58
　Jesus Christ on, 57
　prolongation of, 191–94
　purpose of, 195–96
　sacredness of, 130, 139–40, 198,
　　229
Life Script (Wade), 154
life support treatment. *See also*
　　end-of-life care
　burden of, 191, 193, 196
　the *Directives* on, 234
　informed consent and, 194–95
　ordinary and extraordinary,
　　191–94, 234
　withdrawal of, 86, 190–96, 202,
　　234
lifeboat ethics, 117
lifestyle, 58–59
liver transplantation, 119
living donors, 144–45, 158, 227–28
living wills, 195
lobotomy, 162, 163, 164, 175
love
　community and, 35–36
　contraception and, 133
　John Paul II on, 122
　of neighbors, 144
　principles of, 23–25
lying, 22, 82, 83, 114

M
magisterium, 62, 63–64, 220
malpractice, 83, 85, 192
managed care, 89
Maritain, Jacques, 50

market system. *See* capitalism;
　　free-market system
marriage
　artificial reproduction and, 129
　contraception and, 134
　the *Directives* on, 229–30
　Jesus Christ on, 123
　John Paul II on, 122
　Second Vatican Council on,
　　123, 229
　sexuality and, 28, 122–24, 139
　United Nations's *Declaration*
　　on, 244
Marx, Karl, 92
Marxism, 90
Maslow, Abraham, 38–40
masturbation, 239–40n29
material cooperation, 21–22
material goods, 35, 37
McShane, Gerald, 137
meaning, 168
Medicaid, 80
medical errors, 84–85
medical futility, 191
medical model, 78–80, 82, 162–64
medical professional. *See* health
　　care professionals;
　　physicians
medical records, 68
medical review boards, 84
Medicare, 80, 104
medicine. *See also* health care
　commercialization of, 75
　Hippocratic tradition of, 46, 58
　humanization of, 75
meditation, 59
Menninger Foundation, 162
mental health, 49–50
　freedom and, 161, 167–68, 171,
　　172, 175
　lifestyle and, 59
　optimal, 160, 161
　research and, 114
　spirituality and, 168
mental illness, 159–77. *See also*
　　psychotherapy
　case studies on, 176–77
　electroconvulsive therapy for,
　　162, 163–64
　informed consent in, 163, 164
　levels of, 49
　medical model for, 162–64
　vs. physical disease, 56, 57,
　　159–60
　society and, 159–60
　subjectivity of, 56
　therapy for, 161–68
mental retardation, 33, 160
mercy killing. *See* euthanasia
miscarriage, 129, 211
misleading information, 22, 83
monopolies, 88–89, 94
monotheistic religions, 48, 188
*The Moral Norms of Humanae
　　Vitae*, 138
"Moral Principles Concerning
　　Infants with Anencephaly,"
　　132

moralism, 50
morality
    of actions, 48, 50, 62
    choice and, 62
    divine command, 6
    freedom and, 50
    legal, 6
    natural law on, 11
    objective vs. subjective, 138–39
Moses, 56
motherhood, 245
mothers, surrogate, 231
motivation, 10, 165
Mullerian ducts, 147
murder, 187, 188–89
mutations, genetic, 150–54

N
Nash, Molly, 150
National Commission for the Pro-
    tection of Human Subjects of
    Biomedical and Behavioral
    Research, 98–99
National Conference of Catholic
    Bishops, 63. See also United
    States Conference of
    Catholic Bishops
National Council of Catholic
    Bishops, 132. See also Ethical
    and Religious Directives for
    Catholic Health Care Facilities
national health care, 94–95, 104
National Institute of Medicine,
    84–85
nationality, 244
natural family planning, 134–35,
    229–30
natural law, 1, 7, 8–12, 143, 157
nature. See also human nature
    Art perfects nature, 141
    exploitation of, 60
    human dominion over, 59–60,
        141–43
    principle of stewardship and
        creativity and, 26–27
    stewardship of, 59–60
Nazi experiments, 106
needs
    basic, 40
    biological, 38–39, 45, 51, 168
    common good and, 95–96
    creative, 39, 45, 51
    culture and, 32, 39
    decision making and, 33, 40, 41
    dependency, 172–73
    health care allocation and, 92
    Maslow on, 38–40
    priorities in, 38–40
    psychological, 39, 45, 51
    responsibility for meeting,
        92–93
    satisfying, 32–33, 38, 40
    social, 39, 45, 51
    spiritual, 39
    values and, 38
    of wards, 112
neighbors, love of, 144
nervous system, 52

neurosis, 160, 167, 168
The Nicomachean Ethics (Aristotle),
    3
Nietzsche, Friedrich, 69
nonmaleficence, 5
norms
    application of, 65–66
    case study on, 13
    Catholic influence on, 13
    common good and, 3
    culture and, 100
    general, 17
    hope and, 26
    legal, 6–7, 100
    love and, 25
    of natural law, 8–9
    for research, 98–99, 108–15
    stewardship and, 60
    utilitarianism on, 5
Nuremberg statement on
    research, 109
nurses, 96, 97–98
nutrition, artificial, 191, 195–96,
    233, 234

O
object
    intended, 20
    moral, 9, 10, 11, 19
obligations, 79
occupations, productive, 73
Old Testament, 57
opinion polls, 2
organ donors
    anencephalic infants as, 184–85
    death and, 182–83, 199–200
    the Directives on, 234–35
    infants as, 235
    living, 144–45, 158, 227–28
organ systems, 51–52
organ transplantation, 143–46
    animals for, 146
    case studies on, 119, 158, 202
    the Directives on, 227–28,
        234–35
    John Paul II on, 144, 145
    organ sales for, 145, 199–200
    triage in, 116, 118–19, 146
organisms, development of,
    125–28
original sin, 179
ought, 2, 3, 61
overpopulation, 117–18
ovulation, 134, 137

P
pain, 5, 27, 197–98, 232
parental relationships, 78, 215,
    246
partial brain death, 184–86
participatory model, 90
partnerships, 235–37
passivity, 79
pastoral care, 203–13
    case studies on, 213
    the Directives on, 219–20,
        223–26
    healing and, 206–8, 213

health care team and, 97
    lay ministers and, 209–10, 213,
        219–20, 224
    for non-Catholics, 225–26
    program for, 101
    vs. psychotherapy, 205, 213
    purpose of, 203–4
    trust in, 205–6
The Pastoral Constitution of the
    Church in the Modern World,
    36, 61, 63
paternalism, 85, 186
patient care teams. See health care
    teams
patient-centered health care, 96
patients. See also physician-
    patient relationships
    best interests of, 194, 195, 227
    decision making by, 97, 194–95
    the Directives on, 222
    passivity of, 79
    patient's bill of rights, 68–69, 227
Paul, Saint
    on baptism, 180
    on death, 57, 58, 179, 180, 219
    on marriage and celibacy, 124
    on sin, 57, 179
    on virtues, 16–17
Paul VI, 28, 133
PCEMR (President's Commission
    for the Study of Ethical
    Problems in Medicine and
    Biomedical and Behavioral
    Research), 98–99
peer relations, 83–85, 97, 98
peer review, 83–84
penance, 224, 225
persistent vegetative states,
    195–96
person. See also personhood
    community and, 34–36
    definition of, 31–32, 33
    improving, 156–57
    integration of, 45, 50, 51–52
    rights of, 32–33, 34
personality, 50, 59
personalized sexuality, principle
    of, 27–28
personhood
    Christianity on, 34
    community and, 35
    conception and, 124–25
    definition of, 25, 33, 127–28
    dignity of, 31–32
    growth and, 33
    sexuality and, 121–22
Peter, Saint, 62–63
phenotype, 156
phobias, 27
physician-assisted suicide, 12,
    240n44
physician-patient relationships
    communication in, 80, 81–83
    contracts in, 79
    the Directives on, 226–29
    privacy and confidentiality in,
        82, 83
    truth in, 82, 186–87

validity of, 72
physicians. *See also* health care
    professionals
    autonomy of, 97
    choice of, 67–69
    decision making and, 74, 96, 97
    discipline of, 84, 85
    dying patients and, 186–87
    ethics education and, 97–98
    fees of, 80–81
    ideals of, 74–76
    informed consent and, 66–67
    judgment of, 75–76
    life support treatment and,
        192–93
    medical model and, 78–80, 82
    peer relations of, 83–85, 97, 98
    as priests, 75, 76
    role of, 74, 97
    as scientists, 75, 76
    trust in, 75, 79, 83, 85
physiological addiction, 173
physiological health, 44, 53
Piccione, Joseph, 137
Pius XII, 175, 193
placebos, 112, 113
Plato, 50, 93, 188
pleasure, 5, 26, 27, 172
pluralist model, 88–89, 94
pluripotent cells, 155–56
poliomyelitis vaccines, 109
polytheistic religions, 48
population growth, 117–18
positivism, 6
postindustrial society, 71–72
potentiality, 125, 126
poverty
    charity for, 30
    Christian ethics on, 37
    common good and, 92
    the *Directives* on, 221, 222
    health care and, 87, 103
    pluralist model and, 94
    research and, 110
    welfare system and, 93
power, in society, 72
powers, personal, 25
prayer, 207–8
pre-embryo, 106, 127
pregnancy. *See also* abortion
    ectopic, 131, 132, 231
    rape and, 136–37
prenatal diagnosis, 150–52,
    231–32
prenatal therapy, 153, 231
Presidential Ethical Commission,
    99
President's Commission for the
    Study of Ethical Problems in
    Medicine and Biomedical
    and Behavioral Research
    (PCEMR), 98–99
preventive medicine, 58–59, 69,
    89, 95, 117
pride, 179
priests, physicians as, 75, 76
primary care practitioners, 96
principles, Christian, 15, 17–30

application of, 65–66
case studies on, 30
common good and subsidiar-
    ity, 23, 24
cooperation, 18, 21–22
definition of, 17
double effect, 20–21, 109–10,
    196
faith, 17–23, 30
free and informed consent, 18,
    19
growth through suffering, 26,
    29, 197
hope, 25–29
human dignity, 23–24
inner freedom, 26, 27
love, 23–25
personalized sexuality, 27–28
professional communication,
    18, 22–23
stewardship and creativity,
    26–27, 143
totality and integrity, 23, 25,
    110, 144–45
well-formed conscience, 18–19,
    60–64
privacy. *See also* confidentiality
    in communication, 23
    the *Directives* on, 228
    in group therapy, 168
    patient's bill of rights on, 68
    in physician-patient relation-
        ships, 82, 83
    United Nations's *Declaration*
        on, 244
procreation, 122, 123–24, 129, 230,
    240n29
productive occupations, 73
professional-client relationships,
    81–83, 226–29. *See also* physi-
    cian-patient relationship
professional communication,
    principle of, 18, 22–23
professionals. *See also* health care
    professionals
    autonomy of, 84, 90
    contracts with, 79
    discipline of, 84, 85
    knowledge of, 72, 73
    peer relations of, 83–85
the professions, 71–74, 81
profit, 80–81, 89, 94
On the Prolongation of Life (Pius
    XII), 193
Proportionalism, 11
Protestants, 6–7
proxies
    the *Directives* on, 227
    end-of-life decisions and,
        194–95
    informed consent and, 66,
        111–12
    psychotherapy and, 170, 176
    research and, 111–12
proximate end, 9
prudence, 16, 18, 19
psychoactive drugs, 162–63, 164,
    175

psychoanalysis, 77–78, 82, 164,
    166, 171
psychological addiction, 173
psychological disorders. *See* men-
    tal illness
psychological health. *See* mental
    health
psychological needs, 39, 45, 51
psychological research, 113–14,
    115
psychologism, 49
psychosis, 50, 160, 167
psychosocial development, 165
psychosurgery, 162, 163, 164, 175
psychotherapy, 49–50, 164–67
    dignity and, 175
    ethical issues in, 168–72
    freedom and, 167–69, 170, 171,
        172, 175
    goals of, 166–67, 177
    informed consent for, 169–70,
        175–76
    integrity and, 176
    vs. pastoral care, 213
    as punishment, 168–69
    vs. spiritual care, 205
    values and, 170–72
public hospitals, 104
public policy, 98–100
punishment, 168–69
pure soul, 50

R
Rahner, Karl, 180
randomized clinical trials, 112–13
rape, 136–37, 228
rationalism, ethical, 4
rationalization, 172
Rawls, John, 5
reality, 115
reason, 1–2, 5, 8
reconciliation, sacrament of,
    208–9, 210
reconditioning, 165
reconstruction, 141–58
    genetic, 141, 143
    surgical, 141, 143–48
reductionism, 76–77
reflection, 59
*Reflections on the Encyclical "On
    Human Life" of Pope Paul VI*
    (John Paul II), 133–34
regimen, 58
reincarnation, 36, 48
relativism, moral, 6
religion
    common values of, 36
    on dignity, 36
    Eastern, 36
    monotheistic, 48, 188
    polytheistic, 48
    of reason, 1–2
religious communities, 219
religious humanism, 36, 37
religious legalism, 6–7
reproduction, 121, 137–39
    artificial, 128–29, 230, 239n27
reproductive system, 52

Republic (Plato), 93
research, 105–15
    abuses of, 106
    on AIDS, 113, 119
    animal experimentation for, 41,
        109
    case studies on, 119
    on children, 111–12
    choice in, 115
    for the common good, 110
    definition of, 105–6
    dignity and, 38, 112
    the *Directives* on, 222, 228, 232
    donating bodies for, 199
    double-blind protocols in,
        112–13
    embryo, 106–7, 232
    fetal, 106–7, 232
    funding, 107, 108
    Geneva statement on, 109
    guidelines for, 98–99
    informed consent for, 108,
        110–11, 113
    institutional review boards in,
        107–8
    knowledge from, 108, 109
    nontherapeutic, 108, 232
    norms for, 98–99, 108–15
    Nuremberg statement on, 109
    poverty and, 110
    proxies and, 111–12
    psychological, 113–14, 115
    risk in, 108, 109–10, 111–12, 115
    for scientific progress, 110
    selection of subjects for, 110
    social, 114
    stem cell, ix, 99, 107, 150,
        155–56
    suffering in, 109–10
    terminating participation in,
        113
    therapeutic, 108, 110, 228, 232
    trust in, 114
resource allocation, 105, 115–19
    common good and, 116–17
    the *Directives* on, 221, 222
    global, 115, 117–18
    justice in, 116–17, 118
    micro, 115–17
    triage in, 115–17, 118, 119
respect, 25, 85, 198–99, 222
On Respect for Human Life, 126,
    128–29, 151
respirators, 191
responsibility
    for actions, 66
    addiction and, 174
    for decision making, 61–62,
        65–66
    freedom and, 168–69
    for health, 55–70, 74, 91
    for health care, 87–104
    of health care professionals,
        71–86
    social, 87–104, 221–23
rest, 58
resuscitation, 182–83
revelation, 1, 7, 8

right(s)
    of animals, 41, 109
    of autonomy, 66
    to death, 190
    to health, 37–38, 91
    of patient's, 68–69, 227
    of person, 32–33
    priorities in, 38–40
    research and, 98–99, 105–6
    United Nations's *Declaration*
        on, 243–44
    of wards, 112
risk
    vs. benefit, 108, 109
    case study on, 69
    minimal, 111–12
    in research, 108, 109–10,
        111–12, 115
    values and, 42
Rogers, Carl, 78
Roman Catholic Church. *See*
    Catholic Church
Rousseau, Jean-Jacques, 2

S
sacraments, 208–10, 212, 213,
    224–25
salpingostomy, 131
scandal, 21, 237, 241n45
schools. *See* church teachings;
    education
science. *See also* research
    the *Directives* on, 220
    faith and, 220–21
    reductionism and, 76–77
    values and, 31–32
scientists, physicians as, 75, 76
screening, genetic, 150–52
Scriptures, 207–8
Second Vatican Council
    on abortion and infanticide,
        130
    on conscience, 61
    *Decree on the Apostolate of Lay
        People*, 101
    on marriage, 123, 229
    *The Pastoral Constitution of the
        Church in the Modern World*,
        36, 61, 63
    on teaching authority, 63
    on the three-fold ministry, 102
secular humanism, 2, 93
A Secular Humanist Declaration, 37
self-actualization, 39
self-control, 27
self-criticism, 65
self-determination, 170
self-respect, 25, 75
self-understanding, 49
sensation, 161
sex selection, 148–49, 156
sexuality, 121–29
    ambiguous, 147
    biological drives and, 48
    case studies on, 140
    church teachings on, 28, 139
    contraception and, 133
    definition of, 121

family and, 28, 122, 139, 215
Jesus Christ on, 28
John Paul II on, 28, 121
marriage and, 28, 122–24, 139
meaning of, 121–24
pastoral considerations for,
    137–39
personalized, 27–28
personhood and, 121–22
principle of, 27–28
reassignment of, 146–48
values of, 122–23
sharing, 22–23, 40
shock therapy, 162, 163–64
sin
    acknowledgment of, 210
    community, 215
    conscience and, 61
    death and, 179
    disease and, 50
    God and, 7
    original, 179
    Saint Paul on, 57, 179
skepticism, 2
slavery, 91, 243
sleep, 58
social justice, 37–38, 91–92, 116–17
social needs, 39, 45, 51
social relations, 167
social research, 114
social responsibility, 87–104,
    221–23
social security, 245
social workers, 97
socialism, 89, 90, 93
society. *See also* common good;
    community
    communication and, 44–45
    decision making in, 24, 93–94
    Gospel organization of, 91–93
    human needs and, 92–93
    industrial, 71–72, 117–18
    mental illness and, 159–60
    the person and, 34–36
    postindustrial, 71–72
    power in, 72
    psychoanalysis and, 171
    sex selection and, 149
    sick, 93
    subsidiarity and, 24, 93–96
    United Nations's *Declaration*
        on, 246
sociopathy, 168
sonography, 151, 152
soul, 50, 126. *See also* body–soul
    dualism
specialists, 96
spiritual care, 97, 101, 203–13,
    223–26. *See also* pastoral care
spirituality
    the *Directives* on, 223–26
    functional integrity and, 52
    health and, 50, 53, 59
    illness and, 206–7
    material goods and, 35, 37
    mental health and, 168
    needs of, 39
    wholeness of, 57

The Splendor of Truth (John Paul II), 9, 10–11
standard of living, 118, 245
stem cell research, ix, 99, 107, 150, 155–56
sterilization, 22, 135–36, 232, 240n44
stewardship
    collaboration and, 222
    the *Directives* on, 221, 238–39n10
    of health, 59–60, 69
    human reconstruction and, 143, 157
    of nature, 59–60
stewardship and creativity, principle of, 26–27
stipends, 80–81
stress, 58–59
structure vs. functions, 125
subsidiarity, 24, 92–93, 116
suffering
    of animals, 41
    death and, 29, 179–80
    the *Directives* on, 219, 234
    euthanasia and, 189
    growth through, 26, 29, 197
    in research, 109–10
suicide, 188, 202
    physician-assisted, 12, 240n44
Summa Theologica (Thomas Aquinas), 9, 10, 195
superego, 170
Supreme Court, on assisted suicide, 12
surgical reconstruction, 141, 143–48
    psychosurgery, 162, 163, 164
surgical sterilization, 135–36
surrogate mothers, 231
swine flu vaccines, 109
symbols, 44–45, 49
syngamy, 126
Synod Bishops, 138

T
teachings. *See* church teachings
teams. *See* health care teams
technology
    the *Directives* on, 220, 233
    emphasis of, 58
    ethical guidelines and, 98
    as exploitation of nature, 60
    humanization of, 73
    principle of stewardship and creativity and, 26–27
    as a priority, 89, 94
    professionals and, 72, 73
teleogism, 11–12
teleology, 8, 26–27
temperance, 16, 26, 27
Ten Commandments, 7
theological virtues, 16
therapy
    the *Directives* on, 228
    family, 167
    group, 167–68
    prenatal, 153, 231

refusal of, 68, 189–90, 228
vs. research, 108
Third Reich, 6
Thomas Aquinas, Saint
    on actions, 9–10
    on animal organisms, 125
    on circumstances, 9, 10
    on double effect, 20
    on natural law reasoning, 8–9
    on needs, 40
    on the purpose of life, 195
    Summa Theologica, 9, 10, 195
totalitarianism, 93
totality and integrity, principle of, 23, 25, 110, 144–45
totipotent cells, 150, 155
touch, 207–8
transference, 78
transplantation. *See* organ transplantation
transsexuals, 146
transvestism, 147–48
treatment. *See* therapy
treatment refusal, 68, 189–90, 228
triage
    in organ transplantation, 116, 118–19, 146
    in resource allocation, 115–17, 118, 119
trust
    in communication, 22, 23
    healing and, 75
    in pastoral care, 205–6
    in patient care teams, 85
    in physicians, 75, 79, 83, 85
    in psychoanalysis, 78
    in research, 114
truth
    dying patients and, 186–87
    in physician-patient relationships, 82, 186–87
    right to, 68–69
tube feeding. *See also* artificial nutrition
Tuskegee syphilis study, 98, 106
twins, identical, 127, 150, 158

U
ultimate end, 9, 10, 11
unconsciousness, 211
understanding, 67, 164
Uniform Anatomical Gift Act, 199
uninsured persons, 222
United Kingdom, Warnock Commission, 106
United Nations's *Declaration*. *See* *Universal Declaration of Human Rights of the United Nations*
United States Conference of Catholic Bishops, 218
Universal Declaration of Human Rights of the United Nations, x, 15, 243–46
    on community, 246
    on confidentiality and privacy, 244
    on dignity, 41, 243

on education, 245–46
on equality, 243–44
on freedom, 243, 244–45
on governments, 245
on health, 245
on health and health care, 245
laws, 243–44
on marriage, 244
on the right to health, 91
on rights, 243–44
social justice and, 37–38
universal health care, 87, 103
the universe, 142
USCCB Committee on Pro-Life Activities, 233
utilitarianism, 3, 5

V
values, 2, 3, 4, 15–17
    actions and, 32
    community, 36–38, 40
    in decision making, 62
    hierarchy of, 25, 51–52
    innate, 8
    needs and, 38
    priorities in, 38–40
    psychotherapy and, 170–72
    risk and, 42
    science and, 31–32
    secular humanistic, 37
    of sexuality, 122–23
vegetative organisms, 125–26
venereal disease, 136
Veritatis Splendor (John Paul II), 9, 10–11
viability, 132
Viaticum, 209, 213, 225
violence, 228
virginity, 122
virtues, 16, 26, 27

W
Wade, Nicholas, 154
wakes, 199
wards, 112. *See also* proxies
Warnock Commission, 106
wealth, 92
welfare, 35, 93
well-formed conscience principle, 18–19, 60–64. *See also* conscience
wholeness, 43, 50, 57
why circumstances, 9–10
will, 7, 47, 52, 56
Willowbrook experiments, 106
wills, living, 195
withdrawal of care. *See* life support treatment
Wolffian ducts, 147
World Health Organization, 31, 45, 109

Z
zygote, 124, 126, 127